Practical Guide to History Taking, Physical Exam, and Functioning in the Hospital and Clinic

a LANGE medical book

Practical Guide to History Taking, Physical Exam, and Functioning in the Hospital and Clinic

Editor

Charlie Goldberg, MD
Clinical Professor of Medicine
Associate Dean of Graduate Medical Education
University of California, San Diego School of Medicine
San Diego, California

1 2 3 4 5 6 7 8 9   DSS   29 28 27 26 25 24

ISBN 978-1-264-27803-9
MHID 1-264-27803-9

This book was set in Minion Pro by KnowledgeWorks Global Ltd.
The editors were Michael Weitz and Kim J. Davis.
The production supervisor was Catherine Saggese.
Project management was provided by Tasneem Kauser of KnowledgeWorks Global Ltd.
The cover illustration was by Catherine Cichon, MD, MPH.

This book is printed on acid-free paper.

Library of Congress Cataloging-in-Publication Data

Names: Goldberg, Charlie, editor.
Title: Practical guide to history taking, physical exam, and functioning in
    the hospital and clinic / editor, Charlie Goldberg.
Other titles: Lange medical book.
Description: New York : McGraw Hill, [2025] | Series: Lange medical book |
    Includes bibliographical references and index. | Summary: "The focus of
    this book is to describe foundational skills needed in order to provide
    clinical care"— Provided by publisher.
Identifiers: LCCN 2023057603 (print) | LCCN 2023057604 (ebook) | ISBN
    9781264278039 (paperback ; alk. paper) | ISBN 9781264278046 (ebook)
Subjects: MESH: Medical History Taking—methods | Physical
    Examination—methods | Clinical Medicine—methods
Classification: LCC RC65 (print) | LCC RC65 (ebook) | NLM WB 290 | DDC
    616.07/51—dc23/eng/20240311
LC record available at https://lccn.loc.gov/2023057603
LC ebook record available at https://lccn.loc.gov/2023057604

McGraw Hill books are available at special quantity discounts to use as premiums and sales promotions or for use in corporate training programs. To contact a representative, please visit the Contact Us pages at www.mhprofessional.com.

I am grateful for the love and support provided by my wife and sons: Teddy, Aaron, and Max. Forever gratitude to my mom and dad for their guidance and for launching me in the right direction. Thanks also to Jan Thompson, for her efforts on the original Practical Guide website.

Finally, thanks to the students, trainees, patients, and colleagues at UC San Diego and the VA San Diego Healthcare System, who have made teaching and learning such a great and rewarding gig!

Contents

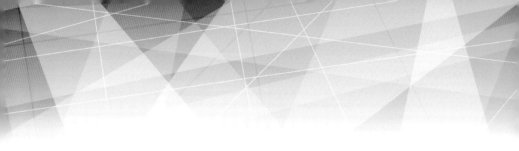

Contributors

Jessica Bailis, PsyD
Clinical Psychologist, UC San Diego Health
  Sciences, College Mental Health Program,
  San Diego, California

Savita G. Bhakta, MD, DFAPA
Associate Clinical Professor of Psychiatry,
  University of California San Diego,
  School of Medicine; Director,
  College Mental Health Program;
  Physician Wellness Director,
  Department of Psychiatry,
  UC San Diego Health System,
  San Diego, California

Jill Blumenthal, MD, MAS
Clinical Professor of Medicine;
  Division of Infectious Diseases and
  Global Public Health Director,
  Owen Clinic PrEP Program
  Co-Medical Director Gender Health
  Program, University of California,
  San Diego, San Diego, California

Stacy Charat, MD
Clinical Professor of Medicine, Division of
  General Internal Medicine, University of
  California, San Diego, School of Medicine;
  Staff Physician, VA San Diego
  Healthcare System,
  San Diego, California

Catherine Cichon, MD, MPH
Clinical Fellow in Infectious Diseases,
  Division of Infectious Diseases,
  University of Nebraska Medical Center,
  Omaha, Nebraska

Charley Coffey, MD, FACS
Clinical Professor of Otolaryngology—Head and
  Neck Surgery, University of California,
  San Diego School of Medicine; Chief of
  Otolaryngology–Head and Neck Surgery,
  UCSD Healthcare and VA San Diego
  Healthcare System,
  San Diego, California

Julia Cormano, MD
Associate Clinical Professor of Obstetrics,
  Gynecology, and Reproductive Medicine;
  Obstetrics and Gynecology Clerkship
  Director, University of California
  San Diego School of Medicine,
  San Diego, California

Sean J. Evans, MD
Clinical Professor of Neurosciences and
  Associate Dean for Undergraduate Medical
  Education, University of California
  San Diego School of Medicine,
  San Diego, California

Charlie Goldberg, MD
Clinical Professor of Medicine and Associate
  Dean for Graduate Medical Education,
  University of California, San Diego
  School of Medicine, Staff Physician,
  VA San Diego Healthcare System,
  San Diego, California

Jean Guan, MD
Assistant Professor of Clinical Medicine,
University of Missouri School of Medicine,
Springfield Clinical Campus,
Springfield, Missouri

Roopali Gupta, MD
Clinical Professor of Medicine; Program
Director, Geriatric Medicine Fellowship,
Division of Geriatrics, Gerontology and
Palliative Medicine, University of California,
San Diego School of Medicine,
San Diego, California

Leonie Heyworth, MD, MPH
Deputy Director for Clinical Services,
Telehealth Services, Office of Connected
Care, US Department of Veterans Affairs;
Associate Clinical Professor of Medicine,
University of California, San Diego
School of Medicine,
San Diego, California

Michal "Kalli" Hose, MD
Clinical Professor of Medicine, University of
California, San Diego, School of Medicine;
Staff Physician and Director,
VA Primary Care Musculoskeletal Clinic,
VA San Diego Healthcare System,
San Diego, California

Simerjot K. Jassal, MD, MAS
Clinical Professor of Medicine, University of
California, San Diego School of Medicine;
Program Director, University of California,
San Diego Internal Medicine Residency
Program, San Diego, California; Staff
Physician, VA San Diego Healthcare System,
San Diego, California

Maya Michelle Kumar, MD, FAAP, FRCPC
Associate Clinical Professor of Pediatrics,
Division of Adolescent and Young Adult
Medicine, University of California, San
Diego; Adolescent Medicine Physician,
Rady Children's Hospital San Diego,
San Diego, California

Brian K. Kwan, MD, SFHM
Clinical Professor of Medicine, University of
California, San Diego; Co-Clerkship Director,
Internal Medicine, University of California,
San Diego School of Medicine,
San Diego, California;
Staff Physician, VA San Diego
Healthcare System,
San Diego, California

Jeffrey E. Lee, MD
Clinical Professor of Ophthalmology;
Ophthalmology Residency Program Director,
University of California, San Diego,
School of Medicine; Chief of Ophthalmology,
UC San Diego Medical Center,
San Diego, California

**Michelle Leff, MD, IBCLC, NABBLM-C,
FAAP**
Clinical Professor of Pediatrics, University of
California, San Diego School of Medicine;
Newborn Hospitalist, San Diego, California

Anna P. Quan, MD
Clinical Professor of Medicine, University of
California, San Diego School of Medicine;
Primary Care Section Chief, Sorrento Valley
VA Clinic; Co-Director, Musculoskeletal
Clinic, VA San Diego Healthcare System,
San Diego, California

Jeremy A. Schneider, MD
Associate Clinical Professor of Dermatology,
UC San Diego School of Medicine; Director,
Inpatient Dermatology Consult Service,
UC San Diego Health,
San Diego, California

Vanessa P. Scott, MD, MSc
Assistant Clinical Professor of Pediatrics,
University of California, San Diego
School of Medicine,
San Diego, California

Meghan Sebasky, MD
Clinical Professor of Medicine; Co-Director,
 Internal Medicine Clerkship,
 University of California, San Diego
 School of Medicine,
 San Diego, California

Rebecca E. Sell, MD
Clinical Professor of Medicine, Division of
 Pulmonary and Critical Care Medicine,
 University of Washington School of Medicine,
 Seattle, Washington

Emily "EB" Sladek, MD, CMD
Associate Clinical Professor of Medicine,
 Division of Geriatrics, Gerontology, and
 Palliative Care, University of California,
 San Diego School of Medicine; Medical
 Director, Community Living Center; Chief,
 Geriatrics Section,
 VA San Diego Healthcare System,
 San Diego, California

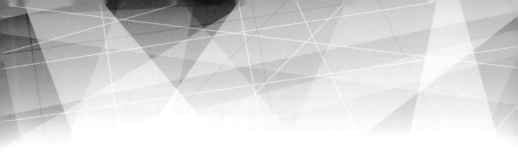

Preface

When performed well, the clinical exam (history and physical) feeds the diagnostic reasoning, testing, and therapeutic decision-making process. It is the key entry point when interacting with patients and drives much of the care that follows.

However, the data accumulated is only useful when it is done in an accurate and complete fashion. The focus of this book is to describe foundational skills that you will need in order to provide clinical care. Achieving competence requires practice, feedback, and refinement.

Why Obtain a History and Perform a Physical Exam?

It seems important to take this on from the outset, as time pressure, technology, and questioning about what constitutes an appropriate exam and why we do it have drawn increasing attention. Our goal in this book is to teach about elements that have value. Doing something "just because" makes no sense and is not a good use of time or other resources. By the same token, thoughtful and skilled interactions with patients can provide an effective road map for guiding clinical care. These person-to-person interactions are also moments of connection which remind us that human beings are at the center of healthcare. Furthermore, while technology offers great information and insights, indiscriminate use can drive up costs and provide less than helpful guidance. And even a powerful tool like AI is dependent on core data to drive its recommendations. If that information (including the clinical exam) is incorrect, the subsequent guidance can be misleading (ie. garbage in, garbage out).

We are also living in a moment of increasing distance from one another, with the US Surgeon General, Dr. Vivek Murthy, noting that, "Loneliness and isolation represent profound threats to our health and well-being." In a sense, medicine too is suffering from a crisis created by clinical distance and disconnection. Physicians value one-on-one interactions, yet many aspects of the healthcare system create barriers between ourselves, patients, and colleagues. Technology (eg, the electronic medical record, instant messaging) provides tools that simultaneously enhance our ability to deliver elements of care, while also acting as distractions that can create distance between all of us. Healthcare organizations, reimbursement, and compensation can prioritize productivity over presence.

Seen in this context, the clinical exam is a tangible way of truly being with another person while collecting key information. Humans are delightfully quirky, such that the way in which they describe symptoms often requires an open and tuned in human ear to truly understand and contextualize their stories. Physical connection, providing comfort and healing through touch, can only be delivered when you are next to another living soul. This provides additional impetus to learn and utilize core bedside skills, which can be applied in a pragmatic fashion to the care that you deliver. This will also help you to become better doctors and afford you with defined moments that rejuvenate and humanize. Helping others through medicine is an immensely rewarding activity and being connected to someone, hearing their stories, and guiding their care in a hands-on manner is a unique privilege that we should all hold onto tightly.

We recognize that point-of-care ultrasound (POCUS) has a role as a complementary skill in further identifying and characterizing exam findings. Interested learners are directed to the growing number of resources that capably cover this area.

DESIGN OF THIS BOOK

This book has been assembled with an eye toward clinical relevance. By approaching clinical medicine in a practical and demystified fashion, the significance of the material should be readily apparent and the underlying principles more clearly understood. In particular:

- Every section is constructed to answer the question: "What do I really need to know about this area?" The material is presented in a concise, bulleted fashion that is easy to read and follow. The focus is on "meat and potatoes" skills and approaches, which should be readily applicable during clinical encounters.
- Exam techniques are described in step-by-step detail. Special maneuvers that are occasionally utilized are also described, as well as when they should be implemented. Photos and illustrations are incorporated to make the descriptions and techniques easier to understand and apply.
- There are chapters dedicated to every major organ system. In addition, care of specific patient groups is covered, including 3 chapters dedicated to pediatrics (infant, toddler/child, and adolescence). There are also separate chapters covering LGBTQ+ health and geriatrics.
- The rationale for each aspect of the examination is addressed, and where appropriate, relevant physiology and pathophysiology are discussed.
- Every chapter contains "Pearls" to draw attention to particularly noteworthy elements.
- Following many exam descriptions, "Findings and Their Meaning" are provided, which highlight common abnormalities that might be identified as well as their clinical significance. Images of exam findings accompany many of these sections.
- The techniques and approaches described are evidence-based where possible. Expert experience is also utilized to shape the messaging and approaches. The presentation style is meant to be pleasantly rigorous, one that makes the information accessible and more easily applied.
- Tables and charts are used throughout to allow the reader to more easily identify key points and make connections between findings and common diagnoses.
- Many chapters have novel features (eg, "Quiz Yourself" questions for the neuro exam, diagnostic charts for mental status).
- Unique clinical illustrations by Dr. Catherine Cichon further highlight the link between historical information, exam findings, and common disorders.
- Most chapters have "Telehealth Tips" highlighting the ways in which this growing modality might be utilized to evaluate specific organ systems and symptoms. There is also a chapter dedicated to telehealth that provides core information that is broadly applicable to typical telehealth visits as well as other uses of communication technology to enhance the delivery of care.

- Checklists at the end of each chapter highlight the core aspects of each organ system exam and the order in which they can be performed. A chapter dedicated to "Putting it All Together" provides guidance about how to sequence a comprehensive exam so that the flow is optimized.
- Chapters dedicated to oral presentations and documentation are included, to assist students in developing skills that will help them to function and learn in the hospital and outpatient clinical environment.

We hope that this book helps to make the learning process both fun and rewarding. Core behaviors are described that have diagnostic utility and prolonged applicability, even in a technology-driven world. The process of personal improvement should continue until the day you stop practicing medicine. There are always new techniques to learn and unusual findings to incorporate into your personal libraries of medical experience. However, unless you take the time to build a solid foundation, you will never have confidence in the accuracy and value of what you can uncover with a sharp mind, attentive ear, agile fingers, and a few simple tools!

BIBLIOGRAPHY

Diagnosis. *JAMA*. 1901;37:1118 (reprinted in *JAMA*. 2001;286:1944).

Holt-Lunstad J, Perissinotto C. Social isolation and loneliness as medical issues. *N Engl J Med*. 2023;388:193-195.

Huang C, Drazen JM. Artificial intelligence and machine learning in clinical medicine, 2023. *N Engl J Med*. 2023;388:1201-1208.

Mangione S, Basile M, Post S. Out of touch. *JAMA*. 2024; Published online 2/9/24; doi:10.1001/jama.2024.0888

Murthy V. Addressing health worker burnout. The U.S. Surgeon General's advisory on building a thriving health work force. 2022. Accessed June 27, 2023. https://www.hhs.gov/sites/default/files/health-worker-wellbeing-advisory.pdf.

Murthy V. Our epidemic of loneliness and isolation. The U.S. Surgeon General's advisory on the healing effects of social connection and community. 2023. Accessed June 27, 2023. https://www.hhs.gov/sites/default/files/surgeon-general-social-connection-advisory.pdf.

Porter S. Ellipsis. *N Engl J Med*. 2023;388:2311-2313.

Verrees M. Touch me. *JAMA*. 1996;276:1285-1286.

History Taking

Charlie Goldberg, MD

INTRODUCTION

Obtaining an accurate history is the critical first step in determining the etiology of a patient's concern or defining their risk for developing specific disorders. A large percentage of the time, clinicians will be able to make diagnoses based on history alone. The value of the history, of course, depends on the ability to elicit relevant information. This requires being thorough and systematic when interviewing a patient.

In obtaining the history, the doctor functions like a sculptor. The tools are not a hammer or chisel; they are the words and questions used to gather information (**Figure 1-1**). You take a block of marble (ie, a nonspecific symptom) and shape it into something that is recognizable, a diagnostic possibility.

Being thorough and organized enables clinicians to generate a historical foundation that is solid and accurate and will serve as a great backbone for the care that will be provided.

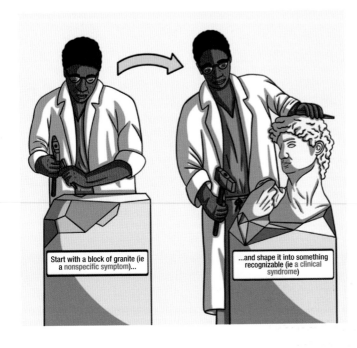

Start with a block of granite (ie a nonspecific symptom)...

...and shape it into something recognizable (ie a clinical syndrome)

FIGURE 1-1 • **Physician as sculptor.** (Reproduced with Permission from Cathy Cichon, MD.)

The patient's answers are the construction material, the bricks of the history-taking trade. The goal is to build a "historical structure" that is substantial, not a house of cards that is incomplete and/or weakened by inaccuracies **(Figure 1-2)**.

The first part of this chapter focuses on key approaches to optimizing interactions with patients. This is followed by a description of how to obtain the history of present illness (HPI). The patient initiates the HPI by describing a symptom, and it is the clinician's responsibility to take this information and use it as a springboard for additional questioning that will help to identify the root cause of the patient's concern. Details for obtaining the rest of a comprehensive history are described after the section on the HPI.

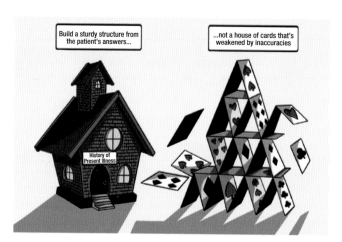

FIGURE 1-2 • **Obtaining a history that is accurate and solid.** (Reproduced with Permission from Cathy Cichon, MD.)

OPTIMIZING YOUR CLINICAL INTERACTIONS

Communicating Effectively

Effectively interacting with a patient requires excellent communication skills. This entails speaking clearly and using terminology that is easily understood. It also requires that the clinician slow down and listen well, providing adequate time for the patient to ask and answer questions, as well as clarifying points when there is confusion. Responding to nonverbal cues (eg, sadness, hesitation indicating reluctance to answer questions) is also critical in order to communicate well and set up a relationship that promotes engagement and trust.

It is very easy to reduce history taking to a task composed of a list of questions to be asked and answered, losing track of the fact that, at its core, this is a dialogue between 2 people. Information needs to be exchanged in a way that maintains the human connection that is at the center of healthcare. Honoring this takes practice, attention to detail, skills, and an appropriate (not infinite) amount of time.

Cultural Awareness and Humility

Every patient has a lifetime of experiences as well as belief systems that they bring to the clinical encounter. Clinicians have these as well. Try not to make assumptions about what someone wants or how they would like it delivered based on their appearance, speech, or other subjective assessments. In addition, it is not possible to know specific aspects about their approach to healthcare (or anything else) without inquiring. When you are confused by a patient's response or uncertain about how to engage in a particular topic, ask them for guidance. After all, they are the experts about their own perspectives and goals.

Previewing the Patient

Many patients have information from previous encounters available in the electronic health record. It is useful to review this prior to interacting, so that you are aware of background information about their health, treatments, known diagnoses, and so on. Doing this in an efficient manner takes practice and experience, which will guide you in terms of what is relevant and where to find it. In addition, it is important to be informed but not overly influenced by what you read. Always confirm key points with the patient and maintain an open mind so that you can draw your own conclusions based on the data that you gather.

Note Taking During the Interview

Early in your career, as you are developing clinical skills, try to avoid typing while you talk. Multitasking in this fashion diminishes the attention that you are paying to data gathering and can negatively impact your ability to connect with the patient. This includes picking up on nonverbal cues that the patient might express and could be missed if you are not fully engaged. Writing notes on a piece of paper is likely less obtrusive and distracting.

Using Interpreters

Getting accurate information requires clear communication that is understood by all parties. Use interpreters when patients speak a language different than your own, including American Sign Language (ASL) for those with hearing impairment. If you are truly fluent in another language, it is fine to proceed without an interpreter. Otherwise, use a trained professional (in person or via phone or live video). Find out what resources are available in your healthcare setting(s). Getting collateral information from family members is fine. However, do not use them as primary translators unless there truly are no other options. Important information might be lost and/or there could be reluctance in sharing personal data.

Bias and History Taking

Implicit biases are negative and positive associations that we maintain about specific groups without being aware of their presence. Bias can impact every aspect of healthcare, including how we interact with patients and colleagues, make clinical decisions, apply therapeutic and diagnostic strategies, and perform research. In addition, bias can impact a patient's willingness to interact with the healthcare system and negatively affect the clinical and learning environment for students, trainees, faculty, and other healthcare workers.

It is very easy to let biases and other unfounded beliefs affect the way in which we ask questions and provide care. This can lead to missed opportunities and uneven approaches based on a patient's appearance, race, ethnicity, or other factors that really should have no impact on the healthcare that we deliver.

The best way of avoiding this is to be aware of bias, admit its role, and adopt standardized strategies to mitigate its impact (eg, asking the same questions of everyone, using nonstigmatizing language).

Patient Autonomy

In some instances, a patient will indicate that they do not wish to discuss a particular issue, even after you have offered a thoughtful explanation as to why exploring this area is important. Respect their decision and move on. This is a key tenet of trauma-informed care, where a patient's life experiences may limit their willingness to engage in aspects of the history or exam. Increased awareness can enable you to engage in a more empathetic and respectful manner, while avoiding inadvertently retraumatizing your patients.

Red Flag Symptoms

Recognizing symptoms that demand urgent assessment (ie, "red flag symptoms") versus those that can be handled in a less time-sensitive fashion comes with knowledge and experience.

- Every organ system has red flag symptoms, with some being "redder" than others based on severity, risk factors, and potential for morbidity or mortality. Those that are new or acute and/or causing significant discomfort or limitations in function tend to be most important. A few examples include the following:
  - A 72-year-old patient with known metastatic prostate cancer who presents with acute low back pain, leg weakness, and urinary incontinence merits emergent evaluation for cauda equina syndrome.
  - In contrast, a 22-year-old, otherwise healthy patient presenting with acute low back pain after lifting something heavy, without associated neurologic or systemic symptoms, is much less concerning for emergent neurologic or musculoskeletal pathology.
- The use of immune-modulating medications (eg, steroids, some chemotherapies) or the presence of certain immune-compromising disorders (eg, untreated HIV infection) creates red flag conditions, as they alter the normal response of the body to injury and infection. In these situations, almost any new symptom merits scrutiny.
- Patients on either end of the age spectrum may have a blunted ability to respond to physiologic stress, such that symptoms related to underlying disorders may not be robust or typical. As such, the bar should be lower for identifying something as a red flag symptom in these groups.
- All patient concerns merit careful consideration, which is achieved by asking the right follow-up questions and performing an appropriate evaluation. That is, you need to perform your due diligence in order to correctly identify red flag issues.

Dealing With Your Own Discomfort

New clinicians may feel uncomfortable with the patient interview for many readily understandable reasons, including:

- This process is, by its very nature, intrusive.
- The patient has been stripped, both literally and figuratively, of the layers that protect them from the physical and psychological probes of the outside world. Furthermore, in order

to be successful, you must ask in-depth questions of a person with whom you essentially have no relationship. This is completely at odds with your normal day-to-day interactions.

- The patient interview must be managed in a way that maintains respect for the patient's dignity and privacy. In fact, early in your career, you perhaps have an advantage over more experienced providers as you are hyperaware that this is not a natural environment.
- Listen to the patient and be aware of all of their responses (verbal and nonverbal). Use these to guide your interactions.

The Setup

- Always introduce yourself to the patient, providing your name and role on the healthcare team. Let them know how you would like to be addressed. Also, ask the patient how they would like you to refer to them, both during the interview as well as in your write-up. This should include preferred pronouns.
- Try to make the environment as private and free of distractions as possible. This may be difficult depending on where the interview is taking place. The emergency department and nonprivate patient rooms are challenging spots.
- Ask the patient if they want family or friends to stay. If the room is crowded and/or they want to talk with you alone, it is acceptable to politely ask visitors to leave.
- If possible, sit down next to the patient while conducting the interview.
- Remove any physical barriers (eg, side rails of beds) that stand between yourself and the patient so that your view of one another is unimpeded. Help to ensure your patient's safety by putting the barriers back in place at the end of the interview.

These simple maneuvers help to put you and the patient on more equal footing. Furthermore, they enhance the notion that you are completely focused on them. You can either disarm or build walls through the speech, posture, and body language that you adopt. Recognize the power of these cues and the impact that they can have on the interview. Paying attention to what may seem like small details as well as always showing kindness and respect can go a long way toward creating an environment that facilitates the exchange of useful information.

If the interview is being conducted in an outpatient setting, it is probably best to allow the patient to wear their clothing while you talk with them. At the conclusion of the discussion, provide them with a gown (as necessary to allow adequate exposure) and leave the room while they undress in preparation for the physical exam.

Managing telehealth encounters is covered in Chapter 24 as well as in tips at the end of each organ specific chapter.

CORE ELEMENTS OF THE HISTORY OF PRESENT ILLNESS

Chief Concern

The patient's reason for presenting to the clinician is often referred to as the *chief complaint*. A less pejorative (ie, referring to "complaints" can generate negative feelings) and more accurate nomenclature is to identify this as their *chief concern* (CC). Sometimes there is more than one CC. Regardless, it represents the jumping off point for the HPI. Sample CCs include "I can't catch my breath" or "I feel so tired."

Initial Question(s)

Ideally, you want to hear the patient describe the concern in their own words. Open-ended questions are a good way to get the ball rolling. These include: "What brings you here?" "How can I help you?" "What seems to be the problem?" Push the patient to be as descriptive as possible. Although it is simplest to focus on a single, dominant problem, patients occasionally identify more than one issue that they wish to address. When this occurs, explore each issue individually using the strategy described below, recognizing that they may derive from a common cause. Physicians often have a very hard time waiting for responses and tolerating silence.

Follow-Up Questions

There are a number of important follow-up questions that are applicable to most symptoms and help to further define their core dimensions. Successful interviewing requires that you avoid medical terminology and make use of a descriptive language that is familiar to the patient. These questions include the following:

- **Onset?**
  - When did the symptom begin and what was happening at that time?
    - This is also a good moment to clarify if the symptom is completely novel or similar to a past problem. If recurrent, what was done previously?
  - It can sometimes be challenging for patients to pin down the time of onset. This is important data for clinicians in determining whether a process is hyperacute (<24 hours), acute (<7 days), subacute (1-4 weeks), or chronic (>4 weeks).
  - Asking the patient (or a friend/family member) when they last felt symptom free or "normal for them" is an alternative approach to trying to accurately characterize when a process began.
- **Duration?**
  - Is the symptom constant/ongoing? If so, how long has it been present?
  - If it's intermittent, how long does each episode last? How frequent are the episodes?
- **Location and radiation?**
  - Is the symptom (eg, pain) located in a specific region of the body? Has it moved since it started (eg, began in umbilical area and now located in right lower quadrant)?
  - Does it radiate to a specific area of the body (eg, travels from the central chest to the shoulder with a deep breath)?
  - NOTE: Some symptoms (eg, fatigue, shortness of breath, sadness, dizziness) do not have an anatomic location.
- **Intensity?**
  - How severe is the problem? Is it more of a nuisance (ie, annoying and in the background), or is it very present and a focus of their attention?
  - Does it interfere with their daily activities? Does it keep them up at night?
  - If it affects their activity level, determine to what degree this occurs. If, for example, they mention shortness of breath with walking, how far can they go without stopping? Try to get them to be as objective as possible when describing distance (eg, up a flight of stairs, across a room, from the parking lot to the supermarket) and when they were last able to perform at that level. Have they given up any activities due to feeling limited (eg, parking closer to store entrances, no longer shopping)?

- If they are describing pain, ask them to describe it from 1 to 10, with 10 being the worst pain of their life. Identify what caused the high level of reference pain so that you know what they are using for comparison (eg, a broken limb).
- **Anything that makes it better or worse?**
  - Does anything make the symptom better or worse? For example, shortness of breath might be provoked by exercise and relieved by rest.
  - If the patient has tried treatments, what were they? Did they have any impact?
- **Characteristics?**
  - Ask them to describe the character of the symptom in terms with which they are familiar.
  - When describing pain, is it like anything else that they have felt in the past? For example, is it knife-like? A sensation of pressure? An ache?
- **Any changes over time?**
  - Has the symptom changed or evolved in any way?
  - How does their present experience of the symptom compare with 1 day, 1 week or 1 month ago (if it has been present over time)?
- **Associated symptoms**
  - Often, patient's notice other symptoms that have popped up around the same time as the dominant problem. These may be related.
  - These can be generalized (eg, fever, chills, aches) or focal (eg, knee or other joint pain).
- **What worries them about the symptom?**
  - This question is not designed to promote self-diagnosis, and sometimes the answer is obvious and thus the question is unnecessary.
  - However, some patients have specific concerns surrounding the cause of their symptoms that are not clear to the clinician. These can be most expeditiously addressed if you are aware of them.
- **Why today?**
  - This question is particularly relevant when a patient chooses to make mention of symptoms or concerns that appear to be long-standing.
  - Is there something new or different today as opposed to every other day when the symptom has been present (eg, worsening or changing in some way)?
  - Has the patient developed a new perception of its relative importance (eg, a friend told them they should get it checked out)?
  - Do they have a specific agenda for today's encounter related to the symptom?

The HPI concludes with a list of pertinent positives and negatives, items drawn from a review of symptoms of the relevant organ systems (see Chapter 2, Review of Systems). Their presence or absence helps to refine the list of possible diagnoses.

OLD CARTS is a commonly used mnemonic to help remember and apply these core questions. It stands for **O**nset, **L**ocation and radiation, **D**uration, **C**haracter, **A**ggravating/**A**lleviating factors, **R**elated symptoms, **T**iming, and **S**everity.

The content of subsequent questions will depend both on what you uncover and your knowledge base and understanding of patients and their illnesses. If, for example, the patient's CC was chest pain, you might have uncovered the following by using the core questions:

The symptom began 1 month ago and only occurs with activity. It rapidly goes away with rest. When it does occur, it feels like a steady pressure focused on the center of the chest that sometimes moves toward their left shoulder. It is roughly a 7 in intensity (on a scale of 1-10). It is worse than when it started, when it felt more like a 2. Over the last week, it has happened a total of 6 times, whereas in the first week, it happened only once. Yesterday it lasted for about 30 seconds, which is a little longer than when it began 1 month ago. During the last 2 episodes, the patient also felt sweaty and nauseous.

The patient is aware that heart problems cause chest pain, as their father had something similar before his heart attack. The fact that it is getting worse, coupled with their father's history, is what made them come to see you today.

The patient has never experienced anything like this previously and has not mentioned this problem to anyone else prior to meeting with you. They have not tried any specific therapies. They deny shortness of breath, paroxysmal nocturnal dyspnea, orthopnea, lower extremity edema, palpitations, cough, fever, chills, abdominal pain, or discomfort elsewhere.

This is quite a lot of information. However, if you were not aware that coronary-based ischemia causes a symptom complex similar to what the patient is describing, you might not have any idea about what further questions to ask. That is okay. With additional experience, exposure, and knowledge, you will learn the appropriate settings for particular lines of questioning.

When clinicians obtain a history, they are continually generating differential diagnoses allowing the patient's answers to direct the logical use of additional questions.

- With each step, the list of probable diagnoses is pared down until a few likely choices are left from what may have been a longer list of possibilities.
- In the patient with chest pain, you may recognize that their story is very consistent with significant symptomatic coronary artery disease. As such, you would ask follow-up questions that help to define a cardiac basis for this concern (eg, history of past myocardial infarctions, risk factors for coronary disease). You would also be aware that other disease states (eg, emphysema) might cause similar symptoms and would therefore ask questions that could lend support to these possible diagnoses (eg, history of smoking or wheezing).
- At the completion of the HPI, you will often have a reasonable idea as to the likely cause(s) of a patient's concern. You may then focus your exam on the search for the presence or absence of physical signs that would lend support to or refute your working diagnosis. This in turn will help direct you in the rational use of adjuvant testing and treatment.

You will undoubtedly forget to ask certain questions, requiring a return visit to the patient's bedside to ask, "Just one more thing." Don't worry; this happens to everyone! You will get more efficient with practice.

After gathering the elements of the HPI, it can be useful to review the key points with the patient, which helps ensure that you have accurately captured their story.

THE REST OF THE HISTORY

The remainder of the history is obtained after completing the HPI. As such, the previously discussed techniques for facilitating the exchange of information apply here as well. If there is no CC (and thus no HPI), you can simply proceed from the outset using the following organizational structure. The extent of additional history taking that is needed is typically based on the clinical environment and CC. Specialty clinics or the emergency department, for example, are places where a focused history is often sufficient (see comments at end of this chapter). Ask those supervising you for guidance.

Past Medical History

- Ask the patient if they have any known medical problems or conditions.
- If you receive little or no response, the following questions can help uncover important past events:
  - Have they ever received medical care? If so, what problems or issues were addressed? Was the care continuous (ie, provided on a regular basis) or episodic?
  - Have they ever undergone procedures, blood tests, x-rays, computed tomography (CT) scans, magnetic resonance imaging (MRI), or other special testing?
  - Have they ever been hospitalized and/or visited an emergency department? If so, for what?
- It is often amazing how many patients forget what would seem to be important medical events or assume that the healthcare system is so interconnected that all clinicians have access to their compete records, regardless of where their care was provided.
- As a student, you will encounter patients who report little past history during your interview yet reveal a complex series of illnesses to your resident or attending! These patients are not purposefully concealing information. They simply need to be prompted by the right questions.

Past Surgical History

- Was the patient ever operated on, even as a child? What year did this occur?
- What was the procedure, and why was it done? Was it successful? Were there any complications?

Review of Systems (ROS)

The review of systems (or symptoms) is a list of questions, arranged by organ system, designed to uncover dysfunction and disease within that area. Details are provided in Chapter 2.

Medications

- Does the patient take any prescription medicines? If so, what are the dose and frequency?
- Do they know what condition(s) is/are being treated?
- Medication nonadherence and confusion are major clinical problems, particularly when regimens are complex or the patients are older, cognitively impaired, have limited resources, or are less engaged. It is important to ascertain whether patients are actually taking medications as prescribed. This can provide critical information, as what may appear to be a failure to respond to a particular therapy might actually be nonadherence to a prescribed regimen.
- Identifying nonadherence requires tact, as you want to encourage honesty without sounding judgmental. It helps to clearly explain that without this information your ability to assess treatment efficacy and make therapeutic adjustments becomes difficult or potentially dangerous.
- If patients are, in fact, missing doses or not taking medications altogether, ask them why this is happening. Perhaps there is an important side effect that they are experiencing, a reasonable fear that can be addressed, cost considerations, strategies to help them remember (eg, use of a pill box), or a more acceptable substitute regimen that could be implemented (eg, a once-daily version of the medicine).

- Ask whether they are taking over-the-counter or "nontraditional" medications? If so, which medications, what are the dose and frequency, and what conditions are they treating? Have these treatments been effective? Are these medicines being prescribed by a practitioner or self-administered?
- Encourage patients to keep an up-to-date medication list and/or print (or write) one out for them.
- If it is unclear which medications are being prescribed or taken, ask the patient to bring them all in when they return to the clinic or to call back or transmit the information electronically. If they are inpatients, ask a family member or friend to do so on their behalf. If that is not possible, see if they can take pictures of the bottles and send them to you.
- This is also a good opportunity to ask about any other doctors and/or health systems that might also be providing care to them.

Allergies and Reactions

- Have they experienced any adverse reactions to medications?
- The exact nature of the reaction should be clearly identified as it can have important clinical implications. Anaphylaxis, for example, is a life-threatening reaction and an absolute contraindication to reexposure to the drug. Other symptoms, however, may not raise the same level of concern, particularly if the agent in question is clearly the treatment of choice.
- Some reported "allergies" are actually common reactions to particular medications (eg, nausea with narcotics) and would not necessarily preclude their use in the future.

Substance Use History

The following history domains (smoking, alcohol, and other substance use) are important, because they may increase a patient's risk for particular disorders and/or guide decision-making about the use of screening strategies (eg, low-dose chest CT to screen for lung cancer in patients with a history of smoking). That said, it is important for this information to be obtained in a nonjudgmental way. Otherwise, patients may be disinclined to provide accurate answers. It might help to state up front that these questions come without judgement, that you ask them of everyone, and that accurate information will help guide healthcare delivery. Your job is to focus on gathering accurate data. Working toward behavior change can (and should) come later.

Smoking

- Has the patient ever smoked cigarettes? If so, how many packs per day and for how many years?
  - The packs per day multiplied by the number of years gives the pack-years, a widely accepted method for smoking quantification.
- If they quit, when did this occur?
- Pipe or cigar smoking and chewing tobacco use should also be noted.

Vaping

- Does the patient vape?
- If so, how much and how often?
- Vaping carries some risk of lung injury (both acute and chronic) as well as nicotine addiction.

Alcohol
- Does the patient drink alcohol? If so, how much per day and what type of drink?
- Encourage patients to be as specific as possible. One drink may mean a 12-oz beer or a 12-oz glass of whiskey, each with different implications.
- If they do not drink on a daily basis, how much do they consume over a week or month?

Other Drug Use
- Any drug use, past or present, should be noted.
- Avoid using the term "recreational" when talking about substance use.

Get in the habit of asking all your patients questions about substance use because it is not possible to accurately determine who is at risk on the basis of appearance, background, or other features. Using these features as triggers for questions often reflects our biases.

Obstetric (as Appropriate)

- Has the patient ever been pregnant? If so, how many times?
- What was the outcome of each pregnancy (eg, full-term delivery, premature or postdate delivery, spontaneous abortion, therapeutic abortion)?

Sexual Activity

- This can be an uncomfortable line of questioning for many clinicians. However, it provides important information and should be pursued.
- As with questions about substance use, you cannot determine on sight who is sexually active (and in what type of activity).
- Key questions to ask include the following:
  - Do they participate in sexual activity? Are their partners persons of the same gender, opposite gender, or both? Do they employ any strategies (eg, use of condoms) to decrease the chances of acquiring or spreading a sexually transmitted infection?
  - Do they use birth control? Are they married or engaged in a long-term relationship? If so, how is the health of their partner?
  - Is there a history of sexually transmitted infections?

Family History

- Do they have children? If so, are they healthy? Do the children live with the patient? If yes, who else lives in the home (eg, partners, spouses, others)?
- Patients should be as specific as possible. Find out the age of onset of the illnesses because this has prognostic importance for the patient. For example, if their parent had a heart attack at age 75, this is less likely to be a marker of genetic predisposition, as compared to a parent that had a similar event at age 40.
- Also ask about any unusual illnesses among relatives or relatives who died suddenly or for unexplained reasons. This may reveal evidence for other heritable conditions.

Screening Tests and Vaccinations

- Has the patient received age-, gender-, and risk factor–appropriate screening tests? This includes assessments for colon, breast, cervical, and lung cancer, as well as screening for specific metabolic disorders (eg, hyperlipidemia, diabetes) as indicated.

If so, how was the testing done (eg, there is more than one way to screen for colon cancer), what were the results, and when was the last assessment performed?

- One-time screen for abdominal aortic aneurysms (AAA) should be offered to men, age 65 to 75, who have ever smoked. Screening is done with ultrasound.
- Women of reproductive age should be screened for intimate partner violence. Multiple screening tools are available for this assessment.
- Adults should be offered depression screening with a validated tool. The Patient Health Questionnaire-2 (PHQ2) is a commonly used 2-question screen that asks the patient the following: How many days over the past 2 weeks have you: (1) been bothered by feeling down, depressed, or hopeless; and (2) had little interest or pleasure in doing things? Positive screens are followed up with additional assessments (eg, PHQ9).
- Anticipate that recommendations about screening tests will change over time. To stay current, episodically review the US Preventive Services Task Force guidelines for additional information and updates.
- If screening tests have not been done, explore why. Were they offered? Declined? Unavailable? This should be done to understand any barriers, including hesitancy, potentially identifying new opportunities to engage.
- Has the patient received age-, gender-, and risk factor–appropriate vaccines? If so, when were they given? If vaccination(s) were not received, explore why. This is done to understand hesitancy or other barriers, potentially identifying new opportunities to engage.

Work, Hobbies and Other Life Domains

- What sort of work does the patient do? Have they always done the same thing? Do they enjoy it?
- If retired, what do they do now on a day-to-day basis?
- Do they have any hobbies? Do they participate in physical activity?
- Where were they born and raised?

Not all of these questions reveal information directly related to the patient's health. However, it is nice to know something nonmedical about your patients. This may help improve the patient-physician bond and relay the sense that you care about them as a person. It also gives you something to refer back to during later visits, letting the patient know that you paid attention and remember them.

Religion and Spirituality

- Identify faith and beliefs and any associated implications for care.

Functional Level

- Assess ability to perform activities of daily living (ADLs) and instrumental activities of daily living (IADLs). These are particularly important for older patients and are discussed further in Chapter 17.

Military Service

- Serving in the armed forces can be an important time in someone's life.
- In addition, inquiring about physical trauma, mental health issues (eg, posttraumatic stress disorder, depression, substance use), military sexual trauma, and unusual exposures (eg, toxins, infections) may reveal important health-related information.

When recounting their history, patients frequently drop clues that suggest issues meriting further exploration. If, for example, they are taking antihypertensive or antianginal medications yet made no mention of cardiovascular disease, additional history taking should be pursued. Furthermore, if at any time you uncover information relevant to the CC do not be afraid to revisit the HPI.

THE FOCUSED HISTORY

Many situations do not require a complete history which includes all of the elements described earlier. Patients often present with a focal concern, such as when they visit an emergency department, see their doctor to address a specific issue, or undergo an evaluation in a specialist's office. In these situations, the CC should be explored as described earlier in this chapter. The extent of additional history taking needed is based on decisions about how this information will help direct diagnostic and therapeutic decision-making.

As an example, an acute sore throat is often the result of an infection (bacterial vs viral), and the focus of history taking and the exam will be on further characterizing this process. On the other hand, acute pharyngitis that is accompanied by generalized adenopathy, fever, rash, and risk factors for acquiring HIV could be the result of acute retroviral infection. Learning when you can be focused and appropriately parsimonious requires experience and an eye for clinical cues and clues that the problem is not "the usual." This awareness will help drive your decision-making about the extent of history and exam needed for particular clinical situations.

TELEHEALTH TIPS

History taking can be obtained via phone or video in a similar fashion as when done in person.

SUMMARY OF SKILLS CHECKLIST

History of Present Illness (HPI)
- ❑ Chief concern
- ❑ Onset
- ❑ Duration
- ❑ Location and radiation
- ❑ Intensity
- ❑ Anything that makes it better or worse
- ❑ Characteristics
- ❑ Associated symptoms
- ❑ Changes over time
- ❑ What does patient believe is wrong
- ❑ Why today

The Rest of the History
- ❑ Past medical history
- ❑ Past surgical history
- ❑ Review of systems
- ❑ Medications
- ❑ Allergies and reactions
- ❑ Smoking use

❑ Vaping use
❑ Alcohol use
❑ Other substance use
❑ Obstetric history
❑ Sexual activity
❑ Family history
❑ Screening tests and vaccinations
❑ Work, hobbies, other
❑ Religion/spirituality
❑ Functional level (ADLs and IADLs)
❑ Military service

BIBLIOGRAPHY

Avorn J, Everitt DE, Baker MW. The neglected medical history and therapeutic choices for abdominal pain: a nationwide study of 799 physicians and nurses. *Arch Intern Med.* 1991;151:694-698.

Bingham J. On being a patient: a complaint against "complaints." *Ann Intern Med.* 2003;138:73-74.

Centers for Disease Control and Prevention. Vaccination recommendations. Accessed December 30, 2022. https://www.cdc.gov/vaccines/.

Goddu P, O'Conor KJ, Lanzkron S, et al. Do words matter? Stigmatizing language and the transmission of bias in the medical record. *J Gen Intern Med.* 2018; 33(5):685-691.

Goldberg C. UCSD's practical guide to clinical medicine: history of present illness. Accessed December 27, 2022. https://meded.ucsd.edu/clinicalmed/history.html.

Goldberg C. UCSD's Practical guide to clinical medicine: the rest of the history. Accessed December 27, 2022. https://meded.ucsd.edu/clinicalmed/rest.html.

Gonzalez CM, Lypson ML, Sukhera J. Twelve tips for teaching implicit bias recognition and management. *Med Teach.*2021;43:1368-1373.

Hampton JR, Harrison MJF, Mitchell JRA, Prichard JS, Seymour C. Relative contributions of history-taking, physical examination, and laboratory investigation to diagnosis and management of medical outpatients. *Br Med J.* 1975;2:486-489.

Henderson MC, Tierney LM Jr, Smetana GW, eds. *The Patient History: An Evidence-Based Approach to Differential Diagnosis.* McGraw Hill; 2012. Accessed December 29, 2022. https://accessmedicine.mhmedical.com/content.aspx?bookid=500&sectionid=41026539.

Keifenheim E, Teufel M, Ip J, et al. Teaching history taking to medical students: a systematic review. *BMC Med Educ.* 2015;15(159):2-12.

Nieblas-Bedolla E, Christophers B, Nkinsi NT, et al. Changing how race is portrayed in medical education: recommendations from medical students. *Acad Med.* 2020;95(12):1802-1806.

Oboler SK, LaForce M. The periodic physical examination in asymptomatic adults. *Ann Intern Med.* 1989;110:214-226.

Paley L, Zornitzki T, Cohen J, et al. Utility of clinical examination in the diagnosis of emergency department patients admitted to the department of medicine of an academic hospital. *Arch Intern Med.* 2011;171(15):1396-1397.

Peterson MC, Holbrook JH, Von Hales D, Smith NL, Staker LV. Contributions of the history, physical examination and laboratory investigation in making medical diagnoses. *West J Med.* 1992;156:163-165.

Rich EC, Crowson TW, Harris IB. The diagnostic value of the medical history: perceptions of internal medicine physicians. *Arch Intern Med.* 1987;147:1957-1960.

Sabin J. Tackling implicit bias in health care. *N Engl J Med.* 2022;387:105-107.

Sandler G. The importance of the history in the medical clinic and the cost of unnecessary tests. *Am Heart J.* 1980;100:928-931.

Taylor D. You are now entering a guilt free zone. *N Engl J Med.* 2020;383(22):2103-2105.

US Preventive Services Task Forces. Recommendations for screening tests. Accessed December 30, 2022. https://www.uspreventiveservicestaskforce.org/uspstf/.

2

Review of Systems

Charlie Goldberg, MD

The review of systems (or symptoms) (ROS) is a list of questions, arranged by organ system, designed to uncover dysfunction and disease within that area. It can be applied in several ways:

- As a screening tool asked of every patient that the clinician encounters
- Asked only of patients who have specific risk factors or symptoms or who present with certain clinical scenarios

Is it appropriate (as is frequently done) to perform the same ROS on all patients as a screening tool? Using the ROS in this fashion would make sense if all of the following hold true:

- The questions have the potential to uncover an array of common and important clinical conditions.
- These disorders would go unrecognized if the patient was not specifically prompted.
- The identification of these conditions through an ROS would have a positive impact on morbidity and/or mortality.

There is no evidence to support these assumptions. In fact, positive responses to a broadly applied screening ROS are often of unclear significance and may even create problems by generating a wave of additional questions (and testing) that can be of low yield. For these reasons, it is better to incorporate a more targeted and thoughtful approach to ROS questions based on patient-specific characteristics, risk factors, clinical scenarios, and symptoms. For example:

- ROS questions designed to uncover occult disease of the prostate can be asked of men over 50.
- A cardiovascular ROS can be used when caring for patients who have risk factors for atherosclerotic disease, such as diabetes and hypertension.
- A multisystem ROS can be used when patients present with nonspecific symptoms, such as fever without focality, fatigue, or weight loss.

If a patient feels well and has neither risk factors nor symptoms, then no ROS would be necessary. This approach is likely to be both more efficient and revealing.

It is important to recognize that positive responses to an ROS query will require follow-up questions. For example, if a patient responds "yes" to an ROS question about chest pain, you will then need to ask additional questions to further define the core dimensions of this symptom. These are described in the history of present illness (HPI) section of Chapter 1.

There is no ROS gold standard. The breadth of questions that follows is based on commonly occurring illnesses and symptoms. There is planned redundancy because the same symptoms often apply to multiple organ systems (eg, chest pain could be of cardiac, pulmonary, gastrointestinal, or musculoskeletal etiology). The reason for gaining familiarity with these ROS questions is so that you can use them during situations where you believe they are appropriate. With experience and consideration, you will identify the questions that fit your clinical needs and gain facility with how to apply them in a way that is consistent with your overall patient care strategy.

Realize that uncovering unusual or regional illnesses (ie, those common to certain areas of the world, such as Lyme disease or malaria) might require different ROS questions. In addition, many subspecialty fields use an expanded ROS that is specific to the conditions that they commonly evaluate and treat. When working in these environments, check with the specialists and/or review field-specific references to learn about any additional questions to use and why they are asked.

Each category listed below begins with a specific question as to whether the patient has any known problems in that organ system. This is a way of catching issues that might not have been mentioned during history taking.

General

- Weight loss?
- Weight gain?
- Fatigued and/or tired?
- Problems sleeping?
- Fevers or sweats?
- Feeling well or poorly in general?

Head and Neck

- Any known head and neck conditions?
- Sore throat?
- Oral ulcers, sores, or masses?
- Tooth problems?
- Changes in hearing?
- Ear pain or discharge?
- Nasal congestion or discharge?
- Change in voice, such as volume or character?

Vision

- Any known eye problems?
- Changes in vision, such as blurriness, double vision, or decline in acuity?
- Eye redness or discharge?
- Eye pain?
- Eye discoloration?
- Growths, swelling, or abnormalities around the eye (eg, lids)?

Pulmonary

- Any known pulmonary problems?
- Chest pain or pressure?
- Shortness of breath (SOB)? At baseline or with exertion?
- Cough?
- Hemoptysis?
- Wheezing?
- Snoring or witnessed apnea when sleeping?

Cardiovascular

- Any known cardiovascular problems?
- Chest pain or pressure?
- Shortness of breath? At baseline or with exertion?
- Inability to lie flat due to SOB (ie, orthopnea)?
- Sudden awakening due to SOB (ie, paradoxical nocturnal dyspnea [PND])?
- Lower extremity swelling (edema)?
- Sudden loss of consciousness (syncope) or near loss of consciousness (presyncope)?
- Lightheadedness?
- Awareness of heart beating strongly or irregularly or hear racing?
- Pain in legs with activity that resolves with rest (ie, claudication)?
- Nonhealing wounds in legs, feet, or elsewhere?

Gastrointestinal (GI)

- Any known GI problems?
- Heartburn (reflux)?
- Abdominal pain?
- Dysphagia (problems swallowing; eg, food getting stuck or otherwise not going down normally)?
- Odynophagia (pain with swallowing)?
- Nausea and/or vomiting?
- Abdominal swelling or distention?
- Jaundice?
- Melena (black stools)?
- Diarrhea?
- Constipation or other change in bowel movement pattern?
- Change in stool character, consistency or shape?
- Vomiting blood (hematemesis)?
- Bloody stools (hematochezia)?
- Any positive results on prior colorectal cancer screening? If so, what was done?

Genitourinary (GU)

- Any known GU problems?
- Bloody or discolored urine?
- Incontinence?
- Pain with urination (dysuria)?
- Urinary frequency?

- Urinary urgency?
- Nocturia?
- Decreased force of urinary stream?
- Difficulty starting or stopping urination?
- Difficulty getting or maintaining erections?
- Sexually active?
- Number of partners?
- Use of birth control?
- Any problems or challenges with sexual activity?
- Penile mass or ulcer?
- Testicular pain or mass?
- Fertility issues?

Obstetrics and Gynecology (OB/GYN)
- Any known OB/GYN problems?
- Vaginal bleeding?
- Vaginal discharge?
- Duration and frequency of typical menstruation?
- Changes in menstruation (eg, duration or amount of bleeding)?
- Pregnancies? If yes, outcome(s)?
- Fertility issues?
- Abnormal Pap smears? If yes, how were they handled?
- Sexually active?
- Any problems or challenges with sexual activity?
- Number of partners?
- Use of birth control?
- Pelvic or vaginal pain?
- Breast pain, mass, or discharge?

Musculoskeletal (MSK) and Rheumatologic
- Any known MSK or rheumatologic problems?
- Joint pain?
- Joint swelling?
- Low back pain?
- Neck pain?
- Muscle aches?
- Fatigue?
- Fevers, sweats, and/or chills?

Neurologic
- Any known neurologic problems?
- Seizures?
- Numbness?
- Weakness?
- Dizziness?
- Balance or gait problems?

- Tremor?
- Headache?
- Confusion?

Infectious Diseases (ID)

- Any known ID problems?
- Fevers?
- Chills?
- Sweats?
- Immunocompromised (eg, HIV, use of immunosuppressive medications, cancer, other disorders affecting immune system function)?

Hematology and Oncology

- Any known hematology or oncology problems (eg, cancer or blood disorders)?
- Unusual bleeding or bruising?
- History of deep vein thrombosis or pulmonary embolism?
- Adenopathy (discrete swelling in lymph nodes)?
- Fevers, chills, or sweats?
- Weight loss?
- Fatigue?

Endocrine

- Any known endocrine problems?
- Polyuria (excessive urination) or polydipsia (excessive drinking)?
- Weight gain?
- Weight loss?
- Fractures?

Mental Health (Psychiatric)

- Any known mental health problems?
- Feeling sad, depressed, and/or hopeless?
- Low level of interest in participating in activities?
- Alcohol use?
- Other substance use?
- Anxious?
- Excessive energy?
- Not sleeping or sleeping too much?
- Too happy (to extent that others are worried)?
- Memory problems?
- Confused?
- Agitated?

Skin and Hair (Dermatologic)

- Any known dermatologic problems?
- Skin growths changing in size, shape or color?
- New pigmented lesion? Existing pigmented lesion changing in size, shape, symmetry, color? Bleeding from lesion?
- Nail problems or concerns?

- Rashes?
- Skin ulcers?
- Blisters?
- Nonhealing wounds?
- Itching?
- Hair loss or other problems?

TELEHEALTH TIPS

ROS questioning during a telehealth encounter would follow the same format as during an in-person interview.

BIBLIOGRAPHY

Anderson M, Klink K, Cohrssen A. What is causing this patient's vaginal symptoms? In: Simel D, Drummond R, eds. *The Rational Clinical Exam.* McGraw-Hill; 2009:691-707.

Barry M, Tseng CW. Moving to more evidence-based primary care encounters: a farewell to the review of systems. *JAMA.* 2022;328(15):1495-1496.

Bastian L, Smith CM, Nanda K. Is this patient peri-menopausal? *JAMA.* 2003;289(7):895-902.

Bent S, Nallamothu BK, Simel DL, et al. Does this woman have an acute uncomplicated urinary tract infection? *JAMA.* 2002;287(20):2701-2710.

Bradford J, O'Donoghue MW. Blurred vision. *N Engl J Med.* 2000;343(8):556-562.

Chunilal SD, Eikelboom J, Attia J, et al. Does this patient have pulmonary embolism? In: Simel D, Drummond R, eds. *The Rational Clinical Exam.* McGraw-Hill; 2009:561-575.

Cuker A, Connors JM, Katz JT, et al. A bloody mystery. *N Engl J Med.* 2009;361(19):1887-1894.

DeGowin R. Review of systems. In: *DeGgowin's Diagnostic Examination.* 7th ed. McGraw Hill; 2000:29-31.

Detsky AS, Smalley P, Chang J. Is this patient malnourished? In: Simel D, Drummond R, eds. *The Rational Clinical Exam.* McGraw-Hill; 2009:371-382.

Detsky ME, McDonald DR, Baerlocher MO, et al. Does this patient with headache have a migraine or need neuroimaging? *JAMA.* 2006;296(10):1274-1283.

Deyo R, Weinstein JN. Low back pain. *N Engl J Med.* 2001;344(5):363-370.

Froehling DA, Silverstein M, Mohr D, Beatty C. Does this dizzy patient have a serious form of vertigo? In: Simel D, Drummond R, eds. *The Rational Clinical Exam.* McGraw-Hill; 2009:709-718.

Gross G. *Review of Systems.* Maine Medical Center, Department of Internal Medicine; November 1989.

Hoffbrand BI. Away with the system review: a plea for parsimony. *BMJ.* 1989;298:817-819.

Khan NA, Rahim SA, Anand SS, et al. Does the clinical examination predict lower extremity peripheral arterial disease? *JAMA.* 2006;295(5):536-546.

Klompas M. Does this patient have an acute thoracic aortic dissection? In: Simel D, Drummond R, eds. *The Rational Clinical Exam.* McGraw-Hill; 2009:659-674.

Margaretten ME, Kohlwes J, Moore D, et al. Does this adult patient have septic arthritis? *JAMA.* 2007;297(13):1478-1488.

Metlay J, Kapoor W, Fine M. Does this patient have community-acquired pneumonia? Diagnosing pneumonia by history and physical examination. In: Simel D, Drummond R, eds. *The Rational Clinical Exam*. McGraw-Hill; 2009:527-537.

Panju A, Hemmelgarn B, Guyatt G, Simel D. Is this patient having a myocardial infarction? In: Simel D, Drummond R, eds. *The Rational Clinical Exam*. McGraw-Hill; 2009:461-476.

Rao G, Fisch L, Srinivasan S, et al. Does this patient have Parkinson disease? In: Simel D, Drummond R, eds. *The Rational Clinical Exam*. McGraw-Hill; 2009:505-514.

Sharpe M, Wilks D. Fatigue. ABC of psychological medicine. *BMJ*. 2002;325:480-483.

Silen W. *Cope's Early Diagnosis of the Acute Abdomen*. 22nd ed. Oxford University Press; 2010.

Swartz MH. Review of systems. In: *Swartz Textbook of Physical Diagnosis: History and Examination*. 4th ed. WB Saunders; 2002:28-30.

Trowbridge R, Rutkowski N, Shojania K. Does this patient have acute cholecystitis? In: Simel D, Drummond R, eds. *The Rational Clinical Exam*. McGraw-Hill; 2009:137-147.

Wagner J, McKinne W, Carpenter J. Does this patient have appendicitis? In: Simel D, Drummond R, eds. *The Rational Clinical Exam*. McGraw-Hill; 2009:53-63.

Wang C, FitzGerald J, Schulzer M, Mak E, Ayas N. Does this dyspneic patient in the emergency department have congestive heart failure? In: Simel D, Drummond R, eds. *The Rational Clinical Exam*. McGraw-Hill; 2009:195-213.

Wells PS, Own C, Doucette S, Fergusson D, Tran H. Does this patient have deep vein thrombosis? In: Simel D, Drummond R, eds. *The Rational Clinical Exam*. McGraw-Hill; 2009:235-246.

Whited JD, Grichnik J. Does this patient have a mole or a melanoma? In: Simel D, Drummond R, eds. *The Rational Clinical Exam*. McGraw-Hill; 2009:383-394.

Williams J, Noel P, Cordes J, Ramirez G, Pignone M. Is this patient clinically depressed? In: Simel D, Drummond R, eds. *The Rational Clinical Exam*. McGraw-Hill; 2009:247-263.

Williams J, Simel D. Does this patient have sinusitis? Diagnosing acute sinusitis by history and physical examination. In: Simel D, Drummond R, eds. *The Rational Clinical Exam*. McGraw-Hill; 2009:593-603.

3

Vital Signs

Charlie Goldberg, MD

INTRODUCTION

Vital signs (aka "vitals") include the measurement of temperature, respiratory rate, pulse, blood pressure, and oxygen saturation. These numbers provide critical information (hence the name "vitals") about a patient's state of health. In particular, vital signs:

- Can point to the existence of an acute medical problem.
- Are a means of rapidly quantifying the magnitude of an illness and how well the body is coping with the resultant physiologic stress. Often, the more deranged the vitals, the sicker is the patient.
- Are a marker of chronic disease states. For example, hypertension is defined as chronically elevated blood pressure.

Most patients will have had their vital signs measured by a nurse or healthcare assistant before you see them. However, these values are of such great importance that you should get in the habit of repeating them yourself if they are very abnormal. As noted later in this chapter, there is significant potential for measurement error, so repeat determinations can provide critical information.

In the outpatient/elective visit setting, the patient should have had the opportunity to rest for approximately 5 minutes so that the values are not affected by the exertion required to walk to the exam room. All measurements are made while the patient is seated (or lying in bed if hospitalized or presenting with acute symptoms).

Observation

Start by looking at the patient in their entirety, if possible, from an out-of-the-way perch. Do they seem anxious, in pain, or upset? What about their dress and hygiene? Remember, the exam begins as soon as you lay eyes on the patient.

TEMPERATURE

- This can be done via oral, ear, rectal, or nontouch sensors.
- Temperature is measured in either Celsius or Fahrenheit, with a fever defined as greater than 38 to 38.5°C or 101 to 101.5°F.
- Temperature measurement is of greatest importance when there is concern about infection or other acute inflammatory states.

RESPIRATORY RATE

- Respirations are recorded as breaths per minute.
- They should be counted for at least 30 seconds because the total number of breaths in a 15-second period is small and any miscounting can result in relatively large errors when multiplied by 4.
- Try to measure the respiratory rate as surreptitiously as possible so that the patient does not consciously alter their rate of breathing, which can happen if they feel they are being watched. This can be done by observing the rise and fall of the patient's chest area while you appear to be taking their pulse.
- Normal respiratory rate (RR) is between 12 and 20 breaths per minute.
- In general, RR is not relevant information for the routine examination. However, particularly in the setting of acute illness, it can be a useful marker of disease severity and compensation. Increases in RR measured over time help to identify clinical deterioration, especially for hospitalized patients who can be assessed serially.

> PEARL: Identifying new tachypnea is an important clinical clue that is often missed because clinicians fail to measure the respiratory rate. When present, it always merits an explanation.

Findings and Their Meaning: Tachypnea (Fast Respiratory Rate)

- Tachypnea can be a response to hypoxemia or hypercarbia, often the result of acute or chronic cardio-pulmonary conditions.
- Can be related to physiologic stress elsewhere in the body (eg, sepsis, hyperthyroidism, pain).
- Can be part of respiratory compensation for metabolic acidosis (eg, diabetic ketoacidosis).
- Can be related to anxiety, fear, or other sources of stress.

Findings and Their Meaning: Bradypnea (Low Respiratory Rate)

- Low RR can result from acutely impaired central stimulation, as from overdose (eg, narcotics), head trauma, profound metabolic disturbances (eg, advanced kidney or liver disease, hypothyroidism), or other severe processes that depress core brain functions.
- Obstructive sleep apnea can lead to low RR, although the decrease or cessation of breathing (in severe settings) is followed by spontaneous resumption, often with elevated respiratory rate. This is typically diagnosed by a sleep study. It can also be identified clinically when previously undiagnosed patients are hospitalized for other reasons and are observed while sleeping.

PULSE

- Pulse rate is typically determined electronically by the same device that measures blood pressure. This suffices in most clinical environments. Pulse can also be easily assessed manually, useful when no machine is available or when there is a need for the clinician to make this determination independently (e.g. if the patient is tachycardic, bradycardic, or otherwise ill).
- Pulse can be measured at any place on the body where there is a large artery (eg, radial, carotid, or femoral artery, or by listening over the heart). For the sake of convenience, it is generally done by palpating the radial impulse.
- Place the tips of your index and middle fingers just proximal to the patient's wrist on the thumb side, orienting them so that they are both aligned over the length of the vessel (**Figure 3-1**).

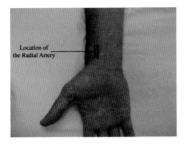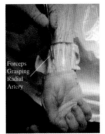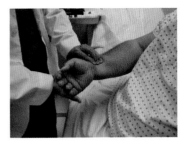

FIGURE 3-1 • **Location and technique for measuring the radial pulse.** (Photos from *Practical Guide to Clinical Medicine: Vital Signs*. Available from: https://meded.ucsd.edu/clinicalmed/vital.html.)

- Frequently, you can see transmitted pulsations on careful visual inspection of this region, which may help in locating the radial artery.
- Press lightly at first, adding pressure if there is a lot of subcutaneous fat or you are unable to detect a pulse.
- If you push too hard, you might occlude the vessel and mistake your own pulse for that of the patient.
- Upper extremity peripheral vascular disease is uncommon, so the radial artery should be readily palpable in most patients.

Heart rate is dependent on the function of the electrical conducting system. The impulse starts in the sinoatrial node, traverses the atria, and passes through the atrioventricular (AV) node, down the bundle of His, through the bundle branches, and out to the ventricles through the Purkinje system. This path of electrical activation causes the atria to contract, followed by the ventricles (**Figure 3-2**), which optimizes cardiac performance.

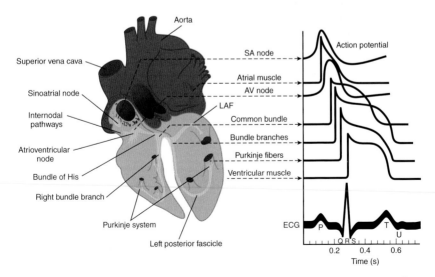

FIGURE 3-2 • **The electrical conduction system of the heart.** (Reproduced with permission from Barrett KE, Barman SM, Brooks HL, Yuan JX-J, eds. *Ganong's Review of Medical Physiology*. 26th ed. New York: McGraw Hill; 2019.)

During assessment of the pulse, the key elements to note are the rate, rhythm, and volume. Each is described separately, though in reality, the assessments are done simultaneously.

Rate

- Measure the rate of the pulse (recorded in beats per minute [bpm]). Count for 30 seconds and multiply by 2 (or 15 seconds × 4).
- If the rate is particularly slow or fast, it is best to measure for a full 60 seconds in order to minimize the impact of any error in recording over shorter periods of time. The normal rate is between 60 and 100 (**Figure 3-3**).

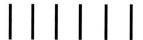

FIGURE 3-3 • **Normal rate, regular rhythm.** (Illustration from *Practical Guide to Clinical Medicine: Cardiovascular Exam.* Available from: https://meded.ucsd.edu/clinicalmed/heart.html.)

Findings and Their Meaning: Tachycardia (>100 bpm)

- An ECG or cardiac monitor is often used to definitively measure the rate (fast or slow). It also identifies the rhythm (information to follow)
- Sinus tachycardia: The rate is fast and the rhythm regular. Some potential causes include:
  - Physiologic response to hypovolemia, anemia, both
  - Response to physiological stressor(s), including fever, pain, metabolic disorders, or other acute illnesses/processes
  - Response to anxiety or fear
- Non-sinus tachycardia: Includes atrial fibrillation, atrial flutter and atrio-ventricular nodal reentrant tachycardia (AVNRT). See **Figure 3-4** and "Rhythm" section below for details.

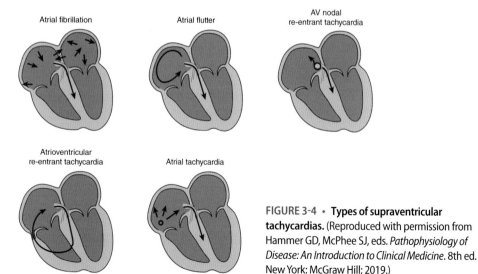

FIGURE 3-4 • **Types of supraventricular tachycardias.** (Reproduced with permission from Hammer GD, McPhee SJ, eds. *Pathophysiology of Disease: An Introduction to Clinical Medicine.* 8th ed. New York: McGraw Hill; 2019.)

- The rhythm can be more or less regular (AVNRT, atrial flutter) or irregularly irregular (atrial fibrillation).
- Symptoms vary, depending on the rate as well as whether perfusion/blood pressure is affected.

Findings and Their Meaning: Bradycardia (<60 bpm)

- Rates between 40 and 60 may be normal in patients who are very fit. They will typically describe themselves as being active and have no symptoms related to the bradycardia.
- Pathologic bradycardia can be from conduction system disease (eg, sick sinus syndrome, third-degree heart block), medications, hypoxia, metabolic disorders (eg, hypothyroidism), and other processes.
- When pathologic, bradycardia is often associated with symptoms including exercise intolerance, fatigue, heart failure, presyncope, or syncope. The severity of symptoms is based on degree of bradycardia, ability to compensate, and impact of low heart rate on blood pressure and perfusion.

Rhythm

- In the normal setting, the heart rate is quite regular, with a consistent amount of time between beats (see Figure 3-3).

Findings and Their Meaning: Irregular Rhythm

- If the rhythm is entirely chaotic with no discernable pattern, it is referred to as irregularly irregular and likely represents atrial fibrillation (**Figure 3-5**).
- Extra beats can be added into the normal pattern, in which case the rhythm is described as regularly irregular. This may occur, for example, when impulses originating from the ventricle are interposed at regular junctures on the normal rhythm.
- If the pulse is irregular, consider verifying the rate by listening over the heart (see Chapter 6, Cardiovascular exam). This is because certain rhythm disturbances do not allow adequate ventricular filling with each beat. The resultant systole may generate a rather small stroke volume whose impulse is not easily palpable in the periphery.

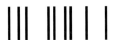

FIGURE 3-5 • **Irregularly irregular rhythm: atrial fibrillation.** (Illustration from *Practical Guide to Clinical Medicine: Cardiovascular Exam.* Available from: https://meded.ucsd.edu/clinicalmed/heart.html.)

Pulse Volume

- Note if the pulse volume (ie, the subjective sense of the impulse's fullness) feels normal. This may be a reflection of changes in stroke volume.

Findings and Their Meaning: Increased or Decreased Pulse Volume

- In the setting of hypovolemia, for example, the pulse can feel of lower amplitude, described as weak or thready. When caring for ill or unstable patients, palpating the pulse and noting the volume can provide insights about perfusion status.
- Volume can be increased if there are particularly vigorous contractions, as can occur with conditions where preload is high and ventricular performance preserved (eg, compensated aortic insufficiency; see Chapter 6: Cardiovascular Exam).

- There may even be beat-to-beat variation in the volume, occurring occasionally with systolic heart failure or cardiac tamponade.

BLOOD PRESSURE

- Blood pressure (BP) readings in hospitals and clinics are typically obtained using digital equipment.
- It is still relevant to learn how to use manual cuffs, as clinicians occasionally need to check the validity of digital readings (eg, when BP is high or low) or an electronic device may not be available. The technique is described for both.

Positioning the Patient

- Appropriate positioning is critical in order to obtain accurate measurements. Patients should be seated for 5 minutes, with the back supported, the feet on floor, legs uncrossed, arm supported at level of heart, wearing nonconstricting clothes, and with the cuff placed on skin. Errors in any of these steps, which may be additive, can lead to inaccurate measurements (**Figure 3-6**).

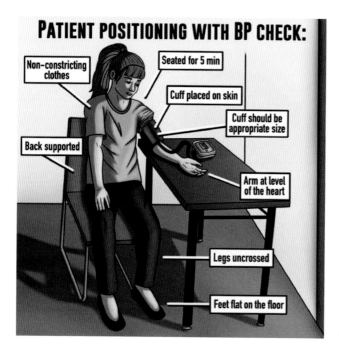

FIGURE 3-6 • Patient positioning when measuring blood pressure (BP). (Reproduced with permission from Cathy Cichon, MD.)

Cuff Selection (for Manual or Digital Measurements)

- The size of the BP cuff will affect the accuracy of the readings. The inflatable bladder, which can be felt through the vinyl covering of the cuff, should reach roughly 80% around the circumference of the arm while its width should cover roughly 40% (**Figure 3-7**).
- If the cuff is too small, the readings may be artificially elevated. The opposite occurs if the cuff is too large.
- Most healthcare settings have several size cuffs available to accommodate different-sized patients.

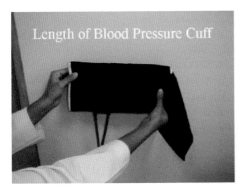
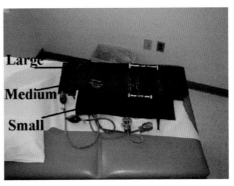

FIGURE 3-7 • **Selecting the correct size cuff.** (Photos from *Practical Guide to Clinical Medicine: Vital Signs.* Available from: https://meded.ucsd.edu/clinicalmed/vital.html.)

Positioning the Cuff

- The cuff should be placed directly on the skin.
- The antecubital fossa should be easily accessible. The brachial artery is located in the medial one-third of the fossa, although it does not have to be directly palpated (**Figure 3-8**).
- Wrap the cuff around the patient's upper arm so that the line marked "artery" is roughly over the brachial artery, located toward the medial aspect of the antecubital fossa.
- The placement does not have to be exact.
- The automatic measuring device (if that is being used) can now be activated. A digital reading (typically pulse and BP) should show up on the screen pretty quickly.

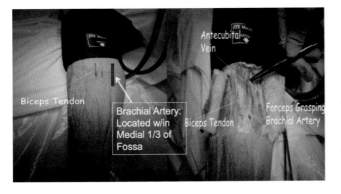

FIGURE 3-8 • **Positioning the blood pressure cuff.** (Photo from *Practical Guide to Clinical Medicine: Vital Signs.* Available from: https://meded.ucsd.edu/clinicalmed/vital.html.)

Special Testing: Obtaining a Manual BP Reading

- Put on your stethoscope. Use the bell because it is slightly better for detecting the low-pitched sounds associated with measuring BP. Place the bell over the brachial artery area and hold it in place with one of your hands (**Figure 3-9**).
- With your other hand, turn the valve on the pumping bulb clockwise (may be counter-clockwise in some cuffs) until it no longer moves. This is the position that allows air to enter and remain in the bladder.

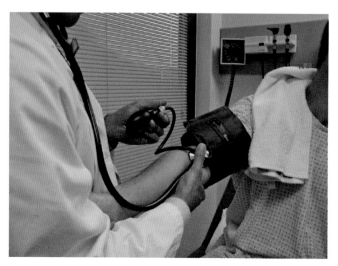

FIGURE 3-9 • Hand positioning when using a manual blood pressure cuff. (Photo from *Practical Guide to Clinical Medicine: Vital Signs*. Available from: https://meded.ucsd.edu/clinicalmed/vital.html.)

- Pump the bulb until you have generated 160 mmHg on the manometer. This is greater than the upper limit of normal for systolic blood pressure (SBP).
- Then listen. You should not hear any sound if you have inflated to a value above the SBP. If you do hear sound, it means that you have underestimated the SBP. Pump up an additional 20 mmHg and repeat. If you again immediately hear sound, pump up an additional 20 mmHg and repeat.
  - Alternatively, you can inflate the cuff while simultaneously palpating the radial artery. Make note of the reading on the gauge when the pulse is no longer present. This is the SBP. Inflate to approximately 10 mmHg above the point where the pulse disappeared.
- Then turn the valve in a counterclockwise direction (allowing air to escape the bladder), listen over the brachial artery, and slowly deflate the cuff (ie, a few mmHg per second) while watching the pressure gauge.
- The first sound that you hear reflects the flow of blood through the brachial artery. The value on the manometer at this moment is the SBP. Note that although the needle may oscillate prior to this time, it is the sound of blood flow (known as the sounds of Korotkoff) that indicates the SBP.
- Continue listening while you deflate the cuff. The diastolic blood pressure (DBP) is measured when the sound completely disappears. This is the point where the pressure within the vessel is greater than that supplied by the cuff. Listen as the needle drops another 10 mmHg to ensure that you have identified the true DBP.
- The recorded values are written as SBP/DBP.
- Repeated measurements in the same arm can be uncomfortable. Rather than re-inflating multiple times, consider giving the patient a break or measuring BP in their other arm.
- Avoid moving your hands or the head of the stethoscope while you are taking readings because this may produce noise that can obscure the sounds of Korotkoff.

- For the purposes of practice, you can repeat the measurement on the patient's other arm, reversing the position of your hands. The 2 readings should be within 10 to 15 mmHg of each other.
  - Differences greater than this imply that there is differential blood flow to each arm, which can occur in the setting of atherosclerosis or diseases of the aorta (eg, dissection of the thoracic aorta, subclavian artery stenosis).

Findings and Their Meaning: Hypertension

- Normal <120/80 mmHg
- Elevated: SBP 120-129 mmHg and DBP <80 mmHg
- Stage 1 hypertension: SBP 130-139 mmHg or DBP 80-89 mmHg
- Stage 2 hypertension: SBP ≥140 mmHg or DBP ≥90 mmHg

It is worth noting that the BP values that define hypertension have changed over the years and may continue to do so.

Hypertension (HTN) is a common disease, affecting >40% of the US adult population. With the steady increase in obesity rates (a major driver of HTN), it is anticipated that the numbers of those affected will continue to increase.

- The diagnosis of HTN is typically based on 2 readings, done at 2 different settings.
- A single measurement >160/100 mmHg should prompt consideration for medication treatment (ie, you do not necessarily need 2 values indicating stage 2 HTN).
- Lifestyle interventions (eg, managing weight, healthy eating, being active, not smoking, sleeping well) are important and should be incorporated into any treatment plan. In addition, identifying and managing other disorders that synergize with HTN to cause target organ damage (eg, high cholesterol, diabetes) are also critical. A full discussion of treatments is beyond the scope of this chapter and can be found in the American Heart Association guidelines and other references (see the Bibliography at the end of this chapter).
- Home readings (with a validated device) can also be used for the diagnosis and management of HTN.
- Careful attention must be paid to the use of appropriate techniques (described earlier), as measurement error(s) can lead to inaccurate values and diagnoses.

HTN is a common disorder, causing and accelerating many important conditions that have significant morbidity and mortality. These include coronary artery disease, heart failure, left ventricular hypertrophy, aortic aneurysm development, peripheral arterial disease, stroke, chronic kidney disease, and retinopathy. The risk of HTN-induced damage correlates with both the height of BP and the chronicity of elevation. It also synergizes with other risk factors (eg, diabetes, elevated cholesterol) to cause target organ damage.

Most patients with elevated BP suffer from primary HTN, where the elevation in BP is the primary disorder. Secondary HTN occurs when the elevation in BP is secondary to another, treatable condition. Obesity, endocrine disorders (eg, hypo- or hyperthyroidism, hyperaldosteronism, pheochromocytoma, cortisol excess), chronic kidney disease, sleep apnea, renal artery stenosis, and coarctation of the aorta are examples of secondary causes.

Findings and Their Meaning: Hypotension

- Low end of normal BP is approximately 90-100 mmHg for SBP and 60-70 mmHg for DBP.
- The minimal BP required to maintain perfusion varies with the individual patient.
- A young, small person may have a normal SBP of 90 mmHg and feel great, in which case they will often report that this is consistent with their typical readings (if measured previously). Interpretation of low BP values must therefore take into account the clinical situation. To better understand the causes of hypotension, it's useful to first review the physiologic inputs that contribute to blood pressure (**Figure 3-10**).

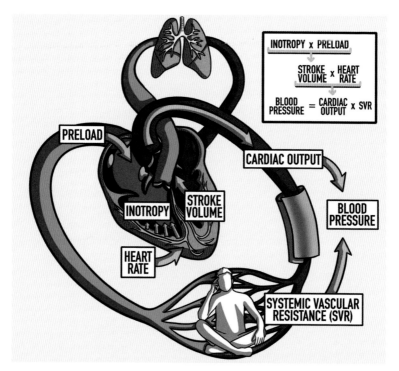

FIGURE 3-10 • **Physiologic contributors to Blood Pressure.** (Reproduced with permission from Cathy Cichon, MD.)

- The body has an ability to compensate and maintain perfusion in the setting of physiologic stress. For example, with blood loss, heart rate and contractility will increase and peripheral vasoconstriction will occur in an effort to maintain BP and perfusion. However, compensatory mechanisms can be overwhelmed if the challenges are too great. Common contributors to hypotension are described in **Figure 3-11**.
- Abrupt decreases in BP to levels significantly lower than baseline will typically generate symptoms of hypoperfusion (eg, feeling weak, dizzy, lightheaded, syncope).

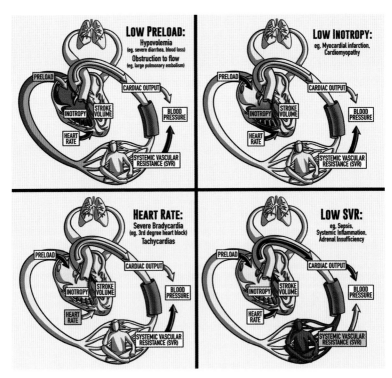

FIGURE 3-11 • **Causes of Hypotension.** (Reproduced with permission from Cathy Cichon, MD.)

Special Testing: Orthostatic (ie, Postural) Measurements of Pulse and Blood Pressure

- This may be part of an assessment for hypovolemia and/or dizziness. It requires first measuring heart rate and BP when the patient is supine and then repeating these measurements after the patient has been standing for a few minutes (**Figure 3-12**). Postural VS can also be obtained sitting if the patient isn't able to safely stand – with the changes evaluated in comparison with the supine position.
- Normally, SBP does not vary by more than approximately 20 mmHg and DBP by more than approximately 10 mmHg when a patient moves from lying to standing.

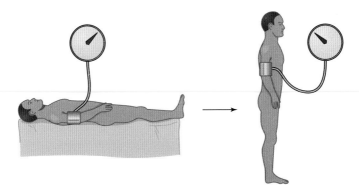

FIGURE 3-12 • **Measuring orthostatic vital signs.** (Reproduced with permission from Neurologic History and Examination. In: Aminoff MJ, Greenberg DA, Simon RP, eds. *Clinical Neurology.* 9th ed. New York: McGraw-Hill; 2015.)

- In the setting of significant volume depletion, a greater drop may be seen. This may also be associated with symptoms of cerebral hypo-perfusion (eg, lightheadedness, presyncope). For example, if a patient is experiencing acute gastrointestinal bleeding, a drop in BP and/or rise in heart rate when moving from lying to standing is a marker of significant blood loss and has important prognostic implications.
- It is also possible to have volume loss without attendant postural changes (ie, the absence of changes does not rule out hypovolemia).
- Orthostatic measurements may also be used to determine if postural dizziness or syncope/presyncope is the result of a decrease in BP.
  - For example, patients who suffer from diabetes may have autonomic nervous system dysfunction and impaired ability to appropriately vasoconstrict when changing positions.
  - If the patient's dizziness/lightheadedness is the result of orthostatic changes, their BP will drop when they move from a lying to standing position and symptoms will be reproduced.
- The 20-mmHg value is a rough guideline. In general, the greater the change in BP, the more likely it is to cause symptoms and be of clinical significance.

OXYGEN SATURATION

- Pulse oximetry (aka "pulse ox") is a noninvasive measurement of hemoglobin saturation (SpO_2) and is often referred to as the fifth vital sign. Normal is ≥95%.
- It is usually obtained through the nail bed by placing the probe on the patient's finger. Nail polish should be removed and the probe should fit (**Figure 3-13**). There are also sensors that can be placed on the earlobes and other peripheral points of the body.
- SpO_2 is a useful indicator of hypoxemia and thus is measured in almost every clinical setting.
- Pulse oximeters are often built into devices that measure other vital signs and also come in versions that are small and portable. They are also part of all intensive care, telemetry unit, emergency department, and anesthesia monitoring systems.

Findings and Their Meaning: Low SpO_2

- Any process that impairs the movement of oxygen through the bronchi, into the alveoli, across the interstitial space, and onto the red blood cells can lower hemoglobin saturation. This can result from a wide range of acute (eg, pulmonary edema, pneumonia, overdose, lower respiratory rate) and chronic conditions (eg, chronic obstructive pulmonary disease).
- It is important to note that the SpO_2 may be normal when there is subtle hypoxemia. Patients who are healthy without baseline gas exchange problems can compensate, with

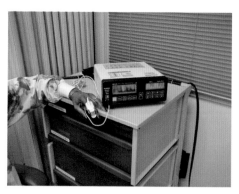

FIGURE 3-13 • **Pulse oximeter.** (Photo from *Practical Guide to Clinical Medicine: Vital Signs*. Available from: https://meded.ucsd.edu/clinicalmed/vital.html.)

enough oxygen made available to saturate their hemoglobin even in the presence of pathology that is impairing gas exchange. Thus, a normal SpO_2 does not exclude important cardiopulmonary disease.

- The SpO_2 does not provide an accurate measurement of ventilation, which is reflected in the partial pressure of carbon dioxide (PCO_2; measured via blood gas analysis).
- Rare disorders of the hemoglobin itself (eg, methemoglobin or carboxyhemoglobin) can impair saturation without there being an issue with gas exchange in the lungs. These are uncommon and are linked to specific exposures. For example, dapsone use can cause production of methemoglobin, and use of indoor heaters with poor ventilation can result in carbon monoxide exposure and carboxyhemoglobin production.
- There has to be good perfusion in order for the saturation to be accurately measured. Hypotension, for example, may cause inaccurate readings. The oximeter displays an arterial pulse tracing, which can be used to assess perfusion.
- Black patients may have inaccuracies in oxygen saturation measurement due to interference from dark skin, leading to readings that are higher than they should be based on the measured partial pressure of oxygen (PO_2).

🖥 TELEHEALTH TIPS

- Vital signs (pulse and BP) can be obtained if the patient has an electronic unit at home and knows how to use it. Ideally, the unit should be one that is newer, calibrated, and recognized by the clinic site as a device that is accurate.
- Patients may also have the ability to take their temperature with a thermometer and oxygen saturation with a pulse oximeter.
- When measuring BP with a home machine, appropriate technique (as described in this chapter) should be followed.
- Measurement of respiratory rate (in particular, if it is very elevated) may also be possible if you can observe the patient's upper chest area on camera.
- General appearance, level of alertness, and ability to converse and answer questions should also be noted.

✓ SUMMARY OF SKILLS CHECKLIST

- ❏ Clean your hands
- ❏ Observe patient
- ❏ Measure temperature
- ❏ Measure respiratory rate
- ❏ Measure pulse, noting: rate, regularity, and volume
- ❏ Measure BP
- ❏ *Special testing: Orthostatic vital signs
- ❏ Measure oxygen saturation
- ❏ Clean your hands

BIBLIOGRAPHY

ACC/AHA Task Force. Guideline for the prevention, detection, evaluation, and management of high blood pressure in adults. *Hypertension*. 2017:1-283.

American College of Cardiology. ACC atherosclerotic cardiovascular disease (ASCVD) risk estimator tool. Accessed May 16, 2023. https://tools.acc.org/ascvd-risk-estimator-plus/#!/calculate/estimate/.

American Heart Association. AHA hypertension guideline toolkit. Accessed December 31, 2022. https://aha-clinical-review.ascendeventmedia.com/books/aha-high-blood-pressure-toolkit/.

Benowitz NL, Kuyt F, Jacob P. Influence of nicotine on cardiovascular and hormonal effects of cigarette smoking. *Clin Pharmacol Ther.* 1984;36:74-81.

Carey RM, Whelton PK; 2017 ACC/AHA Hypertension Guideline Writing Committee. Prevention, detection, evaluation, and management of high blood pressure in adults: synopsis of the 2017 American College of Cardiology/American Heart Association Hypertension Guideline. *Ann Intern Med.* 2018;168:351-358.

Corley DA, Stefan AM, Wolf M, Cook F, Lee TH. Early indicators of prognosis in upper gastrointestinal hemorrhage. *Am J Gastroenterol.* 1998;93:336-340.

Goldberg C. UCSD's practical guide to clinical medicine (vital signs). Accessed December 31, 2022. https://meded.ucsd.edu/clinicalmed/vital.html.

James PA, Oparil S, Carter BL, et al. 2014 Evidence-based guideline for the management of high blood pressure in adults: report from the panel members appointed to the Eighth Joint National Committee (JNC 8). *JAMA.* 2014;311(5):507-520.

Kollef MH, O'Brien JD, Zuckerman GR, Shannon W. BLEED: a classification tool to predict outcomes in patients with acute upper and lower gastrointestinal hemorrhage. *Crit Care Med.* 1997;25:1125-1132.

Koziol-McLain J, Lowenstein SR, Fuller B. Orthostatic vital signs in emergency department patients. *Ann Emerg Med.* 1991;20:606-610.

Marino P. *Marino's The ICU Book.* 4th ed. Philadelphia: Wolters Kluwer; 2014.

Maxwell MH, Waks AU, Schroth PC, Karam M, Dornfeld LP. Error in blood-pressure measurement due to incorrect cuff size in obese patients. *Lancet.* 1982;2(8288):33-36.

McGee S, Abernethy WB, Simel DL. Is this patient hypovolemic? *JAMA.* 1999;281:1022-1029.

McGrady A, Higgins JT. Effect of repeated measurements of blood pressure on blood pressure in essential hypertension: role of anxiety. *J Behav Med.* 1990;13:93-101.

Ortega R, Hansen CJ, Elterman K, Woo A. Pulse oximetry. *N Engl J Med.* 2011;364:e33.

Reeves RA. Does this patient have hypertension? How to measure blood pressure. *JAMA.* 1995;273:1211-1218.

Russell AE, Wing LMH, Smith SA, et al. Optimal size of cuff bladder for indirect measurement of arterial pressure in adults. *J Hypertens.* 1989;7:607-613.

Scherwitz LW, Evans LA, Hennrikus DJ, Vallbona C. Procedures and discrepancies of blood pressure measurements in two community health centers. *Med Care.* 1982;20:727-738.

Silverberg DS, Shemesh E, Iaina A. The unsupported arm: a cause of falsely raised blood pressure readings. *Br Med J.* 1977;2(6098):1331.

Sjoding M, Dickson RP, Iwashyna TJ, Gay SE, Valley TS. Racial bias in pulse oximetry measurement. *N Engl J Med.* 2020;383:2477-2478.

Smith TD, Clayton D. Individual variation between general practitioners in labeling of hypertension. *BMJ.* 1990;300(6717):74-75.

Taler S. Initial treatment of hypertension. *N Engl J Med.* 2018;378:636-644.

Viol GW, Goebel M, Lorenz GJ, Ing TS. Seating as a variable in clinical blood pressure measurement. *Am Heart J.* 1979;98(6):813-814.

Williams J, Brown S, Conlin P. Blood pressure measurement (videos in clinical medicine). *N Engl J Med.* 2009;360(5):e6.

4

Head and Neck Exam

Charley Coffey, MD

INTRODUCTION

The comprehensive head and neck exam is typically performed when patients have symptoms, concerns, or risk factors for disorders related to this area.

Although students and providers may not necessarily think of the face and neck as a sensitive region in the same context of other portions of our anatomy, they are nonetheless considered very personal space for many people, and the examiner should remain mindful of this. As such, the exam should be approached in a trauma informed fashion, describing each maneuver, the rationale, moving slowly and providing the patient with an opportunity to stop or opt out.

Communicate your actions with the patient simply and clearly throughout the examination, and consider starting with some of the less intimate portions of the examination (eg, observation, cranial nerves) prior to "moving in close" for aspects such as palpation of the neck and the intraoral exam.

Good lighting is critical for proper oral examination. A headlight is optimal, as this allows maximal illumination while freeing both hands for palpation and manipulation of the tissues. If a flashlight or otoscope is used, ensure that it is turned to the brightest setting.

Head and neck review of systems is covered in Chapter 2. See Chapter 1 for directions about how to obtain historical information related to a head and neck concern.

Observation

- The patient should be comfortably seated on the end of the exam table to provide the examiner with easy access to both sides of the head and neck (eg, for palpation of the neck or inspection of the scalp) (**Figure 4-1**).
- During the initial portion of the visit while speaking with the patient, observe the face and neck for any evidence of asymmetry. Are there visible masses, swelling, or skin lesions? Is there any asymmetry of motion, particularly around the eyes, brow, or mouth (areas that are most animated when we speak)?
- Listen to how the patient sounds. Is the voice quality altered? Is it rough, breathy, strained, or muffled? Are there any audible alterations in speech?
- Hair on the face or scalp can make inspection of the underlying skin challenging. If there is concern for cutaneous pathology, such as malignancy, rash, or an autoimmune disorder, a thorough inspection may require using fingers to manipulate the hair and allow for a systematic examination.

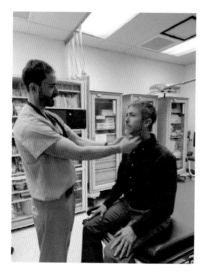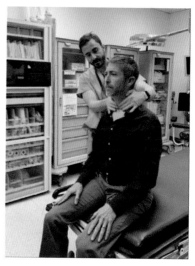

FIGURE 4-1 • **Patient positioning for the head and neck exam.** (Photo by Charley Coffey, MD.)

Findings and Their Meaning: Changes in Speech and Superficial Abnormalities

- Alterations in voice quality could represent pathology of the vocal folds (eg, laryngitis, benign or malignant lesions) or pathology higher in the larynx or pharynx (eg, epiglottitis, tonsillitis).
- Normal speech patterns vary, and breaks in fluency such as hesitance or stuttering are not necessarily pathologic. However, dysarthria (difficulty forming words) can be indicative of central disorders such as stroke or mucosal pathology that affects tongue mobility.
- If cutaneous lesions are present, make careful note of the size, location, distribution, and description. Clinical photography can be a useful adjunct to document the appearance of skin lesions in the medical record.

SELECTED CRANIAL NERVE EXAM

Cranial nerve evaluation is generally performed during the head and neck exam, most commonly focusing on assessment of cranial nerves (CNs) III, IV, V, VI, VII, X, XI, and XII. The neurologic portion can be performed independent of the remainder of the exam or integrated with examinations of each subsite as briefly outlined below. Detailed descriptions of individual CN exam techniques and selected findings and their meaning can be found in the chapters on the neurologic exam (Chapter 12) and ophthalmologic exam (Chapter 5).

- Assess branches of the facial nerve (CN VII) by instructing the patient to elevate the brow, tightly close the eyes, purse lips, and frown. Note any weakness or asymmetry, including which portions of the face are affected.
- Assess facial sensation by using fingertips or gauze to lightly brush the brow (CN V1), cheeks (V2), and chin (V3) on each side. Determine whether there is any subjective loss or decrease in sensation and which portions of the face are affected. If findings are unclear, instruct the patient to close eyes to eliminate visual cues and ask them to indicate each time they are able to detect the light touch.

- Assess extraocular motion (CN III, IV, VI) by instructing the patient to visually track movement of the finger across all fields of view. Systematically assess horizontal, vertical, and diagonal gaze. Advise the patient to let you know if any direction of gaze results in double vision.
- Assess spinal accessory (CN XI) function by asking the patient to raise their arms to the sides and then above the head. Note that a simple shoulder shrug may not be sufficient to detect spinal accessory nerve weakness, but full shoulder abduction provides unequivocal assessment.

PALPATION OF THE NECK

Examination of the neck requires careful palpation to assess for the presence of masses. Although enlarged lymph nodes are the most common finding, a palpable neck mass may also represent pathology of the parotid or submandibular salivary glands, the larynx, the thyroid, or a congenital cyst (eg, thyroglossal duct or branchial cleft cyst).

- Use the sensitive pads of 3 or 4 fingers to palpate each side of the neck. Walk the hands methodically down the neck on each side using firm, steady pressure.
- You may stand in front of or to the side of the patient as you palpate the neck. Alternatively, some examiners palpate while standing behind the patient, with fingers pointed anteriorly. Note that this can be triggering for some patients (ie, hands around neck can simulate a choke hold). If this technique is utilized, the rationale and approach should be explained beforehand, asking permission and providing an opportunity for the patient to opt out. (Figure 4-1).

Lymph nodes are generally distributed symmetrically along both sides of the head and neck, and each lymph node basin drains a specific, corresponding region of the head or neck (**Figure 4-2**). Performing the exam with purposeful attention to each nodal group will help to ensure that subtle findings are not overlooked:

- Pre- and postauricular nodes
  - Location: Anterior to tragus and posterior to the pinna; generally small, superficial nodes
  - Drainage: Pinna and external auditory canal, scalp, parotid gland
- Submandibular/submental nodes
  - Location: Beneath the mandible and chin
  - Drainage: Oral cavity, lips
- Anterior cervical
  - Location: Anterior and deep to the sternocleidomastoid muscle (SCM), from the mastoid to the clavicle
  - Drainage: Oral cavity, pharynx, thyroid, salivary glands, facial skin
- External jugular
  - Location: Overlying (ie, superficial to) the SCM
  - Drainage: Skin of the face and scalp (*not* deep/mucosal tissues)
- Posterior cervical
  - Location: From the posterior border of SCM to the anterior border of the trapezius
  - Drainage: Posterior scalp, pharynx, parotid, thyroid

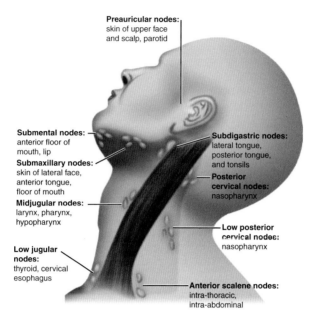

FIGURE 4-2 • **Lymph nodes of the head and neck region.** (Adapted with permission from Hong WK, Bast RB Jr, Hait WN, et al. *Cancer Medicine*. 8th ed. Shelton, CT: BC Decker—People's Medical Publishing House-USA; 2010:959-998.)

- Supraclavicular
  - Location: Fossa just posterior to the clavicle
  - Drainage: Thorax, thyroid, abdomen

If lymph nodes are palpable, assess the size, mobility, relative firmness, and tenderness.

The salivary glands are commonly palpable in the neck. They produce saliva, which is important for chewing and digesting food (**Figure 4-3**).

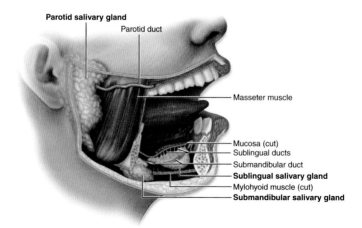

FIGURE 4-3 • **Anatomy of the major salivary glands.** (Reproduced with permission from Mescher AL. *Junqueira's Basic Histology Text and Atlas*. 16th ed. New York: McGraw Hill; 2021.)

- The parotid may be palpable in the upper neck, posterior to the angle of the mandible. The submandibular gland may be palpable high under the mid-portion of the mandible.
- The submandibular glands are often ptotic, and thus more readily palpable, in older individuals.

Findings and Their Meaning: Lymph Node Pathology

Enlarged nodes are common in the setting of infection or malignancy (**Figure 4-4**). The presence of palpable nodes is not necessarily pathologic, especially in young people.

Local Infections

- Understanding nodal drainage patterns may help to better understand the source of underlying pathology. For example, asymmetric left submandibular lymphadenopathy may be the result of a left-sided dental infection or peritonsillar abscess.
- Enlarged nodes associated with infection are usually tender, mobile, and "rubbery" to palpation. They may also feel warm to the touch. These are sometimes referred to as "reactive" nodes or "reactive lymphadenopathy."
- Nodes may remain persistently enlarged following resolution of infection.

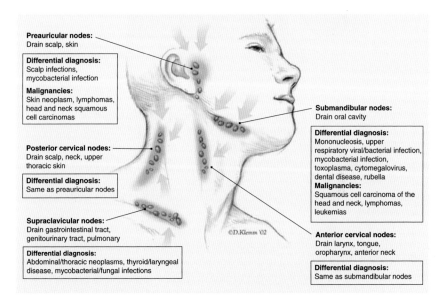

Preauricular nodes:
Drain scalp, skin

Differential diagnosis:
Scalp infections,
mycobacterial infection

Malignancies:
Skin neoplasm, lymphomas,
head and neck squamous
cell carcinomas

Posterior cervical nodes:
Drain scalp, neck, upper
thoracic skin

Differential diagnosis:
Same as preauricular nodes

Supraclavicular nodes:
Drain gastrointestinal tract,
genitourinary tract, pulmonary

Differential diagnosis:
Abdominal/thoracic neoplasms, thyroid/laryngeal
disease, mycobacterial/fungal infections

©D.Klemm '02

Submandibular nodes:
Drain oral cavity

Differential diagnosis:
Mononucleosis, upper
respiratory viral/bacterial infection,
mycobacterial infection,
toxoplasma, cytomegalovirus,
dental disease, rubella
Malignancies:
Squamous cell carcinoma of the
head and neck, lymphomas,
leukemias

Anterior cervical nodes:
Drain larynx, tongue,
oropharynx, anterior neck

Differential diagnosis:
Same as submandibular nodes

FIGURE 4-4 • Common disorders associated with pathologic enlargement of head and neck lymph nodes. (From Bazemore AW, Smucker DR. Lymphadenopathy and malignancy. *Am Fam Physician.* 2002;66:2103–2110. Reproduced with permission from David Klemm.)

Systemic Infections

- Lymphadenopathy in the setting of systemic infections such as HIV, tuberculosis, or mononucleosis is often bilateral and may involve multiple cervical nodal groups.
- Findings of diffuse nodal enlargement may require additional historical information and careful multisystem exam to arrive at a diagnosis. Mononucleosis from Epstein-Barr virus, for example, can cause acute, diffuse adenopathy in the head and neck area (**Figure 4-5**).

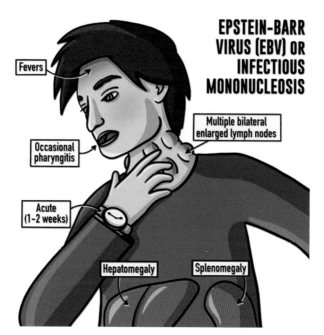

FIGURE 4-5 • **Findings and symptoms associated with mononucleosis.** (Reproduced with permission from Cathy Cichon, MD.)

Malignancy

- Lymph nodes may be involved with cancer, either as manifestation of a primary lymphatic malignancy such as lymphoma or metastasis from a solid tumor.
- Malignant lymphadenopathy of the neck is most commonly associated with primary cancers of the head and neck (mucosal squamous cell carcinoma, thyroid cancer, salivary gland cancer, or melanoma).
- Malignant lymphadenopathy is often nontender, and nodes may be quite firm relative to reactive nodes.
- Similar to local infections, the location of a metastatic node in the neck is frequently a clue to the location of the primary tumor site. For instance, lymphadenopathy of the left anterior cervical chain may lead to discovery of a left tonsil cancer.
- In some instances, the size of a nodal tumor may grow quite out of proportion to the primary tumor (eg, a cutaneous melanoma only several millimeters in size can be associated with bulky lymphadenopathy).
- Malignant nodes may remain mobile or may become fixed or matted together. This is an indication of extranodal extension into the surrounding soft tissues.

> PEARL: Adenopathy is most commonly related to acute, local infections. Distinguishing this from other etiologies (systemic infection, malignancy and autoimmune diseases) is based on the palpable characteristic of the LNs, how they change over time, and the presence of other symptoms and findings.

Findings and Their Meaning: Salivary Gland Pathology

- Asymmetrically enlarged and tender salivary glands may indicate local infection or inflammation (sialadenitis). Firm massage of the affected gland may result in expression of thick or purulent saliva that is visible at the native ductal opening of the affected gland within the mouth (Figure 4-24).

- Bilateral, symmetric enlargement of salivary glands may indicate autoimmune disease, such as Sjögren syndrome, rheumatoid arthritis, or lupus, or viral infection, such as mumps, in regions where vaccination is not prevalent.
- Enlarged glands can also occur with malignancy. This typically occurs more slowly, and the gland tends to feel firm. In the case of parotid tumors, cancer can affect CN VII function, causing asymmetric facial weakness in the distal distribution (can be confused with Bell palsy; see section on neurologic exam from Chapter 12 for details).

EAR EXAM

Observation

The outer ear (auricle, also called the pinna) should be carefully inspected, followed by otoscopic examination of the external auditory canal and tympanic membrane.

Familiarity with the anatomy of the auricle will facilitate description of lesions or abnormal morphology noted on exam (**Figure 4-6**).

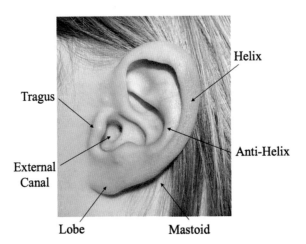

Helix

Tragus

Anti-Helix

External Canal

Lobe   Mastoid

FIGURE 4-6 • **Anatomy of the auricle.** (Photo by Charley Coffey, MD.)

Findings and Their Meaning: Auricle Pathology

- As a sun-exposed area, the auricle is a common location for benign sun-related skin changes (eg, actinic keratoses) and cutaneous malignancies such as basal cell carcinoma, squamous cell carcinoma, and melanoma (**Figure 4-7**).
- Drainage of fluid from the external auditory canal into the auricle (otorrhea) is never physiologic.
- Otorrhea is most commonly associated with bacterial infection of the external auditory canal (otitis externa) or, less commonly, middle ear infection (otitis media) via a perforation in the tympanic membrane.
- Infectious otorrhea is usually thick, turbid, and malodorous. Fluid may be intermixed with white or black fluffy debris indicating fungal infection (otomycosis).

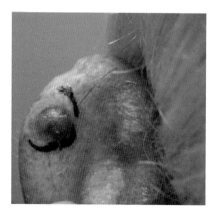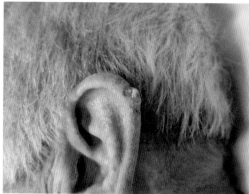

FIGURE 4-7 • **Cutaneous cancers of the auricle. Basal cell carcinoma (left) and squamous cell carcinoma (right).** (Reproduced with permission from Burgin S, ed. *Guidebook to Dermatologic Diagnosis.* New York: McGraw Hill; 2021, Figures 12.53 and 12.54.)

- Otorrhea resulting from otitis externa is usually accompanied by pain and tenderness with manipulation of the auricle. A gentle tug on the earlobe or tragus is painful with otitis externa, but not with otitis media (**Figure 4-8**).

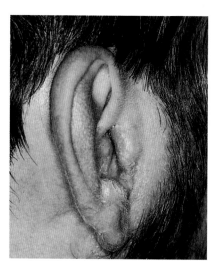

FIGURE 4-8 • **Otitis externa. Note red, edematous auricle, with discharge.** (From Knoop KJ, Stack LB, Storrow AB, Thurman RJ, eds. *The Atlas of Emergency Medicine.* 5th ed. New York: McGraw-Hill; 2021, Figure 5.14. Reproduced with permission from photo contributor: Frank Birinyi, MD.)

- Clear otorrhea is characteristic of cerebrospinal fluid (CSF) leak, which can develop when there is a temporal bone defect between the middle cranial fossa and the auditory canal. CSF otorrhea may develop spontaneously, iatrogenically, or in association with trauma. Traumatic CSF otorrhea may be blood-tinged (ie, transparent pink fluid).
- Malignancy arising in the external auditory canal or temporal bone is a very rare cause of otorrhea.

- A vesicular rash of the auricle is a hallmark of Ramsay Hunt syndrome, or herpes zoster oticus (**Figure 4-9**).
  - Ramsay Hunt syndrome results from reactivation of latent varicella-zoster virus in the geniculate ganglion of the facial nerve (CN VII).
  - The primary symptoms of Ramsay Hunt are pain affecting a defined dermatomal distribution, as with shingles, and unilateral facial paralysis.
  - Formation of vesicles, ear pain (otalgia), and facial paralysis are not necessarily simultaneous.
  - Hearing loss, tinnitus, and vertigo may also be present if there is involvement of the vestibulocochlear nerve (CN VIII).

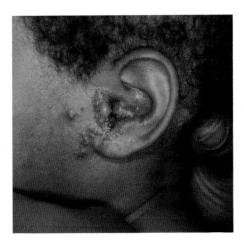

FIGURE 4-9 · Ramsay Hunt syndrome, with visible vesicles from varicella-zoster virus infection.
(From Knoop KJ, Stack LB, Storrow AB, Thurman RJ, eds. *The Atlas of Emergency Medicine.* 5th ed. New York: McGraw-Hill; 2021. Reproduced with permission from photo contributor: David Effron, MD.)

Otoscopy

The otoscope provides simultaneous illumination and magnification of the external auditory canal and tympanic membrane.

- Ensure that the power source is working (battery charged or wall-mounted unit plugged in and turned on) and that the light is at its maximal setting. If using a combination oto-ophthalmoscope, the otoscopic head may need to be twisted into place on the handle.
- The otoscope can be grasped such that the handle points either downward or upward; either technique is acceptable. Positioning the handle upward and forward allows the examiner to use the pinky and fourth finger for stabilization against the patient's temple (**Figure 4-10**). This approach helps to ensure that any sudden movements of the patient's head are immediately translated to the otoscope, thus minimizing the risk of injury or discomfort.
- Affix a disposable speculum to the end of the scope, using the appropriately sized speculum for the adult or pediatric exam. Carefully insert the otoscope into the ear canal *before* looking through the viewing window.
- It is generally easiest to hold the otoscope in the right hand for examination of the right ear, and vice versa on the left. This frees the opposite hand to gently retract the auricle in a posterior-superior direction, which straightens the lateral external canal to assist placement of the speculum.

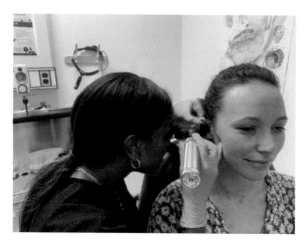

FIGURE 4-10 • Use of the otoscope. (Photo by Charley Coffey, MD.)

- Performing safe otoscopic examination of young children will generally require that the caregiver hold the child upright in the lap with one arm around the child's arms and the head turned to the side and held securely against the adult's chest. Refer to Chapter 20, Toddler and Early Childhood exam, for additional details of pediatric otoscopy.
- Advance the speculum slowly into the canal, directing the otoscope slightly anteriorly (toward the nose) while looking through the viewing window. Avoid excessive movements; the ear canal is sensitive, particularly if there is inflammatory pathology such as otitis externa.
- Once the tympanic membrane (TM) is in view, it is possible to slightly angle the scope tip as needed to examine the majority of the TM (**Figure 4-11**).
- The normal TM appears pale gray and translucent.
- It is frequently possible to partially visualize the ossicles (ear bones) through the TM. The long process of the malleus is visible running vertically from the top to the center of the TM. The short process of the malleus is visible as a prominent projection superiorly.
- The incus may be visible in the superior quadrant, posterior to the malleus.

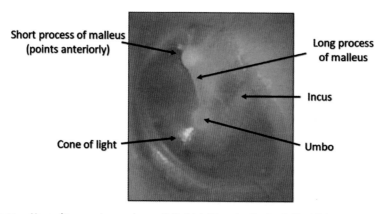

FIGURE 4-11 • Normal tympanic membrane (left side). (Photo by Charley Coffey, MD.)

- The point at which the tip of the malleus ends in the central TM is called the umbo.
- The "cone of light" or "light reflex" is a reflection of the otoscope light normally visible anterior to the umbo. Loss of this reflection indicates a change in the shape of the TM surface (eg, convexity), usually as a result of middle ear pathology.
- A pneumatic otoscope includes a bulb attached via thin tube to the otoscope head. Squeezing the bulb during otoscopy generates a puff of air that results in visible movement of a normal TM. Immobility of the TM with pneumatic otoscopy usually indicates middle ear pathology or TM perforation.

Findings and Their Meaning: Ear Canal and TM Pathology

- In addition to pain, tenderness, and otorrhea, otitis externa (Figure 4-8) is generally characterized by significant edema and erythema of the external auditory canal. The combination of edema and pain can make it difficult or, in some cases, impossible to insert an otoscopic speculum. Use of a smaller-diameter speculum may permit easier exam in these instances.
- Cerumen is generally brown or yellow in color, with consistency ranging from dry and solid to very soft, sticky wax.
  - It is often possible to gently slide the speculum tip around and beyond a small amount of cerumen. If a larger volume of cerumen prevents easy passage of the otoscope, simply back out.
  - Do not attempt to manually remove cerumen unless you have training in the necessary techniques; trauma to the ear canal, TM, or even middle ear can easily result from inexpert instrumentation.
- In contrast to otitis externa, in the setting of otitis media (**Figure 4-12**), the external auditory canal is generally normal in appearance. There is usually pain (otalgia), but the ear canal is nontender for most patients with otitis media.

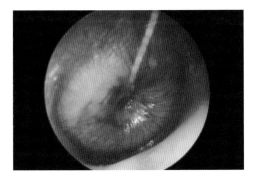

FIGURE 4-12 • **Otitis media.** (From Knoop KJ, Stack LB, Storrow AB, Thurman RJ, eds. *The Atlas of Emergency Medicine.* 5th ed. New York: McGraw-Hill; 2021, Figure 5.3. Reproduced with permission from photo contributor: Richard A. Chole, MD, PhD.)

  - The TM is frequently opaque in otitis media, with loss of normally visible anatomic landmarks (Figure 4-11). The cone of light may be reduced or absent.
  - The TM and adjacent canal may appear erythematous; however, the TM of a crying or screaming child is often erythematous due to vascular blush, and this is thus not a reliable indicator of otitis media in the pediatric exam.
  - An air-fluid line or bubbles may be visible indicators of an effusion within the middle ear. Opaque fluid is indicative of acute otitis media, whereas clear fluid is characteristic of serous otitis media—sterile middle ear effusion (**Figure 4-13**). Effusion results in an immobile TM with pneumatic otoscopy.

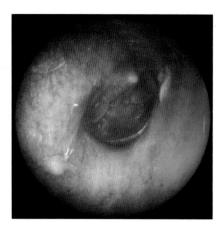

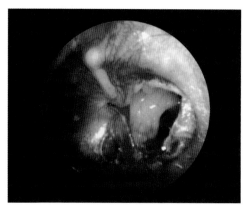

FIGURE 4-13 • Otitis media with effusion (OME) in the right ear: Note multiple air–fluid levels in this slightly retracted, translucent, non-erythematous tympanic membrane. (Used with the Permission from Mikhail V. Komarov/Shutterstock.)

FIGURE 4-14 • Tympanic membrane perforation. (From Knoop KJ, Stack I R, Storrow AB, Thurman RJ, eds. *The Atlas of Emergency Medicine.* 5th ed. New York: McGraw-Hill; 2021, Figure 5.13. Reproduced with permission from photo contributor: Richard A. Chole, MD, PhD.)

- Perforations can range from pinpoint size to near-complete absence of the TM (**Figure 4-14**). Middle ear structures may be clearly visible if the space is well-aerated. Opaque fluid emanating from a TM perforation is evidence of acute or chronic infection.
  - The normal TM consists of 3 layers, including a connective tissue layer covered by epithelium on either side. A TM perforation may heal by formation of a single layer of epithelium to span the defect. This monomer is visible as a transparent area within an otherwise translucent TM. A small, circular monomeric focus in the inferior half of the TM is a common indicator of prior history of pressure equalization tubes in childhood.

> **PEARL:** Examine as many ears as possible to become comfortable with otoscopy techniques, the appearance of the normal TM, and to develop facility in characterizing abnormalities.

Special Testing: Hearing Evaluation

If the patient reports hearing loss, additional physical exam elements may be incorporated. Although formal audiometric testing is required for a comprehensive objective evaluation, some basic exam techniques can help to characterize the nature and degree of loss.

- With the patient's eyes closed, rub your fingers together about 6 inches from one ear and then the other. Note any asymmetry in the patient's ability to detect this sound.
- Ability to discriminate speech can be tested by whispering a series of 2-syllable words while standing about 2 feet behind the patient, while the patient occludes first one and then the other ear canal with a finger.
- A patient with normal hearing should be able to accurately repeat at least 3 out of 6 words.

Tuning Fork Tests

Tuning fork tests of hearing can be used to distinguish **conductive** hearing loss (CHL) from **sensorineural** hearing loss (SNHL) (**Figure 4-15**).

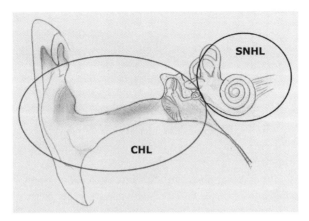

FIGURE 4-15 • **The right external, middle, and inner ears, and the right vestibulocochlear nerve.** Conductive hearing loss (CHL) is due to a lesion in the external or middle ear. Sensorineural hearing loss (SNHL) is due to a lesion in the inner ear, the vestibulocochlear nerve, or the cochlear nuclei in the lateral medulla (not shown). (Drawing by Charles Coffey, MD.)

- The conductive hearing pathway carries sound energy (vibration) from the auricle and external canal to the TM, from which the vibration is transmitted via the ossicles to the cochlea. A disruption of this pathway results in CHL.
- The sensorineural component of hearing includes the cochlea, where mechanical vibration is translated into nerve signals, and the subsequent route of those nerve signals through the auditory nerve, brainstem pathways, and ultimately the auditory cortex. A disruption in any portion of this pathway results in SNHL.
- A 512-Hz tuning fork is favored because this frequency is relatively central within the normal range of human speech.
- Accurate interpretation of the results of tuning fork tests requires that each of 2 tests—the Weber and Rinne tests—are performed and that they are interpreted in the context of the patient's symptoms (ie, from which side the patient subjectively experiences hearing loss) (**Figure 4-16**).

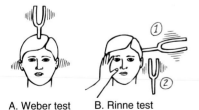

A. Weber test   B. Rinne test

FIGURE 4-16 • **Weber and Rinne tests.** (Reproduced with permission from Suneja M, Szot JF, LeBlond RF, Brown DD. *DeGowin's Diagnostic Examination*. 11th ed. New York: McGraw Hill; 2020.)

Weber Test

The Weber test directly compares hearing on the right and left sides by presenting a sound in the midline. It answers the question, "Does this person have asymmetric hearing loss?"

- Strike a 512-Hz tuning fork on the palm of the hand and then place the stem on the midline of the patient's scalp. Alternately, cover the stem with the finger of a clean glove and place it on one of the maxillary central incisors.
- The sound will be evenly transmitted through the dense bones of the skull and should arrive at the inner ear (cochlea) simultaneously.

Findings and Their Meaning: Interpreting Weber Test Results

- A patient with normal hearing on both sides should perceive the sound as arising in the midline or as being roughly equal in intensity on both sides. A normal Weber test is referred to as "midline."
- If there is unilateral CHL (eg, obstruction of one external auditory canal), the sound will be perceived as louder on that side. This is because the obstruction prevents any competing sounds from the external environment from reaching the inner ear, and thus the tuning fork vibration is the sole source of sound on that side and seems amplified. The sound is said to *lateralize* toward the affected side in CHL.
- If there is unilateral SNHL (eg, loss of sensory hair fibers in the cochlea), the sound will be perceived as louder in the contralateral, normal-hearing ear. The sound lateralizes away from the affected side in SNHL.

Rinne Test

The Rinne test evaluates for the presence of CHL on each side. It answers the question, "Does this ear have conductive hearing loss?"

- Strike the tuning fork and place the stem on the hard prominence of the mastoid bone, just behind the auricle. The sound will transmit directly to the cochlea via bone vibration, thus bypassing the conductive pathway. Instruct the patient to notify you when they can no longer hear the sound.
- Once the tuning fork on the mastoid is no longer audible to the patient, remove the still-vibrating tuning fork and hold the tines vertically in the air several centimeters from the external auditory canal. A normal-hearing ear should still be able to hear the sound.

Findings and Their Meaning: Interpreting Rinne Test Results and Putting It All Together

- Sound presented via the air sounds louder to a normal-hearing ear due to the amplifying effects of the conductive pathway (ie, air conduction is greater than bone conduction; "AC > BC").
- If the conductive pathway is interrupted (CHL), the sound is louder when presented via the mastoid because the vibrations directly bypass the impaired conductive mechanisms. This Rinne result is said to be bone conduction greater than air conduction ("BC > AC").
- If there is SNHL, the Rinne test on that side will still demonstrate air conduction greater than bone conduction since both pathways are equally affected.

It is important that both the Weber and Rinne tests be performed to correctly interpret the results.

- A Weber test that lateralizes to one side is an indication of asymmetric hearing loss but does not distinguish CHL from SNHL or identify the affected side.
- The results of a Rinne test will indicate if there is a CHL on one side and thus also allow correct interpretation of the Weber results.

It is important to be aware of several limitations of tuning fork hearing tests:

- Bilateral hearing loss may complicate accurate interpretation of tuning fork findings. For instance, if there is SNHL on both sides but the right side is worse, the Weber test will lateralize to the left (away from the more affected side), but this does not indicate that the left side is normal.
- Mixed hearing loss refers to the presence of both CHL and SNHL in one or both ears. Tuning fork tests can still be useful in mixed loss, but interpretation of the results may be more challenging.
- In the setting of mild CHL, air conduction will still remain greater than bone conduction. It is only once the degree of conductive deficit reaches about 30 dB of hearing loss that the tuning fork test "flips" to abnormal (BC > AC).

A summary of pathologic processes associated with hearing loss is presented in **Table 4-1.**

TABLE 4-1 • Diagnoses at a Glance: Common Causes of Hearing Loss and Associated Clinical Findings		
Disorder	Symptoms	Findings
Conductive Hearing Loss		Weber lateralizes to affected side; Rinne: bone conduction better than air
Middle Ear Process		
Otitis media	Acute ear pain, reduced hearing, sometimes other URI symptoms, fever	Drum can be red, bulging, loss of light reflex; sometimes effusion visible
Chronic serous effusion	Chronically decreased hearing, can be unilateral or bilateral	Effusion behind TM without inflammation
Tympanic membrane perforation	Acute pain, decreased hearing unilateral; if from infection, fever and URI symptoms; if trauma, appropriate history	TM with perforation, sometimes blood (if trauma); red, opaque, loss of light reflex if associated with an acute infection
Otosclerosis	Bony fixation of the stapes footplate; slow unilateral or bilateral hearing loss	No specific findings on otoscopy
Cholesteatoma	Unilateral hearing loss from buildup of desquamated material; develops slowly	Retracted drum; sometimes visible debris through TM
External Canal Obstruction		
Wax	Slow loss, unilateral or bilateral, no pain or other symptoms	Brown waxy material in external canal; can partially or fully obstruct
Bony growth (exostosis)	Slow loss, unilateral or bilateral, often history of ocean swimming	Evidence of bony encroachment into canal (covered w/normal skin); degree of obstruction variable
Otitis externa	Acute loss, typically unilateral, discomfort and swelling of area around external canal	Swelling of external canal; tender with palpation of area, tragus, manipulation; degree of occlusion variable (can be complete)

(Continued)

TABLE 4-1 • Diagnoses at a Glance: Common Causes of Hearing Loss and Associated Clinical Findings (Continued)		
Disorder	Symptoms	Findings
Sensorineural Hearing Loss		Weber lateralizes to normal side; Rinne: air conduction better than bone
Chronic exposure to loud sound	Slowly progressive loss, bilateral, sometimes clear history of exposure to loud sounds	No external findings
Presbycusis (age-related hearing loss)	Slowly progressive loss, increases with age >65, bilateral	No external findings
Ménière disease	Often unilateral, tinnitus, waxes and wanes over months, vertigo can last for hours	No external findings
Sudden sensorineural hearing loss	Acute, sudden, unilateral, painless loss; sometimes sense of fullness, tinnitus, or dizziness	No external findings
Labyrinthitis	Often URI prior, abrupt, N, V, dizziness, gait problems, unilateral hearing loss; can last days	No external findings; if vertigo, difficulty walking/moving
Acoustic neuroma	Subacute, unilateral progressive hearing loss, sometimes dizziness	No external findings
Ototoxic medications	Exposure to medications known to cause nerve damage; typically bilateral; sometimes tinnitus; often dose and duration related; most common agents include: aminoglycosides, cisplatin, NSAIDs, loop diuretics	No external findings
Autoimmune disorder (lupus, MS, relapsing polychondritis, GCA, PAN, other)	Unilateral or bilateral loss; Systemic symptoms consistent with primary disorder	Findings consistent with underlying autoimmune disorder
Stroke	Acute, unilateral loss, other stroke symptoms in nearby anatomic structures	No external ear findings; Acute neurologic deficits consistent with damage to the affected areas of the brain

Abbreviations: GCA, giant cell arteritis; MS, multiple sclerosis; N, nausea; NSAIDs, nonsteroidal anti-inflammatory drugs; PAN, polyarteritis nodosa; TM, tympanic membrane; URI, upper respiratory infection; V, vomiting.

NASAL EXAM

Observation

- Inspect the external aspect of the nose for asymmetry or deviations from the normally straight contour of the nasal dorsum (**Figure 4-17**).

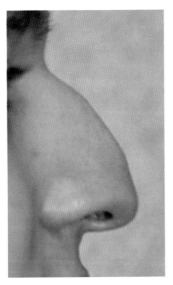
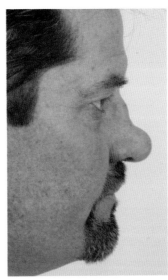

FIGURE 4-17 • **Dorsal hump (left) and saddle nose (right).** (Left photo by Deborah Watson, MD. Right photo from Loscalzo J, Fauci AS, Kasper DL, et al, eds. *Harrison's Principles of Internal Medicine.* 21st ed. New York: McGraw Hill; 2022, Figure 366-1. Reproduced with permission from Marcela Ferrada, MD.)

- If the patient reports difficulty breathing through the nose, assess air movement through each side independently: have the patient hold one nostril closed while breathing deeply through the nose, and ask whether one side feels more open or restricted than the other.
- Look into each nostril. Use of a nasal speculum and headlight provides the most optimal view, but an otoscope can also be used (**Figure 4-18**).

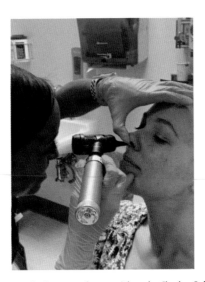

FIGURE 4-18 • **Use of the otoscope for intranasal exam.** (Photo by Charley Coffey, MD.)

- Note the color, location, and appearance of the nasal septum and inferior turbinate on each side. The septum runs vertically along the midline, while the turbinates appear as rounded shelves (inferior turbinate) or protuberances (middle turbinate) extending from the lateral nasal wall (**Figure 4-19**).

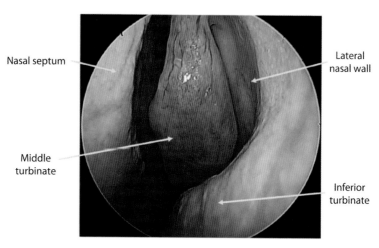

Nasal septum

Lateral nasal wall

Middle turbinate

Inferior turbinate

FIGURE 4-19 · **Intranasal exam (left side).** (Photo by Carol Yan, MD.)

Findings and Their Meaning: Nasal Pathology

There is a range of pathologic and physiologic factors that can affect the appearance of the nasal dorsum:

- External curvature of the nasal dorsum is most often the consequence of prior nasal bone fracture(s). Obstructed nasal breathing is commonly associated with this finding.
- A dorsal hump is most often a normal developmental feature but can also be the result of prior trauma. This finding is most prominent when viewed in profile and generally does not affect breathing (Figure 4-17).
- A depressed or caved-in profile of the nasal dorsum is the consequence of loss of the underlying septal cartilage framework and can be due to granulomatous disease (granulomatosis with polyangiitis), infection (congenital syphilis), drug abuse (cocaine), or trauma resulting in septal hematoma and subsequent necrosis. The resulting defect is referred to as a saddle nose deformity (Figure 4-17).
- Although the nasal septum is a midline vertical structure, in actual practice, the intranasal appearance of the septum is rarely perfectly straight. It is common for the septum to deviate primarily to one side or to have an S-shaped deviation resulting in bilateral obstruction. Septal deviation does not necessarily result in obstructed nasal breathing.
- The soft tissue components of the nasal turbinates and septum change in size throughout the day, which can result in dynamic changes in the intranasal exam as well as airflow and symptoms of nasal obstruction or congestion. This phenomenon is called the "nasal cycle."

- Weakening of the cartilages that provide form to the nasal ala (rim, or "wing") can result in collapse of the nostril with inspiration. This so-called "nasal valve collapse" can be readily observed on physical exam and may contribute to nasal obstruction independent of intranasal causes such as septal deviation or turbinate hypertrophy.
- In the setting of acute rhinosinusitis, the nasal mucosa may appear red and edematous. Thick, opaque mucus may be observed to track over the surface of the inferior turbinate and along the nasal floor toward the pharynx (**Figure 4-20**).

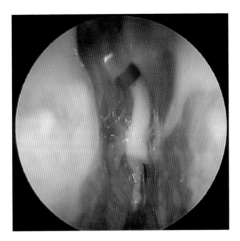

FIGURE 4-20 • **Acute rhinosinusitis (intranasal appearance, left side).** (Photo by Carol Yan, MD.)

Special Testing: Olfaction

Loss of the sensation of smell may result from a range of pathologies including nasal obstruction, mucosal alteration, central neurologic lesions, and postviral syndromes (eg, COVID-19), among others. Loss of smell may be partial (hyposmia) or complete (anosmia). Patients reporting decreased or loss of smell sensation may merit evaluation of olfactory function.

- Intranasal examination should include particular attention to any signs of upper respiratory tract infection or obstruction.
- Basic olfactory testing may be accomplished by assessing the patient's ability to detect the odor of a distinctive substance placed in close proximity. Those with intact olfactory function should be able to detect coffee grounds, mint, or wintergreen oil when the substance is placed 10 cm away from the face with eyes closed.
- More objective assessment is most often accomplished by use of the self-administered University of Pennsylvania Smell Identification Test (UPSIT) or threshold and discrimination testing using a commercially available series of dilutions of several distinctive odorants.

PARANASAL SINUSES

Routine examination of the sinuses is not required but should be included when a patient experiences signs or symptoms of infection or in the setting of facial trauma.

- The paranasal sinuses (most often referred to as simply "sinuses") are a series of pneumatized cavities within the facial skeleton that communicate with the nasal airway (**Figure 4-21**).
- The respiratory mucosa that lines the sinuses filters antigens and particulates from inspired air and warms and humidifies air before it reaches the lower airways. These air-filled spaces may also serve as "crumple zones" to absorb and dissipate energy from facial impacts, thus protecting the eyes and brain.

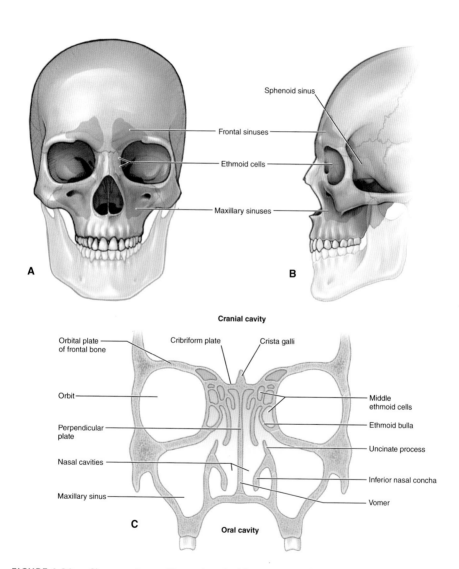

FIGURE 4-21 · **Sinus anatomy.** (Reproduced with permission from Morton DA, Foreman KB, Albertine KH. *The Big Picture: Gross Anatomy, Medical Course & Step 1 Review*. 2nd ed. New York: McGraw Hill; 2019.)

Special Testing: Sinus Exam

- The maxillary and frontal sinuses are somewhat accessible to external exam, whereas the ethmoid and sphenoid sinuses are not (Figure 4-21).
- If there is concern for acute rhinosinusitis, manual palpation overlying the maxillary sinuses (inferior to the infraorbital rim) or the frontal sinuses (superior to the supraorbital rim) may elicit pain. Firm tapping of the upper teeth may also elicit pain due to the proximity of the tooth roots to the maxillary sinuses.
- Intranasal exam in the setting of acute rhinosinusitis may demonstrate characteristic inflammatory findings as described in the preceding section. Rounded, pale polypoid mucosal change may also be visible via intranasal exam in a subset of patients who have rhinosinusitis with nasal polyps (**Figure 4-22**).
- Transillumination
  - The light of an otoscope placed directly over the maxillary sinus in a dark room should be visible intraorally as a glow on the hard palate (**Figure 4-23**).
  - This transillumination is not visible in the setting of maxillary sinusitis due to inflammatory thickening of the mucosa and fluid accumulation within the sinus.

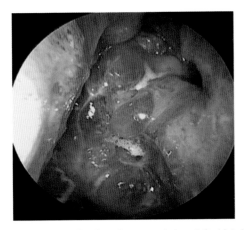

FIGURE 4-22 • **Rhinosinusitis with nasal polyps (intranasal view, left side).** (Photo by Carol Yan, MD.)

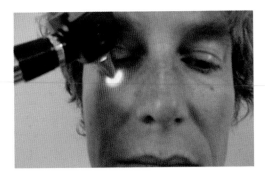
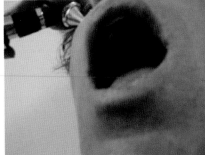

FIGURE 4-23 • **Transillumination of maxillary sinus (normal).** (Photo from *Practical Guide Clinical Medicine: Head and Neck Exam.* Available from: https://meded.ucsd.edu/clinicalmed/head.html.)

ORAL CAVITY EXAM

Anatomy

The oral cavity includes the lips, tongue, floor of mouth, buccal surfaces, gingiva, teeth, and the hard palate (**Figure 4-24**).

- The salivary glands empty into the mouth via ducts that terminate at slightly raised papillae. The ostia of the submandibular (ie, Wharton's) ducts are located in the anterior floor of mouth on either side of the lingual frenulum, whereas the parotid (ie, Stensen's) ducts terminate in the buccal mucosa adjacent to the second maxillary molar.
- Although closely associated with the oral cavity, the oropharynx is a distinct region with different anatomic and pathologic considerations. Using a systematic approach to examine first the oral cavity and then the oropharynx is the best means to ensure that important findings are not overlooked.

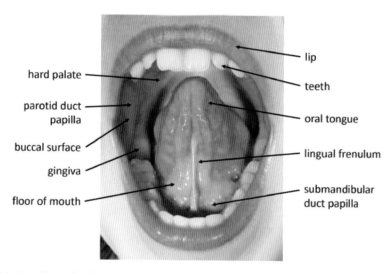

FIGURE 4-24 · **Normal oral anatomy.** (Photo by Charley Coffey, MD.)

Exam

Examination of the oral cavity requires good illumination and the ability to manipulate the tissues for thorough inspection. Ensure that the patient is seated at a comfortable height for you to easily see the entire mouth.

- An otoscope or flashlight is adequate for oral examination, although if available, a headlight is even better due to improved line-of-sight illumination and the freedom to use 2 hands for the exam.
- Either a tongue blade or gloved fingers can be used to gently retract the tongue and cheeks for thorough examination of the mucosal surfaces and teeth. Working around the mouth in a systematic 4-quadrant fashion can help ensure a thorough exam of all mucosal surfaces.
- Firm massage of each of the major salivary glands will usually elicit visible flow of clear saliva from the ostium of the respective duct. In the setting of acute infection or inflammation (sialadenitis), viscous, opaque fluid or debris may be observed.

If submandibular salivary stones are present, they are sometimes palpable as firm foci along the course of the submandibular duct in the floor of the mouth.

● Lightly brush each side of the tongue with gauze or a tongue blade to assess function of the lingual branch of the mandibular nerve (V3). Absent or decreased light touch sensation may indicate injury, the most common cause of which is oral surgery such as wisdom tooth extraction. Loss of sensation along the teeth or adjacent gingiva indicates dysfunction of the superior or inferior alveolar branches of V2 or V3, respectively.

Findings and Their Meaning: Oral Cavity Pathology

A broad range of mucosal findings can be observed in the oral cavity, ranging from benign lesions to malignancies. The size, distribution, specific location, and visible characteristics should be carefully noted.

● Concern for malignancy is elevated with mass lesions or those associated with significant ulceration or pain. Oral premalignant lesions may appear as painless, thickened white patches (leukoplakia) or red patches (erythroplakia) (**Figure 4-25**).

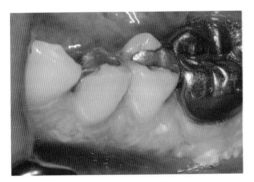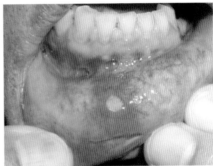

FIGURE 4-25 • **Leukoplakia (left) and aphthous ulcer (right).** (Left photo reproduced with permission from Soutor C, Hordinsky MK. *Clinical Dermatology: Diagnosis and Management of Common Disorders.* 2nd ed. New York: McGraw Hill; 2022, Figure 33-47A. Right photo from Usatine RP, Smith MA, Mayeaux EJ Jr, Chumley HS. *The Color Atlas and Synopsis of Family Medicine.* 3rd ed. New York: McGraw Hill; 2019, Figure 43-3. Reproduced with permission from Richard P. Usatine, MD.)

● Aphthous ulcers are small, shallow, punched out lesions usually arising on the lips or buccal mucosa. They are painful but, unlike neoplastic lesions, are transient, generally resolving within a week. The etiology of aphthous ulcers is not well understood. Presence of fever, lymphadenopathy, or other mucosal or skin lesions should prompt evaluation for systemic disorders (Figure 4-25).

● Geographic tongue is a benign inflammatory condition characterized by loss of papilla on the tongue resulting in distinct patches or islands that appear red with slightly raised borders, often resembling the appearance of a map.

● Oral thrush develops with candidal overgrowth of the oral mucosa. Thrush most commonly appears as white, slightly raised patches that can be wiped off, leaving red areas that may bleed slightly. Thrush may also be associated with a symmetric, smooth geometric red patch of the central tongue (median rhomboid glossitis) or painful cracking at the corners of the lips (angular chelitis). Thrush is often associated with relative

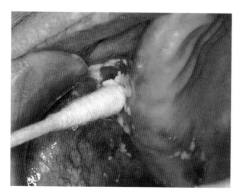 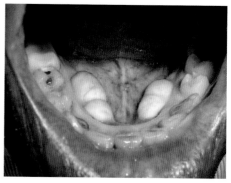

FIGURE 4-26 • Thrush (left) and tori mandibularis (right). (Left photo reproduced with permission from Soutor C, Hordinsky MK. *Clinical Dermatology: Diagnosis and Management of Common Disorders.* 2nd ed. New York: McGraw Hill; 2022, Figure 33-27. Right photo from Usatine RP, Smith MA, Mayeaux EJ Jr, Chumley HS. *The Color Atlas and Synopsis of Family Medicine.* 3rd ed. New York: McGraw Hill; 2019, Figure 35-2. Reproduced with permission from Richard P. Usatine, MD.)

immunosuppression and may develop in the setting of diabetes, HIV, inhaled or systemic steroids, prolonged antibiotics, radiation, or denture use (**Figure 4-26**).

- Oral lichen planus is an idiopathic autoimmune lesion characterized by diffuse white, lacy patches most often affecting the buccal mucosa, tongue, and floor of mouth. Lesions are most often thin and painless but can become red, swollen, tender, and erosive in some cases.
- Oral tori are benign bony growths of the maxilla or mandible. Tori usually arise in the central hard palate (tori palatinus) or the lingual surface of the mandible (tori mandibularis). They are slow growing, nonpainful, and generally do not cause problems unless they become large enough to interfere with normal oral function (Figure 4-26).
- Deviation of the tongue to one side when the patient is asked to stick the tongue straight out may be a sign of CN XII (hypoglossal) dysfunction. Injury of CN XII will result in tongue deviation toward the side of the affected nerve (ie, deviation to the left indicates left CN XII paresis).
- Peripheral nerve injury may result in visible fasciculations, and over time, the affected side will develop visible atrophy. Isolated CN XII dysfunction is most commonly the result of injury, including iatrogenic injury during upper neck surgery, although it may also result from tumor, radiation damage, or carotid artery dissection.

Dental Exam

Dental health has significant implications for overall health.

- Inequalities in access means that many individuals may not receive basic dental care even if they are able to access medical care.
- Dental health can impact nutrition as well as appearance, which can affect self-esteem, employability, and social acceptance.
- Dental disease can lead to local complications such as neck abscess or jaw osteomyelitis or systemic complications such as infective endocarditis.

A basic dental exam can be completed simultaneously with the oral exam. Gloved hands, gauze, tongue depressor, and good lighting are critical.

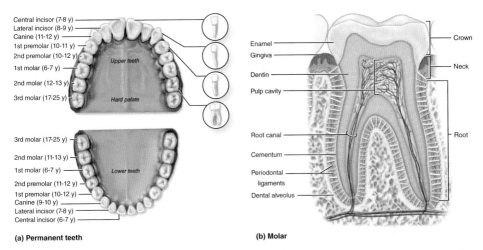

(a) Permanent teeth

(b) Molar

FIGURE 4-27 • Normal dental anatomy. (Reproduced with permission from Mescher AL. *Junqueira's Basic Histology Text and Atlas.* 16th ed. New York: McGraw Hill; 2021.)

- Adults have 32 teeth evenly divided between the 4 quadrants (maxillary/mandibular; left/right). A minority will be missing the most posterior molars, whereas others will have undergone extraction of these third molars, or "wisdom" teeth (**Figure 4-27**).
- Make note of the general dental appearance, including missing or broken teeth or obvious dental caries. Note the presence and condition of any dental work (fillings, crowns, partial dentures).
- Inspect the gingiva for evidence of pain, swelling, or infection.

Findings and Their Meaning: Dental Pathology

- Cavities are the result of chronic decay resulting in a hole in the enamel. They are usually asymptomatic unless more progressive erosion has resulted in exposure of the dental pulp (**Figure 4-28**).

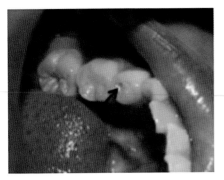
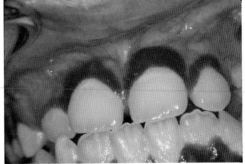

FIGURE 4-28 • Cavity (left) and gum disease (right). (Reproduced with permission from King TE, Wheeler MB, eds. *Medical Management of Vulnerable and Underserved Patients: Principles, Practice, and Populations.* 2nd ed. New York: McGraw Hill; 2016, Figures 41-5 and 41-6.)

- Pain upon palpation of a tooth may be indicative of an underlying abscess involving the root.
- Healthy gingiva should be nontender, pale pink, firm, and fit closely around the teeth.

Bleeding, red, swollen, or tender gingiva is characteristic of gingivitis, which can also be associated with loose teeth (Figure 4-28).

- Gingival hyperplasia may also be related to use of certain medications, including anticonvulsants such as phenytoin, immunosuppressants such as cyclosporin and tacrolimus, or calcium channel blockers such as nifedipine. In contrast to inflammatory gingivitis, medication-induced gingival enlargement is usually nontender, firm, pink, and not associated with bleeding.

PEARL: Given the challenges related to lack of access to dental care for all and the frequency of issues, physicians often have primary responsibility for diagnosing and treating commonly occurring tooth pathology.

OROPHARYNX EXAM

Anatomy

The oropharynx is comprised of the soft palate, uvula, palatine tonsils, posterior and lateral pharyngeal walls, and the base of tongue (**Figure 4-29**). At rest, the palate and pharyngeal walls are relaxed to allow easy movement of air between the nasal cavity and lower airways with respiration. Constriction of muscles in the palate and pharynx closes off this opening to redirect airflow through the mouth during speech and to aid propulsion of food and liquids inferiorly during swallowing.

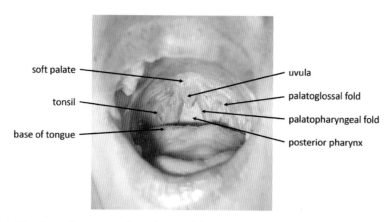

soft palate —
tonsil —
base of tongue —
uvula
palatoglossal fold
palatopharyngeal fold
posterior pharynx

FIGURE 4-29 • **Normal anatomy of oropharynx.** (Photo by Charley Coffey, MD.)

Exam

- Following examination of the oral cavity, direct attention posteriorly to the oropharynx. Note any lesions or asymmetry.
- Size and position of the tongue may limit visualization of the oropharynx. Gentle depression of the tongue with a tongue blade or gloved finger can improve the view. Asking the patient to say "aah" will elevate the palate, further aiding inspection.

- Palpation of the base of tongue and tonsils is important when a mass lesion is suspected based on the history. The patient should be cautioned that this maneuver may elicit gag but reassured that it will be brief. Gently grasp and retract the tongue with gauze while using the index finger to sweep firmly along the tonsils and base of tongue, paying careful attention for any evidence of ulceration, mass, or tenderness.

> PEARL: Performing a careful examination the mouth and oropharynx requires good lighting, gloved hands, a tongue depressor and methodical evaluation (looking and palpating) of both anatomic regions.

Findings and Their Meaning: Oropharynx Pathology

- Enlarged palatine tonsils are commonly observed in children and adolescents, whereas involution or atrophy of the tonsils is more common in adults. History of chronic or frequent infection may result in a "cryptic" appearance characterized by numerous deep pockets on the tonsil surface.
- Accumulation of food particles and squamous debris in these crypts can result in tonsiliths (tonsil "stones") visible as white matter lodged within tonsillar crypts. These are harmless and generally painless but can contribute to bad breath.
- Enlarged tonsils and a large base of tongue in patients with a history of snoring or prolonged pauses in breathing while sleeping may indicate obstructive sleep apnea (OSA). This may be further evaluated by sleep testing to assess the presence and severity of OSA.
- Asymmetric enlargement of one tonsil in an adult can be a sign of malignancy, most commonly squamous cell carcinoma or lymphoma. Referral for additional evaluation is indicated.
- In the setting of pharyngeal infection (pharyngitis, or the synonymous "tonsillitis"), the tonsils or pharyngeal walls may become covered with a thick yellow or white exudate (**Figure 4-30**). Erythema of the pharynx may also accompany infection, but this is a subjective and less specific finding and should not be considered pathologic in the absence of other signs or symptoms of infection or inflammation.

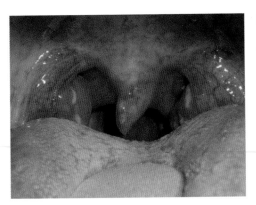 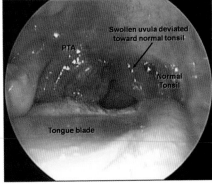

FIGURE 4-30 • **Pharyngitis (left) and peritonsillar abscess (PTA) (right).** (Left photo from Usatine RP, Smith MA, Mayeaux EJ Jr, Chumley HS. *The Color Atlas and Synopsis of Family Medicine.* 3rd ed. New York: McGraw Hill; 2019, Figure 37-1. Reproduced with permission from Richard P. Usatine, MD. Right photo reproduced with permission from Tintinalli JE, Ma OJ, Yealy DM, et al, eds. *Tintinalli's Emergency Medicine: A Comprehensive Study Guide.* 9th ed. New York: McGraw Hill; 2020, Figure 246-1.)

- Acute asymmetric swelling of one side of the pharynx accompanied by deviation of the uvula toward the opposite side is characteristic of peritonsillar abscess, an infectious complication generally accompanied by significant pain and difficulty swallowing (Figure 4-30).
- Flaccid paralysis of one-half of the soft palate with deviation of the uvula to the opposite side during palatal elevation is seen with CN X (vagal) paralysis. Stimulation of the ipsilateral soft palate will fail to elicit a gag reflex due to loss of efferent innervation. In contrast, CN IX (glossopharyngeal) injury will result in absent gag reflex due to interruption of afferent pathways. In practice, isolated CN IX dysfunction is very rare, but rather most commonly associated with other lower cranial neuropathies.
- Failure of the palate to seal off the oropharynx from the nasopharynx (velopharyngeal insufficiency [VPI]) results in a hypernasal speech quality and nasal regurgitation of liquids when swallowing. These clinical findings are heard rather than seen. VPI may occur as a result of stroke, surgical resection, or congenital causes such as cleft palate.

THYROID EXAM

Anatomy

The thyroid gland sits in the central neck overlying the cricoid cartilage and upper trachea, about 3 to 4 cm inferior to the notch of the thyroid cartilage (**Figure 4-31**). The normal thyroid gland is not visible in most people, but thyroid pathology may be apparent by exam.

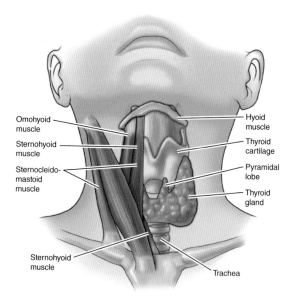

FIGURE 4-31 • **Normal thyroid anatomy.** (Reproduced with permission from Lalwani AK, ed. *Current Diagnosis & Treatment Otolaryngology—Head and Neck Surgery*. 4th ed. New York: McGraw Hill; 2020.)

Exam

- Ask the patient to swallow (offer a glass of water if their mouth is dry) while you carefully observe the lower central neck. Although a normal gland will not be visible, an enlarged or asymmetric gland may elevate noticeably with the surrounding structures while swallowing.

- Palpation of the thyroid can be performed while facing the patient, with the examiner directly in front or off to the side (Figure 4-1). Some practitioners examine the thyroid while standing behind the patient, with hands reaching around the neck (Figure 4-1). See earlier comments in the neck palpation section regarding potential for this maneuver to be triggering.
- Place your hands on either side of the patient's neck with fingertips resting to either side of midline and the little fingers just superior to the clavicles. Gently walk the fingers upward and downward, feeling for any evidence of asymmetric mass or thyroid gland enlargement below the level of the thyroid cartilage.
- Asking the patient to swallow again may help to discern subtle findings as the tissues move beneath your fingers. The normal gland is often difficult to feel, so do not be discouraged if you cannot identify it.

Findings and Their Meaning: Thyroid Pathology

- If the thyroid is enlarged, does it seem to be unilateral or bilateral? Does the gland seem diffusely enlarged, or are there one or more focal, firm nodules palpable? Benign or malignant thyroid nodules and thyroid goiter are generally nontender, whereas the gland may be tender in the setting of thyroiditis.
- If there is a mass lesion, determine whether it seems freely mobile or fixed to surrounding tissues or structures. Be certain to perform a careful lymph node exam as described earlier if malignancy is suspected.

TELEHEALTH TIPS

- Historical information can be obtained in the usual fashion.
- Asymmetry in the face is most easily identified by having the patient look directly at the camera, allowing you to compare left to right.
- Hearing concerns can be further explored as follows:
  - Ask the patient to listen to audio (by headphones or ear buds) using one ear and then the other, which can allow comparison and identify differences. This may provide insight as to the magnitude of asymmetric hearing loss.
  - Ask the patient to hum. In the setting of acute SNHL, it will sound louder in the normal ear. With CHL, it will sound louder in the affected ear.
- Chronic hearing loss is common, particularly in older patients. Hearing loss may be readily apparent based on the patient's ability to interact in the telehealth environment. If severe, it can interfere with the ability to conduct the visit. Further evaluation requires evaluation with an audiologist.
- Good lighting is critical for a head and neck tele-examination. Ideally, the light source is behind the patient's device shining toward their face or whatever body surface is facing the camera. Lighting coming from behind the patient and shining into the camera reduces clarity.
- Acute or chronic external abnormalities (eg, bumps, lumps, growths, areas of pain or swelling) might be visible via the telehealth camera. You can ask the patient to further characterize the area in question by having them comment on whether it is warm or painful. Can they move it around (eg, like a "pea under the skin"), or is it stuck and associated with other bumps (eg, multiple lymph nodes)? Placing the camera directly in front of the neck will allow comparison of right and left sides for asymmetry.

- Teeth, gum, cheek, or tongue abnormalities might be explored by having the patient expose the area in question to the camera. It might also help if you direct the patient to use both of their hands to pull down gums (to see teeth) or pull their cheeks out of the way. Grasping the tongue can be facilitated by using a hand towel or napkin to hold it (otherwise, it is slippery). The patient might also enlist the help of a friend or family member to maneuver the camera if they are using both hands to facilitate exposure.
- For dental issues, you can ask the patient to tap on specific teeth with a spoon, noting if any tooth in particular has pain, which is a common finding if there is a dental infection.
- Looking at the back of the patient's throat can be challenging or impossible to accomplish via telehealth without a telehealth-compatible tongue depressor.
- If there are complaints related to chewing or swallowing, ask the patient to demonstrate while on camera, allowing you to observe and gain insight into the magnitude of the problem.
- Issues with speech may be apparent during your dialogue. A friend or family member might be able to confirm any recent changes.
- As with all other telehealth aspects of the exam, it is important to recognize the limits of what you can accomplish. Those with concerning symptoms or findings usually need to be referred for in-person evaluation with appropriate urgency.

☑ SUMMARY OF SKILLS CHECKLIST

- ❏ Clean your hands.
- ❏ Position patient, seated on exam table.
- ❏ Observe head, face, and scalp.
- ❏ Assess facial symmetry, expression (CN VII), sensation (CN V), and extraocular motion (CN III, IV, VI).
- ❏ Assess spinal accessory (CN XI) function via shoulder abduction.
- ❏ Listen to voice, speech, and respiration.
- ❏ Palpate lymph nodes and major salivary glands.
- ❏ Inspect the external ears and perform otoscopy.
- ❏ Assess auditory function (CN VIII).
  - Perform Weber and Rinne tests *if* there is concern for hearing loss.
- ❏ Examine the external nose and perform anterior rhinoscopy.
  - Perform basic olfactory testing *if* patient reports hyposmia or anosmia.
- ❏ Palpate the frontal and maxillary sinuses.
  - Assess maxillary transillumination *if* concern for rhinosinusitis.
- ❏ Inspect the oral cavity, including teeth, using light and tongue depressor or gloved finger.
- ❏ Assess tongue mobility (CN XII), palate mobility, and gag reflex (CN IX, X).
- ❏ Inspect the oropharynx.
  - Palpate the base of tongue and tonsils *if* there is concern for tumor.
- ❏ Observe and palpate the thyroid.
- ❏ Clean your hands.

BIBLIOGRAPHY

Centor R, Samlowski R. Avoiding sore throat morbidity and mortality: when is it not "just a sore throat?" *Am Fam Phys.* 2011;83(1):26-28.

Crouch AE, Hohman MH, Moody MP, Andaloro C. Ramsay Hunt syndrome. [Updated 2020 Aug 14]. In: StatPearls [Internet]. Treasure Island, FL: StatPearls Publishing; 2020 Jan. https://www.ncbi.nlm.nih.gov/books/NBK557409/.

Ely J, Hansen MR, Clark EC. Diagnosis of ear pain. *Am Fam Phys.* 2008;77(5):621-628.

Feierabend H, Shahram MN. Hoarseness in adults. *Am Fam Phys.* 2009;80(4):363-370.

Ferrer R. Lymphadenopathy: differential diagnosis and evaluation. *Am Fam Phys.* 1998;58:1313-1320.

George E, Richie MB, Glastonbury CM. Facial nerve palsy: clinical practice and cognitive errors. *Am J Med.* 2020;133:1039-1044.

Goldberg C. Digital Ddx: head and neck symptoms or conditions. Accessed January 28, 2023. http://digitalddx.com/symptoms_list/3/.

Goldberg C. Practical guide to clinical medicine: the head and neck exam. Accessed January 28, 2023. https://meded.ucsd.edu/clinicalmed/head.html.

Habermann TM, Steensma DP. Lymphadenopathy. *Mayo Clin Proc.* 2000;75:723-732.

Honigberg M, Westlake AA, Griffin GK, et al. A lump in the neck (adenopathy from syphilis). *N Engl J Med.* 2018;379:e8.

Kuhn M, Heman-Ackah SE, Shaikh JA, Roehm PC. Sudden sensorineural hearing loss: A review of diagnosis, treatment, and prognosis. *Trends Amplif.* 2011;15(3):91-105.

Lee GA, Masharani U. Disorders of the thyroid gland. In: Lalwani AK, ed. *Current Diagnosis & Treatment Otolaryngology: Head and Neck Surgery.* 4th ed. New York: McGraw Hill. Accessed April 15, 2023. https://accessmedicine.mhmedical.com/book.aspx?bookid=2744.

Nieman C, Oh ES. In the clinic: hearing loss. *Ann Intern Med.* 2020;173(11):ITC 81-95.

Plaut M, Valentine MD. Allergic rhinitis. *N Engl J Med.* 2005;353:1934-1944.

Rosenfeld R. Acute sinusitis in adults. *N Engl J Med.* 2016;375:962-970.

Scully C. Apthous ulcerations. *N Engl J Med.* 2006;355:165-172.

Siminoski K, Simel D, Cohen A. Does this patient have a goiter? In: Simel D, Drummond R, eds. *The Rational Clinical Exam.* New York: McGraw-Hill; 2009:277-287.

Wessels M. Streptococcal pharyngitis. *N Engl J Med.* 2011;364:648-655.

Williams JW, Simel DL. Does this patient have sinusitis? Diagnosing acute sinusitis by history and physical examination. In: Simel D, Drummond R, eds. *The Rational Clinical Exam.* New York: McGraw-Hill; 2009:593-603.

5

Eye Exam

Jeffrey E. Lee, MD and Charlie Goldberg, MD

INTRODUCTION

The eye exam is performed when a patient presents with an eye concern, not as part of a screening evaluation. Elements of the evaluation (cranial nerve [CN] assessment) are also covered in the neurologic exam. Many components of the eye exam are relatively straightforward and can be capably performed by nonophthalmologists. It is therefore important to practice as much as possible early in your training, working with asymptomatic patients. The most challenging portion of the exam, direct ophthalmoscopy, is covered at the end of this chapter and takes more time and effort to master, although realize that you can gain a lot of information even if you do not feel comfortable with this component.

ASSESSMENT OF VISUAL ACUITY

Assessing visual acuity is critical in determining the severity of an eye concern. For this reason, it is often referred to as the vital sign of the eye. It is the important first step when evaluating an eye issue and when describing concerns to a consultant.

- Assessment can be done with either a standard Snellen wall chart read with the patient standing at a distance of 20 feet or using a specially designed pocket card held at 14 inches (**Figure 5-1**).
- Each eye is tested independently (ie, one eye is covered while the other is used to read). The patient should be allowed to wear their updated corrective lenses (glasses or contact lenses), and the results are referred to as "best corrected vision."
- You do not need to assess the patient's ability to read every line on the chart. If they have no complaints, rapidly skip down to the smaller characters.
- The numbers at the end of the line provide an indication of the patient's visual acuity compared with normal subjects. The larger the denominator, the worse is the acuity. For example, 20/200 means that the patient can see at 20 feet what a normal individual can at 200 feet (ie, their vision is poor).
- If the patient is unable to read any of the lines (a huge red flag if this is a new symptom), a gross estimate of what they are capable of seeing should be determined (eg, ability to detect light, a waving hand, or number of fingers placed in front of them).

> **PEARL:** Visual acuity is the vital sign of the eye. It is easy to check and is the first step when evaluating patients with eye concerns.

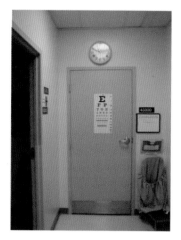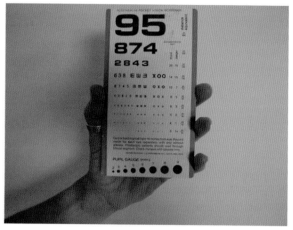

FIGURE 5-1 • **Snellen chart (left) and hand-held acuity card (right).** (Photos from Practical *Guide to Clinical Medicine: Eye Exam.* Available from: https://meded.ucsd.edu/clinicalmed/eyes.html.)

Special Test: Pinhole Testing

Pinhole testing can determine if an acuity problem is the result of refractive error (ie, correctable with glasses) or due to another process. The pinholes only allow the passage of light that is perpendicular to the lens and thus does not need to be bent prior to being focused onto the retina.

- Instruct the patient to view the Snellen chart with the pinholes up (**Figure 5-2**).
- Then repeat with the pinholes down (Figure 5-2).
- If the deficit corrects with the pinholes in place, the acuity issue is most likely related to a refractive problem.

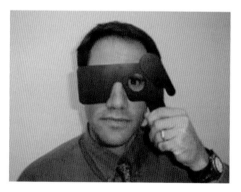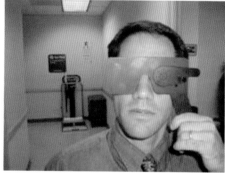

FIGURE 5-2 • **Pinhole testing.** (Photos from Practical *Guide to Clinical Medicine: Eye Exam.* Available from: https://meded.ucsd.edu/clinicalmed/eyes.html.)

OBSERVATION

Positioning the Patient

When performing the rest of the exam, make sure that you are in a comfortable position. It helps if the patient is seated at a height such that their eyes are essentially on the same level as your own when you are standing or seated in front of them.

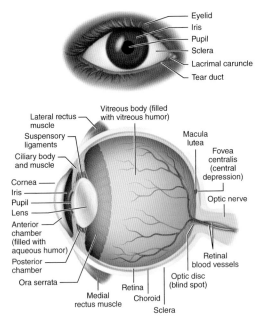

FIGURE 5-3 • **Eye anatomy.** (Reproduced with permission from Huppert LA, Dyster TG. *Huppert's Notes: Pathophysiology and Clinical Pearls for Internal Medicine.* New York: McGraw Hill; 2021.)

Observation of External Structures

Understanding the functional anatomy of the eye is important, both for examining structures and when identifying pathology (**Figure 5-3**). The key structures to note are lids, lashes, pupils, iris, and sclera.

- The pupil is the central dark portion and is actually a hole that allows light to enter the eye and reach the retina. Muscles (not visible) control the size of the opening. The pupils should appear symmetrically positioned (more to follow).
- The iris surrounds the pupil and is colored.
- The normal sclera is white and surrounds the iris and pupil.
- The sclera is covered by a thin transparent membrane known as the conjunctiva, which reflects back onto the underside of the eyelids. Normally, the conjunctiva is transparent except for the fine blood vessels that run through it (**Figure 5-4**).

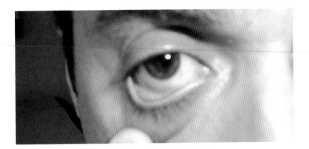

FIGURE 5-4 • **Normal appearing sclera and conjunctiva.** (Photo from *Practical Guide to Clinical Medicine: Eye Exam.* Available from: https://meded.ucsd.edu/clinicalmed/eyes.html.)

- Both eyelids should cover approximately the same amount of eyeball. CN VII controls the muscles that close the eyelid. CN III and the sympathetic nervous system control the muscles that keep the lid open (more to follows).

Findings and Their Meaning: Scleral Discoloration

- In the setting of liver or blood disorders (hemolysis) that cause hyperbilirubinemia, the sclera may appear yellow, referred to as icterus (**Figure 5-5**).
- Identifying the cause requires history, exam, and labs directed toward uncovering disorders of the liver (more common) or blood.

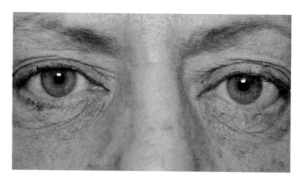

FIGURE 5-5 • **Icteric sclera.** (From Knoop KJ, Stack LB, Storrow AB, Thurman RJ, eds. *The Atlas of Emergency Medicine*. 5th ed. New York: McGraw-Hill; 2021, Figure 27.21. Reproduced with permission from photo contributor: Lawrence B. Stack, MD.)

Findings and Their Meaning: Conjunctival Abnormalities

When infected or inflamed, the conjunctiva can appear quite red, a condition known as conjunctivitis. Visual acuity is typically preserved. Etiologies are usually infectious (viral, bacterial) or allergic.

- Viral etiologies are common, causing 80% of infection-related conjunctivitis in adults. They are acute, unilateral, or bilateral; can cause a local gritty sensation; and are typically associated with watery discharge (**Figure 5-6**). Viral conjunctivitis is often related to

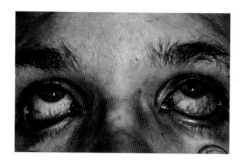
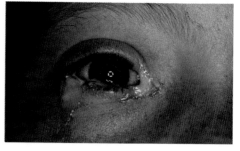

FIGURE 5-6 • **Bilateral, conjunctival inflammation, consistent with viral conjunctivitis (left). Conjunctival inflammation and purulent discharge consistent with bacterial conjunctivitis (right).** (From Knoop KJ, Stack LB, Storrow AB, Thurman RJ, eds. *The Atlas of Emergency Medicine*. 5th ed. New York: McGraw-Hill; 2021, Figures 2.11 and 2.8. Left photo: Reproduced with permission from photo contributor: Kevin J. Knoop, MD, MS. Right photo: Reproduced with permission from photo contributor: Frank Birinyi, MD.)

a viral upper respiratory tract infection, with symptoms that can include cough, nasal congestion, sore throat, fatigue, and postnasal drip.

- Bacterial etiologies usually are acute, cause a sense of local irritation, are more likely to be unilateral, and have intense redness and opaque discharge (compared with viral) (Figure 5-6).
- Allergic conjunctivitis tends to be subacute or chronic, itchy, and bilateral; has less intense redness compared with infectious etiologies; watery discharge; and is sometimes associated with allergic symptoms of the nose or lungs.
- Alternatively, the conjunctiva can appear pale if the patient is very anemic (**Figure 5-7**). By gently applying pressure and pulling down and away on the skin below the lower lid, you can examine the conjunctival reflection, which is the best place to identify if there is pallor.
- Blood can also accumulate underneath the conjunctiva when one of the small blood vessels within it ruptures. This is called a subconjunctival hemorrhage (**Figure 5-8**). This may result from coughing, sneezing, or a direct blow. Much less commonly, it is the result of a bleeding disorder or other unusual process. While dramatic, it is typically self-limited and does not affect vision.

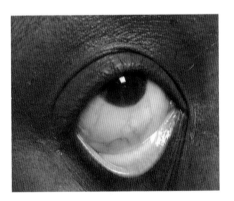

FIGURE 5-7 • **Pale conjunctiva.** (From Knoop KJ, Stack LB, Storrow AB, Thurman RJ, eds. *The Atlas of Emergency Medicine.* 5th ed. New York: McGraw-Hill; 2021, Figure 2.1A. Reproduced with permission from photo contributor: Kevin J. Knoop, MD, MS.)

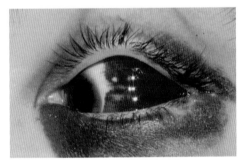

FIGURE 5-8 • **Subconjunctival hemorrhage.** (From Knoop KJ, Stack LB, Storrow AB, Thurman RJ, eds. *The Atlas of Emergency Medicine.* 4th ed. New York, McGraw-Hill; 2016. Reproduced with permission from photo contributor: Dallas E. Peak, MD.)

> PEARL: Common processes affecting the sclera and external structures can be evaluated by any clinician and do not typically affect visual acuity.

Findings and Their Meaning: Eyelid Asymmetry

Damage to the nerves controlling lids (CN III, the sympathetic nervous system and CN VIII) can cause the upper or lower lids on one side to appear asymmetric. In **Figure 5-9**, the image on the left demonstrates a patient with peripheral CN VII dysfunction affecting their left eye. They are unable to completely close the upper eyelid (a sliver of white sclera is still visible). In the image on the right, the patient is unable to fully open their right eyelid (known as ptosis). This is due to CN III dysfunction. For additional information on these disorders, see Chapter 12 on the neurologic exam.

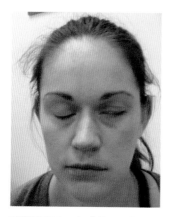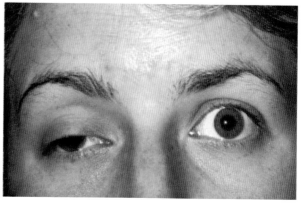

FIGURE 5-9 • Inability to fully close left eye due to CN 7 dysfunction (left). Inability to fully open right eye due to CN3 dysfunction (right). (Left photo: Reproduced with permission from Berkowitz AL. *Clinical Neurology and Neuroanatomy: A Localization-Based Approach.* 2nd ed. New York: McGraw Hill; 2022, Figure 13.5C. Right photo: Reproduced with permission from McKean SC, Ross JJ, Dressler DD, Scheurer DB, eds. *Principles and Practice of Hospital Medicine.* 2nd ed. New York: McGraw Hill; 2017, Figure 83-5.)

EXTRAOCULAR MOVEMENTS

Physiology of Normal Function

Normally, the eyes move in a coordinated fashion. When the left eye moves left, the right eye moves left to a similar degree (and vice versa).

- The brain takes the input from each eye and puts it together to form a single image.
- These coordinated movements depend on 6 extraocular muscles that insert around the eyeballs, allowing them to move in all directions.
- Each muscle is innervated by one of 3 CNs: CNs III (oculomotor), IV (trochlear), and VI (abducens).
- Movements are described as follows (**Figure 5-10**):
  - Elevation (pupil directed upward)
  - Depression (pupil directed downward)
  - Abduction (pupil directed laterally)

Eye Movement Terminology

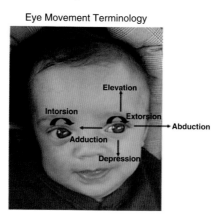

FIGURE 5-10 • **Description of eye movements.** (Photo from *Practical Guide to Clinical Medicine: Eye Exam.* Available from: https://meded.ucsd.edu/clinicalmed/eyes.html.)

- Adduction (pupil directed medially)
- Extorsion (top of eye rotating away from the nose)
- Intorsion (top of eye rotating toward the nose)

The medial and lateral rectus muscles are described first, as their functions are very straightforward (**Figure 5-11**):

- Lateral rectus: abduction (ie, lateral movement along the horizontal plane)
- Medial rectus: adduction (ie, medial movement along the horizontal plane)

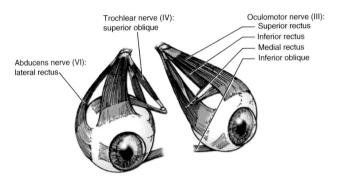

FIGURE 5-11 • **Insertion of extraocular muscles on eyeball.** (Reproduced with permission from Martin JH. *Neuroanatomy: Text and Atlas.* 5th ed. New York: McGraw-Hill; 2021.)

The remaining muscles each cause movement in more than one direction (eg, some combination of elevation/depression, abduction/adduction, intorsion/extorsion). This is because they insert on the eyeball at various angles and, in the case of the superior oblique, through a pulley. Review of the origin and insertion of each muscle sheds light on its actions (Figure 5-11).

Specific actions of the extraocular muscles are described below. The action that the muscle primarily performs is listed first, followed by secondary and then tertiary actions.

- Inferior rectus: depression, extorsion, and adduction
- Superior rectus: elevation, intorsion, and adduction
- Superior oblique: intorsion, depression, and abduction
- Inferior oblique: extorsion, elevation, and abduction

The mnemonic SINRAD may be helpful to remember the movements of these four muscles. All Superior muscles INtort, and all Rectus muscles ADduct.

The muscles, in turn, are innervated by 3 different CNs. Patterns of innervation are as follows:

- CN IV (trochlear): innervates the superior oblique
- CN VI (abducens): innervates the lateral rectus
- CN III (oculomotor): innervates all the remaining muscles (ie, medial rectus, inferior oblique, superior rectus, and inferior rectus)

You can remember this via the following: "SO-4, LR-6, all the rest 3" (ie, superior oblique by CN IV, lateral rectus by CN VI, and all the other extraocular muscles by CN III).

Assessing Extraocular Movements

- Stand in front of the patient. The pupils should appear symmetrically situated within the eye socket.
- Ask the patient to follow your finger with their eyes while keeping their head in one position (**Figure 5-12**).
- Using your finger, trace an imaginary rectangle in front of the patient, making sure that your finger moves far enough out and up/down so that you are able to see all appropriate eye movements (ie, lateral up, lateral down, medial down, medial up). If there is a possible limitation in movement noted, trace the eye back to the center and then move back in the direction of concern.
- Hold your finger at the lateral extremes, which can induce a few beats of nystagmus (normal) and typically leaves no remaining sclera visible between the iris and eyelid.
- At the end, bring your finger directly in toward the patient's nose. This will cause the patient to look cross-eyed and the pupils should constrict, a response referred to as accommodation.
- The eyes should be able to easily and smoothly follow your finger in a coordinated fashion.

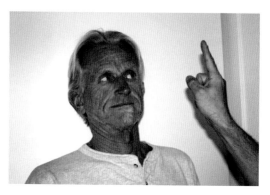

FIGURE 5-12 · **Testing extraocular movements.** (Photo from *Practical Guide to Clinical Medicine: Eye Exam.* Available from: https://meded.ucsd.edu/clinicalmed/eyes.html.)

Findings and Their Meaning: Disorders of Extraocular Movements

- Isolated lesions of a CN or the muscle itself can adversely affect extraocular movement.
- The pupils may appear asymmetric in their position within the eye socket.
- Patients will report diplopia (double vision) when the affected CN or extraocular muscle prevents the eyes from moving in sync with one another. This is because the brain cannot put together the discordant images in a way that forms a single picture. In response, the patient will either assume a head position that attempts to correct for the abnormal eye positioning or close the abnormal eye. In very young children, they will actually suppress vision in one eye to avoid double vision, which can lead to ambylopia (permanently reduced best corrected vision).
- The patient may report other symptoms and have additional findings, based on the underlying cause of the impaired eye movement. Isolated CNs or extraocular muscles can be affected (eg, injury, cancer), or multiple CNs or extraocular muscles can be affected simultaneously (eg, anatomic lesions affecting several CNs or myasthenia gravis).

In the setting of an eye movement problem, isolating which muscle or CN is the culprit can be tricky. When trying to isolate a problem, it can help to check movement in the direction in which that muscle is the primary mover. This can be assessed as follows:

- Superior oblique: depresses the eye when looking medially
- Inferior oblique: elevates the eye when looking medially
- Superior rectus: elevates the eye when looking laterally
- Inferior rectus: depresses the eye when looking laterally
- Medial rectus: adduction when pupil is moving along horizontal plane
- Lateral rectus: abduction when pupil is moving along horizontal plane (**Figure 5-13**)

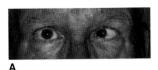 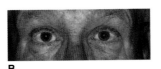 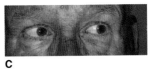

A   **B**   **C**

FIGURE 5-13 • **Right cranial nerve VI palsy. The patient is unable to abduct their right eye. When the patient tries looking to the right (A), they experience double vision, as the right eye cannot move laterally. This is referred to as horizontal diplopia. When the patient looks straight ahead (B) or to the left (C), the gaze normalizes, and typically the double vision will resolve.** (Reproduced with permission from Martin T, Corbett J. *Practical Neuroophthalmology.* New York: McGraw Hill; 2013.)

PEARL: Disorders of eye movements can also be due to problems with the extraocular muscles themselves. When the muscle is injured or trapped as a result of trauma, this can impair the function of the eyes, leading to diplopia.

Describing Diplopia (Double Vision)

- Binocular diplopia resolves when one eye is closed (as with previous examples).
- Monocular diplopia persists with one eye closed. This is usually due to a local anterior segment eye issue such as cataract, corneal scar, or foreign body.

Findings and Their Meaning: Nystagmus

- Nystagmus is the condition of rapid, uncontrolled movements of the eye that can occur in vertical, horizontal, or torsional directions.
- The etiology may be related to vestibular disease (central or peripheral), medications, or other neurologic processes.
- Clues suggestive of central (brain) pathology include persistence, bidirectional nature, rotational movement, vertical movement, and/or the presence of other neurologic findings (eg, hearing loss).

VISUAL FIELD TESTING

The normal visual field for each eye extends out from the patient in all directions, with an area of overlap directly in front. Field cuts refer to specific regions where the patient has lost their ability to see. This occurs when the transmitted visual impulse is interrupted at some point in its path from the eye to the visual cortex in the back of the brain. You would only include a visual field assessment if the patient complained of loss of sight, in particular, "blind spots" or "holes" in their vision. Visual fields can be crudely assessed as follows:

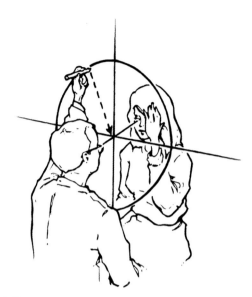

FIGURE 5-14 • **Visual field testing.** (Reproduced with permission from Manish Suneja, Joseph F. Szot, Richard F. LeBlond. Donald D. Brown: *DeGowin's Diagnostic Examination, 11e.* New York: McGraw Hill.)

- The examiner should be nose-to-nose with the patient, separated by approximately 8 to 12 inches (**Figure 5-14**).
- Each eye is checked separately. The examiner closes one eye, and the patient closes the one opposite (occluding is best accomplished with a physical covering such as a hand or occluder). The open eyes should then be staring directly at each another.
- The examiner should move their hand out toward the periphery of their visual field on the side where the eyes are open. The finger should be equidistant from both persons.
- The examiner should then move the wiggling finger in toward them, along an imaginary line drawn between the 2 persons. The patient and examiner should detect the finger at more or less the same time.
- The finger is then moved out to the diagonal corners of the field and moved inward from each of these directions.
- Testing is then done starting at a point in front of the closed eyes. The wiggling finger is moved toward the open eyes.
- The other eye is then tested.

Meaningful interpretation is predicated upon the examiner having normal fields, as they are using themselves for comparison.

If the examiner cannot seem to move their finger to a point that is outside the patient's field, don't worry. It simply means that their fields are normal.

Findings and Their Meaning: Visual Field Defects

Let's review the normal pathways by which visual impulses travel from the eye to the brain as well as the impact of selected lesions.

- The path of fibers from the eye to the occipital lobe is shown in **Figure 5-15**.
- Field deficits resulting from lesions in these paths are noted in the descriptions accompanying Figure 5-15.

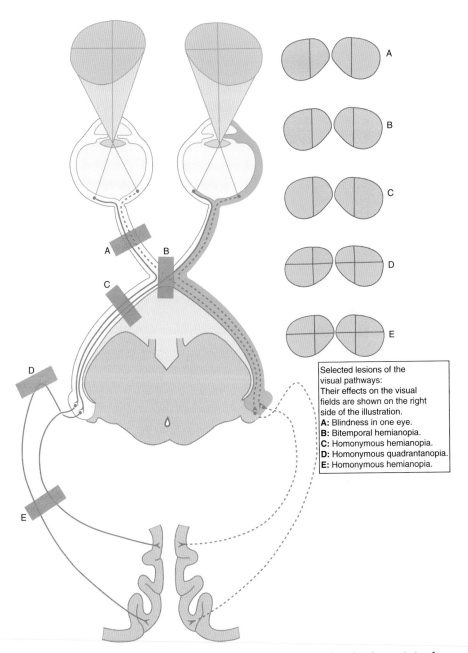

FIGURE 5-15 • **Visual pathways, lesions, and resulting deficits.** (Reproduced with permission from Waxman SG. *Clinical Neuroanatomy.* 29th ed. New York: McGraw Hill; 2020.)

- Loss of vision in one eye is due to a problem only affecting that eye, as with lesion A in Figure 5-15 (optic nerve damage).
- Lesion B in Figure 5-15 would result from a pituitary tumor, affecting the lateral (temporal) fields in both eyes.

- If the same field for both eyes is affected, it is referred to as homonymous (lesions C, D, and E in Figure 5-15). Hemianopia refers to half the visual field being lost (lesions B, C, and E). Quadrantanopia (lesion D) means that a quarter of the visual field is lost.
- Bedside visual field testing can detect large problems, although it is quite possible to have small deficits that are hard to identify with this type of exam. Ophthalmologists use specialized equipment to make these assessments.

PUPILS

Physiology of Pupillary Response

- Response of pupils to light is controlled by the autonomic nervous system.
- Sympathetic activation ("fight or flight") causes the pupils to dilate.
- Parasympathetics cause the pupils to constrict (**Figure 5-16**).
- The normal pupil constricts when the eye is exposed to bright light, known as the direct response. Light presented to the opposite eye also causes constriction, which is referred to as the consensual response.
- Constriction occurs when stimulation of the afferents (ie, sensory nerves carried with CN II) in one eye triggers efferent (carried with CN III) activation and subsequent constriction of the pupils of both eyes.

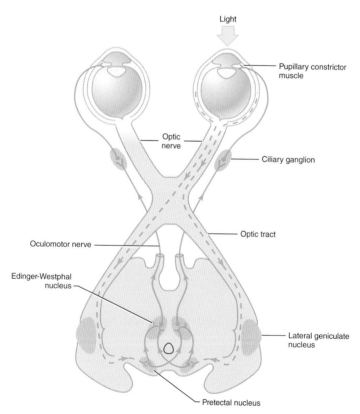

FIGURE 5-16 • **Parasympathetic pathway for pupillary constriction.** (Reproduced with permission from Aminoff M, Greenberg D, Simon R. *Clinical Neurology*. 9th ed. New York: McGraw Hill; 2015.)

- Miosis is when the pupil is abnormally constricted, and mydriasis is when the pupil is abnormally dilated.

Findings and Their Meaning: Anisocoria (Pupils of Unequal Size)

- Normal pupils appear symmetric.
- To assess for symmetry, look directly at the patient's eyes and note whether they are in the same relative position within the eye socket and of equal size and shape.
- When anisocoria is noted, the examiner has to determine which is the abnormal eye (ie, could be either the large or small pupil).
- Pupil asymmetry that is more prominent in the dark suggests that the smaller pupil is abnormal (ie, it fails to dilate). Asymmetry more prominent in the light suggests the larger pupil is abnormal (ie, it fails to constrict) (**Figure 5-17**).
- Prior eye surgery, trauma, or injury to the pupillary dilators/constrictors can result in chronic anisocoria. In these instances, the history should be revealing and there should be no associated acute symptoms. A photo (eg, from driver's license) can be very useful in establishing pupillary appearance at baseline.

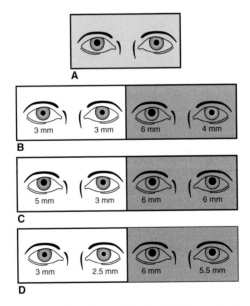

FIGURE 5-17 • **Examining anisocoria in light and dark. (A)** Anisocoria with the larger pupil on the patient's right. **(B)** If the anisocoria is worse in darkness, this suggests that the smaller pupil (on the patient's left) has failed to dilate and is the abnormal pupil. **(C)** If the anisocoria is worse in light, this suggests that the larger pupil (on the patient's right) has failed to constrict and is the abnormal pupil. **(D)** In physiologic anisocoria, subtle anisocoria is generally present in both light and dark. (Reproduced with permission from Martin T, Corbett J. *Practical Neuroophthalmology.* New York: McGraw-Hill Education; 2013.)

Evaluation of Anisocoria

Figure 5-18 provides a flow chart describing the evaluation of anisocoria. **Tables 5-1** and **5-2** provide additional information connected to Figure 5-18.

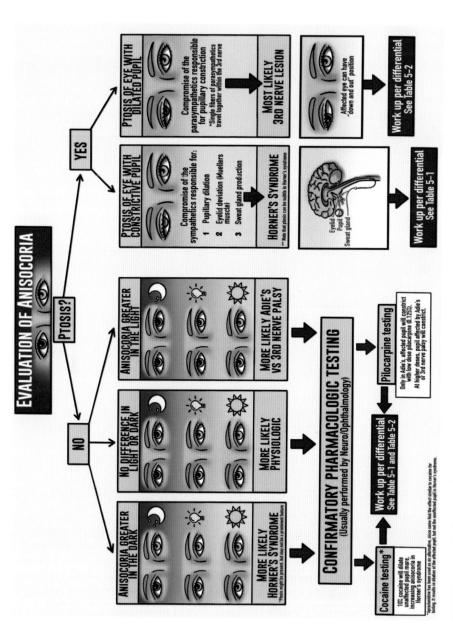

FIGURE 5-18 • **Evaluation of anisocoria.** (Reproduced with permission from Cathy Cichon, MD.)

TABLE 5-1 • Potential Causes of Horner Syndrome: Dysfunction of the Sympathetic Chain Causing Unilateral Ptosis (Droopy Lid), Mydriasis (Dilated Pupil), and Anhidrosis (Impaired Sweating)

First-order neuron lesion	Brainstem stroke, usually accompanied by other symptoms, including: nausea, vomiting, vertigo, dysarthria
Second-order neuron lesion	Apical lung tumor, Neck trauma, Brachial plexus injury, Thoracic surgery
Third-order neuron lesion	Carotid dissection, Cavernous sinus pathology (affecting cranial nerves III, IV, and VI)

TABLE 5-2 • Diagnoses at a Glance: Causes, Symptoms and Findings When One Pupil is Dilated

Cause of Dilated Pupil	Symptoms	Findings
Tumor impinging on cranial nerve (CN) III	• Based on whether primary brain cancer or metastases • Based on whether additional structures affected • Can be acute or subacute	 (Reproduced with permission from McKean SC, Ross JJ, Dressler DD, Scheurer DB, eds. *Principles and Practice of Hospital Medicine*. 2nd ed. New York: McGraw Hill; 2017, Figure 83-5.) • Dilated pupil • Ptosis • Eye is in "down and out" position • Additional findings if additional structures affected
Posterior communicating artery aneurysm (artery located adjacent to CN III)	• Acute or subacute • If unruptured, may only have dilated pupil • Other CN III symptoms based on degree of compression • Sudden severe headache if aneurysm ruptures	• Dilated pupil • Severe discomfort from headache, altered mental status (if ruptured) • Can have other CN III findings based on degree of compression
• Stroke affecting CN III	• Acute onset of symptoms: double vision; may note drooping lid, down and out location of eye • Additional symptoms if other structures also affected by stroke	• Dilated pupil may not be as prominent or may be absent with ischemia (as compared with compression) • Ptosis, down and out position of eye • Other findings based on whether additional structures affected

(Continued)

TABLE 5-2 • Diagnoses at a Glance: Causes, Symptoms and Findings When One Pupil is Dilated (Continued)		
Cause of Dilated Pupil	Symptoms	Findings
• Infection, trauma, bleeding, tumor, or anything that increases intracranial pressure (ICP) • In any of these processes, parasympathetics traveling on the outside of CN III are susceptible to pressure	• Headache, nausea, vomiting, altered mental status • Other neurologic deficits based on acuity, degree of intracranial pressure (ICP) increase, primary process	• Dilated ("blown") pupil; typically nonresponsive to light • Other findings based on primary process, degree of ICP elevation
• Cavernous sinus thrombosis • Often associated with sinus or tooth infection • CNs III, IV, V, and VI all can be affected, as they traverse the cavernous sinus	• Acute onset • Facial and/or tooth pain, fever, chills, nasal congestion/discharge • Nausea, vomiting, altered mental status • Double vision • Facial numbness • Abnormal-appearing eye (eg, proptosis, pain, redness)	• Fever • Facial and/or tooth pain • Impaired extraocular movements • Dilated pupil • Red eye • Proptosis • Facial hypesthesia
• Dilating drops (ie, mydriatic agents) instilled into one eye • Nebulized ipratropium bromide (parasympatholytic) inadvertently striking eye	• Blurred vision in affected eye • Light sensitivity in dilated eye • Any symptoms that lead to eye exam in first place • Shortness of breath, wheezing (if related to ipratropium bromide)	• Dilated eye is nonreactive
• Adie tonic pupil: idiopathic disorder of the parasympathetics	• Photophobia and difficulty adapting to the dark • Blurry vision both for near and far vision and during transitions • Denervation of the affected pupil results in a poor light but better tonic near constriction	• Dilated eye may have slightly oval-shaped pupil given segmental nature of iris dysfunction (denervation)

Assessing Pupillary Response to Light

- Turn down the light in your exam room, which will make the pupils dilate a bit.
- Observe the pupils. Normally, they should appear equal, round, and symmetric in their positioning within the orbit.

- Instruct the patient to look toward a distant area in the room (eg, the corner where the wall and ceiling meet) while keeping both of their eyes open.
- Assess whether each pupil constricts appropriately in response to direct and indirect stimulation as follows:
  - Shine a bright light (flashlight, smart phone light) in one eye and note if the pupil constricts (direct response). The brightness accentuates the response.
  - Then shine a light in the opposite eye while looking at the first eye, noting again whether pupillary constriction occurs (consensual response).
- If you are having trouble detecting any change, have the patient close their eye for several seconds and place your hand over their eyebrows to provide additional shade. This helps to make it as dark as possible, encouraging greater pupillary dilation and therefore accentuating any changes.
- It may be hard to detect the consensual response if the lighting in your room is suboptimal (ie, if it is too dark, you will not be able to see the other eye) or if the patient has dark-colored irises.
- Pupils can differ in size by <1 mm and still be normal. This is called physiologic anisocoria.
- Situations when both pupils are inappropriately dilated or constricted are described in **Tables 5-3** and **5-4**, along with associated symptoms and findings.

> PEARL: If you detect pupillary abnormalities, it can be helpful if the patient has a picture (eg, from a driver's license) so that you can compare current to past appearance in order to determine what is new.

TABLE 5-3 • Diagnoses at a Glance: Causes, Symptoms, and Findings When Both Pupils Are Dilated

Cause of Dilation	Symptoms	Findings
Systemic exposure to sympathetic agonist (eg, cocaine)	• Sweaty, agitated, energized/activated	• Bilateral dilated pupils • Pupils responsive to light (may be sluggish) • Tachycardia, sweaty, hypertensive, agitated
Systemic exposure to parasympatholytic agent (eg, atropine)	• Lightheaded, dizzy, syncope (ie, symptoms meriting use of atropine)	• Bilateral dilated pupils • Bradycardia, hypotension (ie, reason for use of atropine)
Installation of dilating drops (mydriatics) for eye exam	• Blurred vision in both eyes if drops instilled bilaterally. • History consistent with use of mydriatics	• Pupil(s) exposed to mydriatic drops is/are dilated • No response to light
Exposure of eye(s) to parasympatholytic agent (eg, nebulized ipratropium bromide with ill-fitting mask)	• Shortness of breath or wheezing (ie, reason for using nebulizer)	• Nebulizer mask is ill-fitting • Wheezing • Pupil(s) dilated but responsive

TABLE 5-4 • Diagnoses at a Glance: Causes, Symptoms, and Findings When Both Are Pupils Constricted		
Cause of Constriction	Symptoms	Findings
Systemic exposure to narcotics	Lethargy, fatigue, decreased level of consciousness	• Both pupils constricted • Decreased consciousness, often appear acute ill, abnormal vital signs • Not breathing, shallow breathing, decreased respiratory rate
Parasympathetic overactivity with organophosphate toxicity	• Lethargy, fatigue, decreased level of consciousness, shortness of breath, increased secretions, vomiting, diarrhea, urinary incontinence • Consider reason for exposure (eg, suicide attempt, mass poisoning, work-related exposure)	• Both pupils constricted • Acute/severe illness, wheezing, increased secretions, spontaneous urination and defecation
Interruption of midbrain fibers that respond to light (Argyll Robertson pupils): neurosyphilis, Lyme disease, neurosarcoid, other unusual disorders	Lethargy, fatigue, other related to the primary process	• Both pupils constricted

Findings and Their Meaning: Abnormal Pupillary Response

A number of pathologic processes can affect the afferent (sensing) limb, which carries the impulse generated when light is directed toward the affected eye. The result is a relative afferent pupillary defect (RAPD). The Swinging Flashlight Test is used to assess for RAPD (**Figure 5-19**).

- At baseline, both pupils appear symmetric. This is because the afferents from the nonaffected eye are responding appropriately to ambient light.
- Shine your light in the affected eye. No or minimal constriction will occur.
- Then swing the light to the unaffected eye. It should constrict normally.
- Then swing the light back to the affected eye, which will now appear to dilate in response to direct light. This is because it is no longer receiving signals from the normal eye to constrict. Since the affected eye has an abnormal decreased response to direct light, it appears to dilate.
- To confirm this response, swing the light back and forth between the 2 eyes several times.
- When performing the swinging light test on a patient with intact responses, the pupils will consistently appear small.

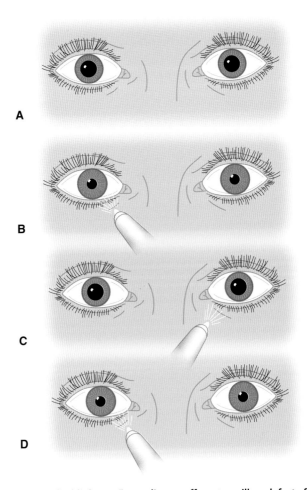

FIGURE 5-19 • "Swinging flashlight test" revealing an afferent pupillary defect of the left eye. **(A)** Pupils are normal and equal before testing. **(B)** Both pupils constrict when light is shined into the normal (right) eye. **(C)** Left eye appears to dilate (ie, does not constrict) in response to direct light. **(D)** Both pupils constrict when light is again directed to the right (normal) eye. (Reproduced with permission from Tintinalli JE, Ma OJ, Yealy DM, et al, eds. *Tintinalli's Emergency Medicine: A Comprehensive Study Guide*. 9th ed. New York: McGraw Hill; 2020.)

Table 5-5 provides a summary of common causes of RAPD, along with symptoms and findings.

TABLE 5-5 • Diagnoses at a Glance: Causes, Symptoms, and Findings Associated With a Relative Afferent Pupillary Defect (RAPD)

Cause	Symptoms	Findings
Optic neuritis • An autoimmune disorder often associated with multiple sclerosis (MS) • 15%-20% of patients with MS will present with optic neuritis • 50% of those with MS will develop optic neuritis at some point during the course of their illness	• Patients typically report the onset of unilateral blurry vision over hours to days • Often accompanied by dull pain that is worse with eye movement • May have other CNS symptoms (eg, weakness, dizziness, sensory deficits) if other regions of the brain or cord are affected	• RAPD of affected eye • Decreased acuity • Abnormal optic disc in one-third of patients • CNS motor and/or sensory findings if other areas of brain or cord affected.
Ischemic optic neuropathy • Etiologies include atherosclerosis as well as vasculitis • Giant cell arteritis (GCA) can involve the contralateral eye and requires emergent treatment to prevent irreversible vision loss	• Patients typically report altitudinal visual field loss • Can be preceded by visual obscurations • In GCA, will have systemic symptoms including headache, jaw pain, unintended weight loss	• RAPD of affected eye • Decreased acuity • Optic disc edema • Visual field deficits that are altitudinal in nature (ie, vision loss is above or below the horizontal midline)
Central retinal artery occlusion • Local thrombosis (associated with typical atherosclerotic risk factors) • Embolic event (eg, from carotid stenosis or atrial fibrillation) • Carotid dissection: From sudden neck flexion/extension (eg. car accident), therapeutic musculoskeletal manipulation, connective tissue disease	• Abrupt, painless, unilateral loss/diminution of vision • Sometimes described as a "curtain dropping" in front of their eye	• RAPD of affected eye • Decreased acuity • Retinal whitening • Usually a retinal cherry-red spot
Severe retinal disease • 80%-90% damaged retina	• Chronic or acute vision loss depending on etiology of retinal injury • Can be painful or painless • Presentation dependent of underlying pathology	• RAPD of affected eye • Decreased acuity

USING THE OPHTHALMOSCOPE

This aspect of the exam is, at least initially, quite awkward. It gets easier with practice. Take some time to play with your scope, paying attention to its assembly, on/off mechanism, and the various lens and light settings. For the purposes of the general exam, we will focus on the simplest settings and most basic techniques for the standard scope (**Figures 5-20** and **5-21**), which will highlight key principles. It is worth noting that there are also scopes that

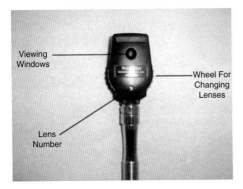
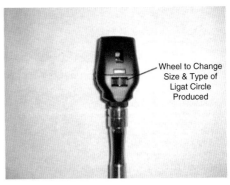

FIGURE 5-20 • Side of scope facing examiner (left) and side of scope facing patient (right). (Photos from *Practical Guide to Clinical Medicine: Eye Exam.* Available from: https://meded.ucsd.edu/ clinicalmed/eyes.html.)

are engineered to allow easier and magnified visualization of the retina (eg. Welch Allyn's Panoptic). These are not described here, though their use is straightforward and can be learned from other resources.

Whichever scope you use, make sure the battery is charged or plugged in (if it is from a wall unit).

Using the Standard Ophthalmoscope (Figures 5-20 and 5-21)

- Use medium circle of light and medium intensity.
- Instruct patient to look toward a distant area (avoid eye roving).
- Place your right eye to patient's right eye, followed by left eye examining left eye.
- Place your hand on their shoulder or forehead.
- Grasp handle near top.
- Start 15 degrees temporal, and find the red reflex.
- Move in slowly. Starting with lens "0," click focus wheel until a retinal structure comes into sharp focus.

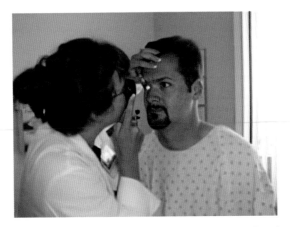

FIGURE 5-21 • Using the standard ophthalmoscope. (Photo from *Practical Guide to Clinical Medicine: Eye Exam.* Available from: https://meded.ucsd.edu/clinicalmed/eyes.html.)

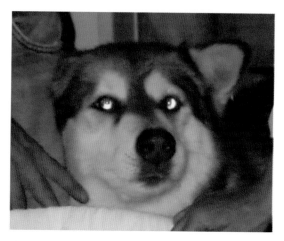

FIGURE 5-22 • **Red reflex.** (Photo from *Practical Guide to Clinical Medicine: Eye Exam.* Available from: https://meded.ucsd.edu/clinicalmed/eyes.html.)

- Evaluate each quadrant of retina systematically.
- If you lose the pupil, back up, find the red reflex, and advance again.
- The red reflex: Looking through the viewing window at the patient's pupil from a distance, you should see a sparkly, orange-red color known as the red reflex (**Figure 5-22**).
  - This is caused by light reflecting off of the retina and is the same phenomenon that produces red eyes in flash photos.
  - Seeing the red reflex indicates that there is nothing interfering with passage of light through all of the structures of the eye, which is then reflected back from the retina.

Findings and Their Meaning: Loss of Red Reflex

- The translucent structures that allow light to pass unimpeded from outside the eye to the retina become opacified, and the red reflex is lost (**Figure 5-23**). This is most commonly associated with cataracts, a process caused by clouding of the lens.
- Interruption of light reaching the retina can be caused by other processes, which will also cause a loss of the red reflex. A few examples include the following:
  - Opacification of the cornea (eg, scarring from prior injury)
  - Bleeding into the vitreous (vitreous hemorrhage)
  - Retinoblastoma (in children)

If there are external symptoms or abnormalities, you can also use the ophthalmoscope as a magnifying lens to examine the external structures of the eye (eg, lids, sclera, conjunctiva, cornea).

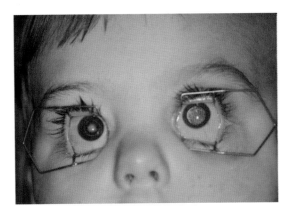

FIGURE 5-23 • **Congenital cataract, right eye. No red reflex on right, normal on left.** (Reproduced with permission from Riordan-Eva P, Augsburger JJ, eds. *Vaughan & Asbury's General Ophthalmology.* 19th ed. New York: McGraw Hill; 2017.)

Visualizing the Retina

- To see the fundus in greater detail, you will need to move very close to the patient, analogous to looking through a keyhole (ie, the closer you are, the more you will see).
  - Your middle finger, the one resting on the low front of the head piece, should be on or near the patient's cheek.
  - Starting with the 0 lens in place, slowly rotate the lens selection wheel. If you change lenses too quickly, you will probably whizz right by the one that gives the sharpest picture, so go slow. In the event that this does not bring anything into focus, try rotating the adjustment wheel in the opposite direction.
  - It does not really matter what number lens is required to achieve the clearest view. This will vary with the refractive error of both you and the patient. The numbers are simply provided for reference (red is to correct myopia/near-sighted, green to correct for hyperopia/far-sighted).
  - Once you are close in and have the retina in clear view, you should only need to change the lens 1 or 2 clicks to keep all structures in focus as you scan across.
- You will only be able to see approximately 15% of the retina at any one time. The initial view will probably be of blood vessels on a random patch of retina.
- The retina has a refractile, orange-red appearance, varying a bit with the skin color and age of the patient. Fundoscopy (looking at the retina) provides important information, as it not only enables you to detect diseases of the eyes but also is the only area of the body where small blood vessels can be studied with relative ease.
- When you first visualize the retina, you will note branching blood vessels. The bigger, darker ones are the veins, and the smaller, brighter red structures are the arteries. These vessels are more obvious in the superior and inferior aspects of the retina, with relative sparing of the temporal and medial regions.
- You will not be able to visualize the entire retina at any one time. Approximately 1 disc diameter should be visible.
  - To view different areas of the retina, you will have to shift the angle with which you peer through the pupil.
  - This requires very small movements.

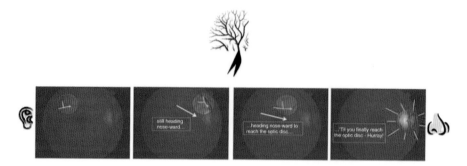

FIGURE 5-24 • **Following retinal vessels to reach the optic disc.** (Photos from *Practical Guide to Clinical Medicine: Eye Exam.* Available from: https://meded.ucsd.edu/clinicalmed/eyes.html.)

- Imagine that the blood vessels are the branches of a tree (**Figure 5-24**):
  - Follow them in a direction that leads to less branching (ie, toward the trunk).
  - This will direct you toward the optic disc, the point at which the vessels enter the retina along with the head of the optic nerve.
- The edges of the optic disc are sharp and well defined in the normal state. It should be a bit more yellow when compared to the rest of the retina (**Figure 5-25**).
- Toward the middle of the optic disc is the optic cup, a distinct circular area from which the blood vessels actually emerge. The disc is not located in the exact center of the retina but rather toward its medial/nasal aspect. Measurements in the eye are made using disc size as a measuring device (eg, a finding may be described as being at 2 o'clock, 2 disc diameters from the center of the disc).
- If you are unable to locate the disc after following the vessels in one direction, simply head the other way.
- The macula is a region located lateral to the optic disc. It looks somewhat darker than the rest of the retina and has no distinct borders.
  - The macula provides the sharpest vision.
  - It can be best visualized by asking the patient to stare directly at the light of the ophthalmoscope while you remain focused on a fixed area of the retina.

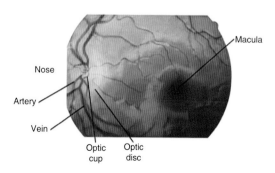

FIGURE 5-25 • **Normal retina.** (Photo from *Practical Guide to Clinical Medicine: Eye Exam.* Available from: https://meded.ucsd.edu/clinicalmed/eyes.html.)

- Try to examine the entire retina systematically, looking up, down, left, and right.
- You will likely have to remind the patient to continue looking straight ahead during your exam, or else the fundus will be in continual motion and you will have no chance of locating anything.
- It is a good idea to periodically give the patient a break (particularly if the exam is taking a while), allowing them to blink in the dark before resuming.
- To view the patient's left eye, hold the scope in your left hand and use your left eye for viewing. Then repeat the process described above.

Findings and Their Meaning: Fundoscopic Abnormalities

- Fundoscopy allows you to visualize disorders that are limited to the eye. Selected examples (photographed through a dilated eye) are shown in **Figure 5-26**.

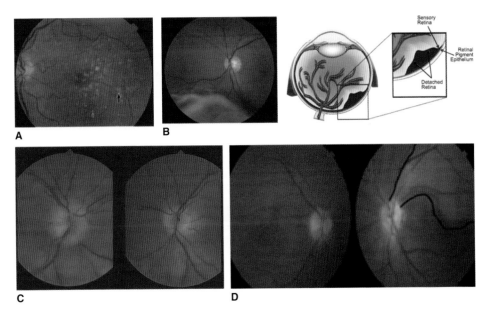

FIGURE 5-26 • Selected examples of retinal pathology. **(A) Age-related macular degeneration.** (Reproduced with permission from Riordan-Eva P, Augsburger JJ, eds. *Vaughan & Asbury's General Ophthalmology*. 19th ed. New York: McGraw Hill; 2017, Figure 10-1A.) **(B) Inferior retinal detachment appears as an elevated sheet of retinal tissue with multiple folds. Illustration demonstrates the separation of neurosensory retina from the underlying retinal pigment epithelium.** (Left photo: Reproduced with permission from Loscalzo J, Fauci AS, Kasper DL, et al, eds. *Harrison's Principles of Internal Medicine*. 21st ed. New York: McGraw Hill; 2022, Figure 32-14. Right illustration: From Knoop KJ, Stack LB, Storrow AB, Thurman RJ, eds. *The Atlas of Emergency Medicine*. 5th ed. New York: McGraw-Hill; 2021, Figure 24.127 (bottom). Reproduced with permission from Robinson M. Ferre, MD.) **(C) Papilledema. Moderate, photo left; mild, photo right.** (Reproduced with permission from Papadakis MA, McPhee SJ, Rabow MW, McQuaid KR, eds. *Current Diagnosis & Treatment 2022*. New York: McGraw Hill; 2022, eFigure 7-67.) **(D) Branch retinal artery occlusion. Left eye with branch retinal arterial occlusion, right eye normal. The ischemic area of the left retina is lighter and bounded by black lines.** (Photo by Dr. Jeff Lee.)

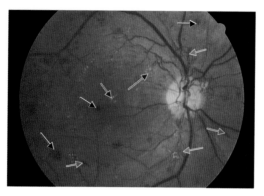

FIGURE 5-27 • **Diabetic retinopathy: Scattered hemorrhages [dot/blot (black arrows) and flame (yellow arrows)]; yellow exudates (blue arrows); and neovascularization, which is growth of fine abnormal vessels in the retina (green arrows).** (Reproduced with permission from Loscalzo J, Fauci AS, Kasper DL, et al, eds. *Harrison's Principles of Internal Medicine*. 21st ed. New York: McGraw Hill; 2022.)

- Fundoscopy also provides an opportunity to gain in-**sights** into systemic diseases (**Figure 5-27**).
  - There are a number of chronic systemic diseases (most commonly hypertension, diabetes, and atherosclerosis) that affect vessels of this size in a relatively slow and silent fashion (Figure 5-27).
  - It is, however, frequently not possible to directly assess the extent of this damage during physical examination as the affected organs (eg, kidneys) are well hidden and their vessels inaccessible.
  - Evaluation of the retina provides an opportunity to directly visualize these processes. Based on this information, clinicians can make informed assumptions as to what is occurring elsewhere in the body.

> **PEARL:** Being able to identify findings on fundoscopy takes a lot of practice. It will take multiple attempts before you are able to identify normal structures with confidence. Practice on as many patients as possible.

> **PEARL:** Remember that a nonophthalmologist can gather a lot of useful information about the eye even without the ophthalmoscopic exam. Make use of all the techniques (eg, assessing visual acuity, observation, pupillary response) described in this chapter to assess all of the other domains of eye function.

Note that it is much easier to examine the retina after the pupil has been pharmacologically dilated. Most providers, with the exception of optometrists and ophthalmologists, do not routinely perform dilated eye exams. This is because dilation takes time and is a bit uncomfortable for the patient as it causes increased light sensitivity that lasts for several hours. Take advantage of any opportunity to perform an examination through a dilated pupil because this is a great way of learning.

🖥 TELEHEALTH TIPS

- Begin with history taking, which can occur in a similar fashion to an in-person exam.
- Acuity assessment can be done in a limited way by asking the patient to read an item that they have on hand at home. They should use glasses if prescribed. You will need to depend on their accurate reporting of any abrupt change or decline in their ability to see.
- Direct observation of the eyes for symmetry and evaluation of external structures can be made by having the patient move close to camera. You can ask them to look left, right, up, and down to enable your ability to see the entire eye.
- The patient can apply pressure and pull down on the area below the lower lid in order to see the lower conjunctiva.
- Extraocular movements can be assessed by having them move close to the camera and follow your finger as you trace a rectangle. Or just have them follow their own finger as it traces a rectangle and you observe.
- Assessing pupillary response to light:
  - Ask the patient to use a flashlight (or light from their phone) and shine it into one eye from the side, while close to and staring into the camera. If the patient has someone else in the room, they can assist with this assessment.
  - This should allow you to see the direct pupillary response (depends on lighting in the room, eye color, and how close they are to the camera).
  - Then have the patient shine the light into the other eye while you are still evaluating the first one (consensual response).
- As with other aspects of the exam, adhere to the principle that urgent concerns (ie, those that carry risks of morbidity or mortality) require in-person evaluations.

✓ SUMMARY OF SKILLS CHECKLIST

- ☐ Clean your hands
- ☐ Observe external structures (lids, sclera, pupil, iris, conjunctiva)
- ☐ Visual acuity
- ☐ Visual fields
- ☐ Extraocular movements
- ☐ Note size, shape, and symmetry of pupils
- ☐ Check pupillary response to light

Using the Ophthalmoscope
- ☐ Red reflex
- ☐ Retinal exam, identifying: optic disc, arteries, veins, color of retina, macula
- ☐ Clean your hands

BIBLIOGRAPHY

Antonetti D, Klein R, Gardner TW. Diabetic retinopathy. *N Engl J Med.* 2012;366:1227-1239.

Balcer E. Optic neuritis. *N Engl J Med.* 2006;354:1273-1280.

Bartalena L, Veronesi G, Krassas GE, et al. Graves ophthalmopathy. *N Engl J Med.* 2009;360:994-1001.

Biswell R. Chapter 6. Cornea. In: Riordan-Eva P, Cunningham ET Jr, eds. *Vaughan & Asbury's General Ophthalmology.* 18th ed. New York: McGraw-Hill; 2011.

Clayton J. Dry eye. *N Engl J Med.* 2018;378(23):2212-2223.

Cronau H, Reddy Kankanala R, Mauger T. Diagnosis and management of red eye in primary care. *Am Fam Phys.* 2010;81(2):137-144.

Cunningham E, Margolis TP. Ocular manifestations of HIV infection. *N Engl J Med.* 1998;339:236-244.

D'Amico D. Primary retinal detachment. *N Engl J Med.* 2008;359:2346-2350.

De Jong P. Age-related macular degeneration. *N Engl J Med.* 2006;355:1474-1485.

Durland M, Barshak M, Sobrin L. Eye infections. *N Engl J Med.* 2023;389:2363-2375.

Goldberg C. Digital DDx: eye symptoms or conditions. Accessed March 25, 2023. http://digitalddx.com/symptoms_list/2/.

Goldberg C. Practical guide to clinical medicine: eye exam. Accessed March 25, 2023. https://meded.ucsd.edu/clinicalmed/eyes.html.

Hollands H, Johnson D, Brox AC, et al. Acute-onset floaters and flashes: is this patient at risk for retinal detachment? *JAMA.* 2009;302(20):2243-2249.

Jager R, Mieler WF, Miller JW. Age related macular degeneration. *N Engl J Med.* 2008;358(24):2606-2617.

Lefebvre D, Reinshagen KL, Yoon MK, et al. An 18-year-old man with diplopia and proptosis of the left eye. *N Engl J Med.* 2018;379:2452-2461.

Leibowitz HM. The red eye. *N Engl J Med.* 2000;343:345-351.

McGee S. Chapter 19: The pupils. *Evidence-Based Physical Diagnosis.* 2nd ed. New York: Saunders; 2007:209-241.

Shingleton BJ. Eye injuries. *N Engl J Med.* 1991;325:408-413.

Shingleton BJ, O'Donoghue MW. Blurred vision. *N Engl J Med.* 2000;343:556-562.

Tan A, Faridah H. The two-minute approach to monocular diplopia. *Malays Fam Physician.* 2010;5(3):115-118.

Vaughan D, Asbury T, Riordan-Eva P. *General Ophthalmology.* 15th ed. Stamford: Appleton and Lange; 1999.

Vinod E, Vaidya A, Cochrane T, et al. Off balance (visual field deficits from CNS lesion). *N Engl J Med.* 2014;370:e37.

Wong T, Scott IU. Retinal vein occlusion. *N Engl J Med.* 2010;363:2135-2144.

Wu G. *Ophthalmology for Primary Care.* Philadelphia: W.B. Saunders Company; 1997.

6

Cardiovascular Exam

Charlie Goldberg, MD

INTRODUCTION

The cardiovascular exam includes evaluation of the heart and peripheral vascular system. It is performed in several settings:

- As part of a screening evaluation for asymptomatic disease in healthy or at-risk populations
- When patients present with symptoms or findings (eg, chest pain, shortness of breath, edema, slow-to-heal extremity wounds) for which cardiovascular disease might be the underlying driver

GETTING STARTED

- The exam space should be quiet, well lit, private, and allow you to adequately expose the chest to facilitate the exam. Sometimes, the situation is not ideal (eg, a busy emergency department), in which case, do the best that you can, and reassess later if/when the physical space changes.
- The patient should rest supine with the upper body elevated to approximately 30 degrees. Most exam tables have an adjustable top. If not, use 2 or 3 pillows.
- Although assessment of pulse and blood pressure is discussed in the vital signs chapter (Chapter 3), they are important elements of the cardiovascular exam. See Chapter 3 for additional information.

Gown Management and Appropriately and Respectfully Examining Your Patients

There are several sources of discomfort related to the physical exam, including:

- People are often uncomfortable, in general, exposing any body part, even more so if it is in a sensitive area.
- In order to perform an accurate exam, exposure is critical.
- The entire process requires touching people with whom you may have little acquaintance.

Keys to performing a sensitive and thorough exam include the following:

- Explain what you are doing (and why) before doing it. Empower the patient to stop the exam or opt out if they are uncomfortable, following the principles of trauma-informed care discussed in the chapters on the breast (Chapter 10) and genital exams (Chapters 9 and 11).
- Expose the minimum amount of skin necessary to do the job; this requires "artful" use of gowns and drapes (**Figure 6-1**).

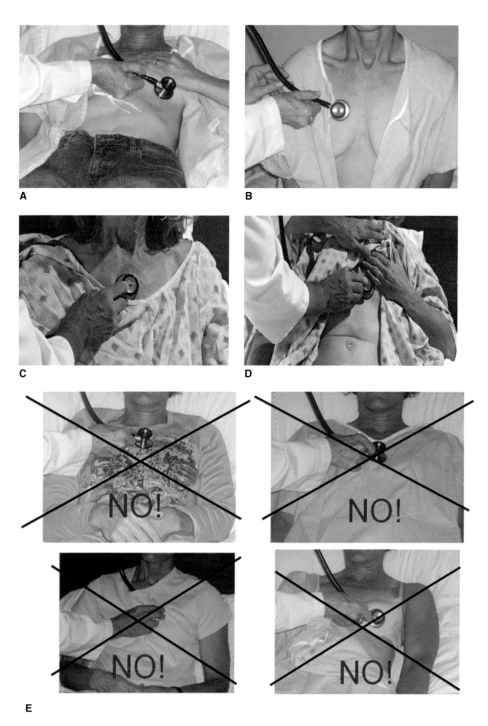

FIGURE 6-1 • Gowning techniques. (A-D) Good exam options for respectfully performing a cardiac exam. **(E) Suboptimal approaches when listening to the heart.** (Photos from *Practical Guide to Clinical Medicine: Cardiovascular Exam*. Available from: https://meded.ucsd.edu/clinicalmed/heart.html.)

- As much as possible, avoid examining through gowns or clothing. It adds another layer between your stethoscope, eyes, hands and the heart, decreasing the chances that you'll appreciate findings.

When examining the heart and lungs of female patients (Figure 6-1):
- Ask the patient to remove their bra prior to examining the chest area.
- Expose the left side of their chest to the extent needed.
- Enlist the patient's assistance, asking them to raise their breast to a position that enhances your ability to listen to and palpate the heart.

> **PEARL:** Thoughtful exposure of the area to be examined is important in order to perform an optimal evaluation.

OBSERVATION

- Note if the patient is in discomfort, having breathing difficulty, sweaty, or otherwise in distress.
- When the chest is exposed, note any scars suggestive of prior surgery. Note any obvious chest deformities.

PALPATION

- Identify the point of maximum impulse (PMI) (**Figure 6-2**):
  - Take the palm of your right hand and place it across the patient's left chest so that it covers the area over the heart. The heel of the hand should rest along the left sternal border with the extended fingers lying below the left nipple.
  - The PMI is generated by the contraction of the apex of the left ventricle, which lies beneath your hand. Using the palm of your hand, note the rough position of the PMI.
  - Try to pin down the precise location of the apical impulse with the tip of your index finger.
  - The normal-sized and functioning ventricle will generate a penny-sized impulse that is best felt in the midclavicular line, roughly at the fifth intercostal space.
  - Occasionally, the PMI will not localize to any one area, which does not necessarily indicate ventricular enlargement or dysfunction. Medical conditions, like obesity or chronic obstructive pulmonary disease, may also limit your ability to identify its precise location.
  - Note whether the PMI is particularly vigorous. Processes associated with ventricular hypercontractility (eg, mitral regurgitation or aortic insufficiency that results in exceptionally large stroke volumes) generate an impulse of increased vigor.

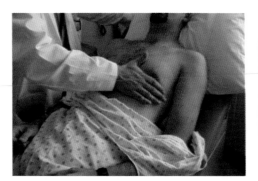 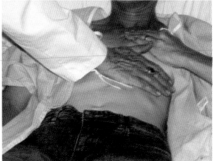

FIGURE 6-2 • Identifying location of the point of maximum impulse. (Photos from *Practical Guide to Clinical Medicine: Cardiovascular Exam.* Available from: https://meded.ucsd.edu/clinicalmed/heart.html.)

Findings and Their Meaning: Displaced PMI

- If the left ventricle becomes dilated (eg, as the result of heart attacks or other pathology affecting the ventricle), the PMI becomes laterally displaced.
- In cases of severe enlargement, the PMI may be located near the axilla.

> **PEARL:** A laterally displaced PMI indicates ventricular enlargement, which is always abnormal.

Findings and Their Meaning: Palpable Thrill

- A thrill is a vibratory sensation produced by turbulent blood flow, generated by valvular abnormalities (insufficiency or stenosis). These also generate characteristic murmurs, described later in this chapter.
- Even in the setting of severe valvular disease, thrills are very uncommon.

Special Testing: Carotid Artery Palpation

This is of value during assessment of aortic valvular and outflow tract disease (**Figure 6-3**) and should be performed after auscultation so that you know whether or not these problems exist. The carotids can be palpated as follows:

- Slide the second and third fingers of either hand along the side of the trachea at the level of the thyroid cartilage.
- The carotid pulsation is palpable just lateral to the groove formed by the trachea and the surrounding soft tissue.
- The pulsations should be easily palpable.
- Do not push on both sides simultaneously as this may compromise cerebral blood flow.

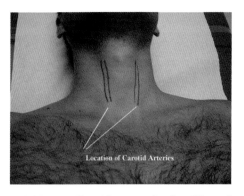 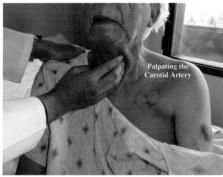

FIGURE 6-3 · Carotid artery palpation. (Photos from *Practical Guide to Clinical Medicine: Cardiovascular Exam*. Available from: https://meded.ucsd.edu/clinicalmed/heart.html.)

Findings and Their Meaning: Abnormalities Identified During Carotid Palpation

- Diminished carotid artery impulse may be caused by very advanced disease, including severe atherosclerosis, aortic stenosis, or very impaired ventricular performance.
- Increased carotid impulse can occur with large stroke volumes, for example, in patients with significant aortic valve insufficiency.

AUSCULTATION

Accurate auscultation is enhanced by placing the stethoscope in direct contact with the patient's skin. To maintain modesty, several approaches to gown management can be employed; see Figure 6-1.

> PEARL: Place your stethoscope directly on the patient's skin when listening to the heart.

General Comments

- Become comfortable with your stethoscope.
- Many brands are available. Read the instructions so you know how to engage the bell (to hear low-pitched sounds) and diaphragm (to hear higher pitched sounds).

> PEARL: Make sure you know how to engage the bell and diaphragm for your stethoscope.

- Adult, pediatric, and newborn sizes exist. Some combine adult and pediatric scopes into a single unit.
- Several are pictured in **Figure 6-4**. Almost any commercially available scope will do the job.

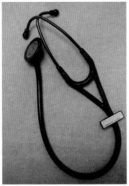

A

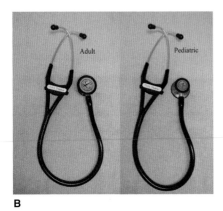

B

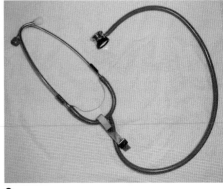

C

FIGURE 6-4 • **Common stethoscope styles. (A) Adult stethoscope: diaphragm and bell incorporated into single side. (B) Combination adult and pediatric stethoscope. (C) Newborn stethoscope.** (Photos from *Practical Guide to Clinical Medicine: Cardiovascular Exam*. Available from: https://meded.ucsd.edu/clinicalmed/heart.html.)

Using Your Stethoscope

- Place the earpieces in your ears, angled toward your nose.
- Place the diaphragm firmly over the second right intercostal space, the region of the aortic valve, and listen.
- Move to the other side of the sternum and listen in the second left intercostal space, the region of the pulmonic valve.
- Move down along the sternum and listen over the left fourth or fifth intercostal space, the region of the tricuspid valve.
- Position the diaphragm over the fourth intercostal space, left midclavicular line, to examine the mitral area.
- These locations are rough approximations and are generally determined by visual estimation (see **Figure 6-5**). In each area:
  - Listen specifically for S1 (closure of atrioventricular valves) and then S2 (closure of the pulmonic and aortic valves).
  - S1 will be loudest over the left fourth intercostal space (mitral/tricuspid valve areas) and S2 loudest along the second right and left intercostal spaces (aortic/pulmonic valve regions).
  - The time between S1 and S2 (systole) is generally shorter than that between S2 and S1 (diastole). This helps you determine which sound is produced by the closure of the mitral/tricuspid and which by the aortic/pulmonic valves and defines when systole and diastole occur.
  - You can palpate the radial artery while you listen to help determine the timing of systole.

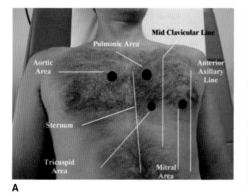 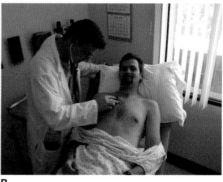

A   **B**

FIGURE 6-5 • **(A & B) Anatomic sites for cardiac auscultation.** (Photos from *Practical Guide to Clinical Medicine: Cardiovascular Exam*. Available from: https://meded.ucsd.edu/clinicalmed/heart.html.)

- In younger patients (younger than approximately 30 years), you can often detect physiologic splitting of S2.
  - S2 is made up of 2 components, aortic (A2) and pulmonic (P2) valve closure.
  - During inspiration, venous return to the right heart is increased and pulmonic valve closure is delayed, allowing you to hear first A2 and then P2.
  - During expiration, the 2 sounds occur closer together and are detected as a single S2 (see **Figure 6-6**).

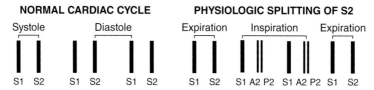

FIGURE 6-6 • **Physiologic splitting of the second heart sound.** (Illustration from *Practical Guide to Clinical Medicine: Cardiovascular Exam*. Available from: https://meded.ucsd.edu/clinicalmed/heart.html.)

Findings and Their Meaning: Extra Heart Sounds

- These can be present in normal patients up to the age of approximately 30 years old. They represent pathology in older patients.
  - An S3 is most commonly associated with heart failure and is caused by blood from the left atrium colliding with blood in an overfilled ventricle during early diastolic filling. It is heard following S2 (**Figure 6-7**).
  - An S4 is created by blood trying to enter a stiff, noncompliant left ventricle during atrial contraction, which happens during late diastole. It is heard before S1 and is most frequently associated with left ventricular hypertrophy, often the result of long-standing hypertension (Figure 6-7). Because an S4 occurs during atrial contraction, it is absent if the patient has atrial fibrillation.

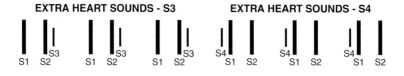

FIGURE 6-7 • **Timing of extra heart sounds during cardiac cycle.** (Illustration from *Practical Guide to Clinical Medicine: Cardiovascular Exam*. Available from: https://meded.ucsd.edu/clinicalmed/heart.html.)

- Both the S3 and S4 are low pitched, detected by listening with the bell of the stethoscope over the apex of the left ventricle (**Figure 6-8**).
- These extra heart sounds are soft, so it will take some practice before you develop the ability to detect them. Positioning the patient on their left side while you listen may be helpful.
- The presence of both an S3 and S4 simultaneously is referred to as a summation gallop.

PEARL: The S3 and S4 are low-pitched extra heart sounds heard best over the apex with the bell. They are most commonly associated with heart failure and hypertension, respectively.

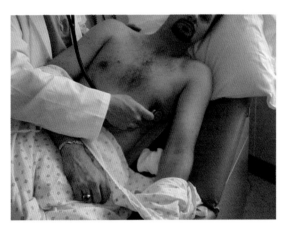

FIGURE 6-8 • Listening for extra heart sounds. (Photo from *Practical Guide to Clinical Medicine: Cardiovascular Exam*. Available from: https://meded.ucsd.edu/clinicalmed/heart.html.)

Findings and Their Meaning: Rubs

Rubs are less common sounds related to pericarditis, where pericardial inflammation generates creaky-scratchy noises.

- The classic rub is actually made up of 3 sounds, associated with atrial contraction, ventricular contraction, and ventricular filling.
- It is rare to hear all 3 components (more commonly, 2 are apparent). They can vary in intensity over the course of the illness. Acute pericarditis is often associated with sharp chest pain that is positional (improves with sitting up and leaning forward) and pleuritic (exacerbated by breathing).
- Pericarditis is most commonly idiopathic and self-limited, such that obtaining studies to define the cause are not typically performed. Many of these are presumed to be viral – although there are a host of other potential etiologies (eg. post cardiac injury, associated with autoimmune disorders like lupus).
- As a result of pericarditis, fluid can accumulate in the pericardial space, known as a pericardial effusion. Rarely, an effusion can generate enough pressure such that the right atrium and ventricle are compressed, impairing filling and decreasing cardiac output. This is referred to as cardiac tamponade, a life-threatening condition that can result in tachycardia, hypotension, diminished heart sounds, and jugular venous distention (described later in this chapter).

MURMURS

Murmurs are continuous sounds that occur during systole or diastole as a result of turbulent blood flow. They fall into 2 broad groups:

- Blood leaking backward across a valve that is supposed to be closed: These are referred to as regurgitant or insufficiency murmurs (eg, mitral regurgitation, aortic insufficiency).
- Blood flow across a valve that will not open fully/normally: These valves suffer from varying degrees of stenosis (eg, aortic stenosis, mitral stenosis).
- Increased blood flow across a normal valve can also cause a murmur, for instance, in high cardiac output states (eg, systemic infection or after exercise).
- Frequently, early in the development of valve pathology, patients are asymptomatic. Over time, symptoms may develop as function becomes impaired.

- Congenital abnormalities (eg, a ventricular septal defect) can also cause murmurs, although they are much less common.

If you hear a murmur, note the following:
- Does it occur during systole or diastole (ie, relationship to S1 and S2)?
- What is the quality of the sound (ie, Does it get louder and then softer? Does it maintain the same intensity throughout? Does it start loud and become soft?)?
- What is the loudness of the sound? The rating system for murmurs is as follows:
  - 1/6: Can only be heard with careful listening
  - 2/6: Readily audible as soon as the stethoscope is applied to the chest
  - 3/6: Louder than 2/6
  - 4/6: As loud as 3/6 but accompanied by a thrill (note earlier comments under palpation)
  - 5/6: Audible even when only the edge of the stethoscope touches the chest
  - 6/6: Audible to the naked ear
- How does the murmur change as you move your stethoscope? Listen in more than 4 places to pick up changes in intensity and quality as you alter your point of auscultation in relation to the specific valves.

> **PEARL:** Murmurs are most commonly caused by regurgitant or stenotic valves. Systolic murmurs are more common than diastolic.

Most murmurs are between 1/6 and 3/6. Louder murmurs generally (but not always) indicate greater pathology.

Identifying Systolic Murmurs

Aortic Stenosis

- Aortic stenosis (AS) tends to be loudest along the upper sternal borders.
- AS has a growling, harsh quality (ie, gets louder and then softer; also referred to as a crescendo-decrescendo or diamond-shaped murmur).
- As the stenosis becomes more severe, the point at which the murmur is loudest (ie, its peak intensity) occurs later in systole (**Figure 6-9**). This is due to the fact that it takes longer to generate the higher ventricular pressure required to push blood through a narrower opening.
- The murmur is often easier to hear when the patient sits up and exhales.
- AS is audible when auscultating over the carotid arteries.
- AS often radiates to the right clavicle, which can be appreciated by listening with the diaphragm of the stethoscope placed directly on the clavicle.

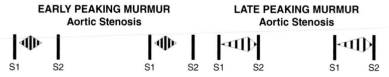

EARLY PEAKING MURMUR
Aortic Stenosis

LATE PEAKING MURMUR
Aortic Stenosis

S1   S2   S1   S2   S1   S2   S1   S2

FIGURE 6-9 • **Timing of aortic stenosis murmur during systole.** (Illustration from *Practical Guide to Clinical Medicine: Cardiovascular Exam.* Available from: https://meded.ucsd.edu/clinicalmed/heart.html.)

- Carotid upstrokes (the quantity and timing of blood flow into the carotids from the left ventricle) can be affected in severe AS:
  - The technique for carotid palpation is as described above, although in this instance, it is performed while you simultaneously listen to the AS murmur.

- Normally, there should be no delay between the onset of the murmur, which marks the beginning of systole, and when you feel the pulsation in the carotid. In the setting of critical (ie, very severe) AS, smaller amounts of blood will be ejected into the carotid, and there may be a lag between when you hear the murmur and feel the impulse.
- This is referred to as diminished and delayed upstrokes (ie, parvus et tardus), as opposed to the full and prompt inflow that occurs in the absence of disease. It is only found in very severe AS.
- Symptoms and findings of AS are summarized in **Figure 6-10**.

> **PEARL:** AS has a softer-louder-softer (rrrRRrrr) quality. The later the murmur peaks in systole, the more severe is the stenosis.

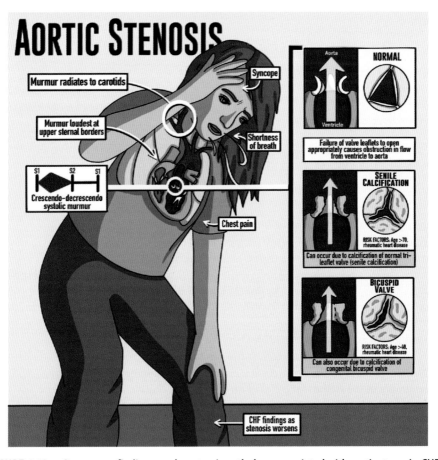

FIGURE 6-10 • Symptoms, findings, and anatomic pathology associated with aortic stenosis. CHF, congestive heart failure. (Reproduced with permission from Cathy Cichon, MD.)

Sub-Aortic Stenosis

A relatively rare condition where the obstruction of flow from the left ventricle into the aorta is caused by an ingrowth of septal tissue in the region below the aortic valve known as the aortic outflow tract. Findings include:

- A crescendo-decrescendo murmur that sounds like AS. As opposed to valvular AS, the murmur tends to be louder along the left lower sternal border and out toward the apex. This makes anatomic sense as the obstruction is located near this region. It does not radiate loudly to the carotids.
- Because the degree of obstruction can vary with ventricular filling, sub-AS is referred to as a dynamic outflow tract obstruction, as opposed to valvular AS, where the degree of obstruction that exists at any point in time is constant. In sub-AS:
  - The murmur gets softer if the ventricle is filled with more blood, as filling pushes the abnormal septum away from the opposite wall, decreasing the amount of obstruction.
  - Conversely, it gets louder if filling is decreased. This phenomenon can be detected on physical exam and is a way of distinguishing between valvular AS and subaortic obstruction.
  - Ask the patient to perform the Valsalva maneuver while you listen, decreasing venous return and making the murmur of sub-AS louder.
  - While listening with your stethoscope, squat down with the patient. This maneuver increases venous return, causing the murmur to become softer. Standing will cause the opposite to occur. You need to listen for approximately 20 seconds after each change in position to appreciate any difference.

Mitral Regurgitation

- The murmur sounds the same throughout systole (**Figure 6-11**).
- Creates a "shhshhing"-type noise, similar to when you pucker your lips and blow through clenched teeth.

MITRAL REGURGITATION

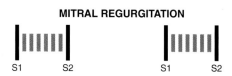

FIGURE 6-11 • **Timing of mitral regurgitation murmur during systole.** (Illustration from *Practical Guide to Clinical Medicine: Cardiovascular Exam.* Available from: https://meded.ucsd.edu/clinicalmed/heart.html.)

- Gets louder as you move your stethoscope towards the axilla.
- Will get even louder if you roll the patient onto their left side while keeping your stethoscope over the mitral area of the chest wall and listening in the same spot after they have moved.
- Gets louder if afterload is suddenly increased, which can be accomplished by having the patient close their hands tightly. Mitral regurgitation is also affected by the volume of blood returning to the heart. Squatting increases venous return, causing a louder sound. Standing decreases venous return, thereby diminishing the intensity of the murmur. These findings are subtle.
- Symptoms and findings are summarized in **Figure 6-12**.

> PEARL: Mitral regurgitation radiates toward the axilla. It tends to maintain a similar intensity throughout systole.

Sometimes murmurs of AS and mitral regurgitation coexist, which can be challenging to sort out on exam. Moving your stethoscope back and forth between the mitral and aortic areas will allow for direct comparison, which may help you decide if more than one type of lesion is present or if the quality of the murmur is the same in both locations, changing only in intensity (ie, consistent with a 1-valve problem).

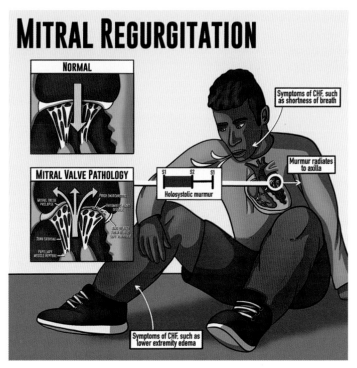

FIGURE 6-12 • Symptoms, findings, and anatomic pathology associated with mitral regurgitation. CHF, congestive heart failure. (Reproduced with permission from Cathy Cichon, MD.)

Tricuspid Regurgitation

- Tricuspid regurgitation (TR) generates a "shshhing"-type murmur, like mitral regurgitation, although it is softer, as right-sided pressures are lower than left.
- TR is louder along the lower left and right sternal borders, areas where the tricuspid valve is best assessed.
- As you move your stethoscope across the precordium toward the axilla, note if there is any change in the character or intensity of the murmur. With TR, it should diminish; with mitral regurgitation, it will increase.
- TR murmurs are also accentuated by inhalation or by applying pressure in the right upper quadrant near the liver, both of which increase venous return and therefore flow across the valve.
- Severe TR may cause visible upstrokes in the right internal jugular vein (also called v waves), as blood flows backward with each systole (see later section on internal jugular vein assessment).

Pulmonic valve murmurs (regurgitation and stenosis) are rare and will not be discussed. Findings associated with most congenital heart disorders are also not reviewed here.

Identifying Diastolic Murmurs

Diastolic murmurs tend to be softer and therefore more difficult to hear than those occurring during systole. This is because diastolic murmurs are not generated by high-pressure ventricular contractions. In adults, they typically represent either aortic regurgitation or mitral stenosis. Given that diastolic murmurs are of lower intensity compared with systolic ones, some clinicians use the following grading system for characterizing them: 1/4 – Barely audible; 2/4 – Faint; 3/4 – Easily heard; 4/4 – Loud.

Aortic Regurgitation (ie, Aortic Insufficiency)

- Aortic regurgitation is best heard along the left parasternal border, as this is the direction of the regurgitant flow.
- It becomes softer over the duration of the murmur (ie, decrescendo) (**Figure 6-13**).

AORTIC INSUFFICIENCY

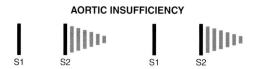

FIGURE 6-13 • **Timing of aortic insufficiency murmur during diastole.** (Illustration from *Practical Guide to Clinical Medicine: Cardiovascular Exam.* Available from: https://meded.ucsd.edu/clinicalmed/heart.html.)

- It can be accentuated by having the patient sit up, lean forward, and exhale while you listen.
- It occasionally accompanies AS, requiring a careful evaluation for regurgitation in patients with AS.
- It often causes the carotid upstrokes to feel extra full, as significant regurgitation increases ventricular preload, resulting in ejection of an augmented stroke volume.
- Pulse pressure (systolic blood pressure minus diastolic blood pressure) widens as chronic aortic insufficiency (AI) worsens.
- Symptoms and findings of AI are presented in **Figure 6-14**.

> **PEARL:** AI murmurs are of lower intensity and easy to miss. AI sounds loudest along the sternal border (the path of regurgitant flow). If AI is significant, carotid upstrokes are often prominent, related to larger stroke volumes.

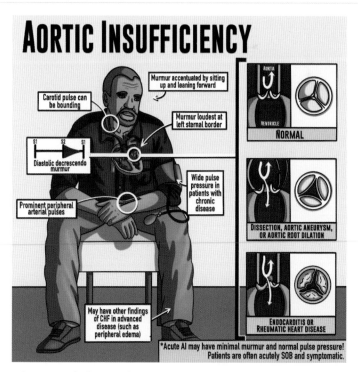

FIGURE 6-14 • **Symptoms, findings, and anatomic pathology associated with aortic insufficiency. CHF,** congestive heart failure; SOB, shortness of breath. (Reproduced with permission from Cathy Cichon, MD.)

Mitral Stenosis

- Mitral stenosis is heard best toward the axilla.
- It can be accentuated by having the patient role onto their left side while you listen with the bell of your stethoscope.
- It is associated with a soft, low-pitched sound preceding the murmur, called the opening snap. This is the noise caused by the calcified valve "snapping" open and is hard to detect.
- With more severe mitral stenosis, the pressure in the left atrium builds up and leads to earlier opening of the mitral valve, resulting in a shorter gap between S2 and the opening snap.
- Mitral stenosis usually occurs secondary to valvular damage associated with rheumatic fever, which is now uncommon.

Auscultation, an Ordered Approach

Try to focus on each sound individually and in a systematic fashion. Ask yourself the following:

- Do I hear S1?
- Do I hear S2?
- What are their relative intensities in each of the major valvular areas?
- Is S2 split physiologically? That is, does the interval between A2 and P2 get wider with inspiration?
- Are there extra sounds before S1 or after S2 (ie, an S4 or S3)?
- Is there a murmur during systole? Is there a murmur during diastole?
- If a murmur is present, how loud is it? What is its character? Where does it radiate? Are there any maneuvers that affect its intensity?

Remember that these sounds are created by mechanical events in the heart. As you listen, remind yourself what is happening to produce each of them (**Figure 6-15**). By linking auscultatory findings with physiology, you can build a case in your mind for a particular lesion.

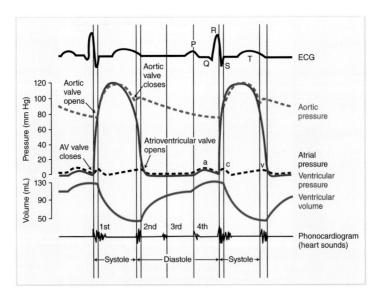

FIGURE 6-15 • **Connection between events in the cardiac cycle and auscultatory findings.** (Reproduced with permission from Kibble JD. *The Big Picture Physiology: Medical Course & Step 1 Review.* 2nd ed. New York: McGraw Hill; 2020.)

PEARL: Correlate your exam with findings from echocardiograms. This is a great way to learn, practice, and verify.

PEARL: Remember the mechanical cardiac events occurring during systole and diastole. This makes it easier to understand the origins of normal and abnormal sounds.

CAROTID ARTERY AUSCULTATION

- Auscultation over the carotid arteries has its greatest utility as part of the assessment of aortic stenosis.
- Place the diaphragm over each carotid and listen for the sound created by the radiating murmur. It occurs during systole, which you can identify by simultaneously palpating the radial artery.
- It can be helpful to ask the patient to hold their breath while you listen, so that you are not distracted by transmitted breath sounds.
- Auscultation can also be performed to assess for bruits, sounds created by turbulent flow associated with atherosclerosis. The presence of a bruit indicates an overall increased risk of atherosclerosis-related events (eg, heart attack and stroke) and might impact decision-making about how aggressively to address cardiovascular risk factors.
- Carotid artery auscultation has limited accuracy for identifying clinically important carotid artery stenosis in asymptomatic patients.

ASSESSMENT OF CENTRAL VENOUS PRESSURE

General Considerations

The internal jugular (IJ) vein is in straight-line communication with the right atrium. It can therefore function as a manometer, with distention indicating elevation of central venous pressure (CVP). This in turn is an important marker of intravascular volume status and related cardiac function and very useful in the diagnosis and assessment of heart failure. It can help differentiate cardiac causes of volume overload from other etiologies (eg, renal or liver disease).

Jugular venous distention can be challenging to assess. This is because the IJ lies deep in the skin and soft tissues and is under much lower pressure than the adjacent, pulsating carotid artery. It takes a sharp eye to identify the relatively weak, transmitted venous impulses. A few things to remember:

- Think anatomically: The right IJ runs between the 2 heads (sternal and clavicular) of the sternocleidomastoid muscle (SCM). The SCM can be identified by asking the patient to turn their head to the left and into your hand while you provide resistance to the movement. The 2 heads form the sides of a small triangle, with the clavicle making up the bottom edge. You cannot actually see the IJ. You are trying to identify impulses from the IJ transmitted to the overlying skin in this area (**Figure 6-16**).
- The external jugular (EJ) vein runs in an oblique direction across the SCM and, in contrast to the IJ, can usually be directly visualized. If the EJ is not readily apparent, have the patient look left and Valsalva.
- EJ distention is not always a reliable indicator of elevated CVP as valves, designed to prevent retrograde blood flow, can exist within this vessel. It also makes several turns prior to connecting with the central venous system and is thus not in a direct line with the right atrium.

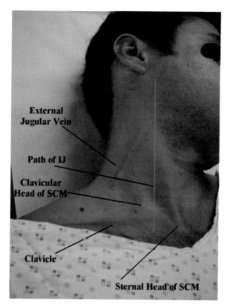

FIGURE 6-16 • Anatomic path of the internal jugular (IJ) vein. SCM, sternocleidomastoid muscle. (Photo from *Practical Guide to Clinical Medicine: Cardiovascular Exam*. Available from: https://meded.ucsd.edu/clinicalmed/heart.html.)

Technique

- Stand on the patient's right side and look at the IJ region while the patient's head is turned to the left.
  - The carotid artery is just medial to the IJ.
  - If you are unsure whether a pulsation is caused by the carotid or the IJ, palpate the patient's radial pulse and use this as a reference.
  - The carotid impulse coincides with the palpated radial artery pulsation. The venous impulse has multiple components, associated with ventricular and atrial events.
  - When these waves are transmitted to the skin, they create a series of flickers that are visible in the overlying skin. In contrast, the carotid causes a single outward pulsation.
  - The carotid is palpable while the IJ is not. The IJ can also be obliterated by applying pressure in the area where it emerges above the clavicle.
- Search along the entire course of the IJ for the top of the pressure wave.
  - If the patient's CVP is markedly elevated, you may not be able to identify the top of the wave unless they are repositioned, with their trunk elevated at 45 degrees or more (or else there will be no identifiable "top" of the column as the entire IJ will be engorged). Conversely, if the CVP is low, the patient's torso may need to be lowered before the IJ becomes visible just above the clavicle.
  - After you have found the top of the wave, you can assess the effect that sitting straight up and lying down can have on the height of the column.
  - Sitting should cause it to appear at a lower point in the neck, while lying has the opposite effect. Realize that these maneuvers do not change the actual value of the CVP. They simply alter the position of the top of the pulsation in relation to other structures in the neck and chest.
- Shine a light tangentially across the neck to accentuate the pulsations.

- Apply steady pressure to the right upper quadrant of the abdomen. This elicits hepatojugular reflux (HJR), which causes blood from the liver to fill out the IJ, making the transmitted pulsations more apparent (and will have no impact on visualized carotid pulsations). The optimal time to detect a change in the height of this column of blood is immediately after you apply hepatic pressure, so make sure to look at the neck when you apply pressure. When the CVP is truly elevated, the finding will persist after releasing pressure.

PEARL: Measuring CVP is an important tool for identifying heart failure and assessing volume status.

Measuring the Height of the CVP

Once you identify jugular venous distention, estimate how high in centimeters the top of the column is above the sternal-manubrial angle (ie, angle of Louis). This is the joint formed where the manubrium connects with the sternum (**Figure 6-17**).

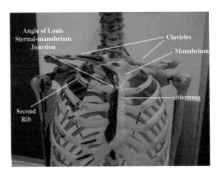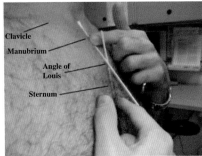

FIGURE 6-17 • **Identifying the sternal-manubrial joint (angle of Louis).** (Photos from *Practical Guide to Clinical Medicine: Cardiovascular Exam*. Available from: https://meded.ucsd.edu/clinicalmed/heart.html.)

- First identify the suprasternal notch, a concavity at the top of the manubrium.
- Then walk your fingers downward until you detect a subtle change in the angle of the bone, which is approximately 4 to 5 cm below the notch. This is roughly at the level of the second intercostal space.
- The vertical distance from the top of the pressure wave in the IJ to this angle is added to 5 cm, the rough vertical distance from the angle to the right atrium (**Figure 6-18**).
- The sum is an estimate of the CVP. The upper limits of normal is 7 to 9 cm when the patient is at approximately a 30-degree angle.

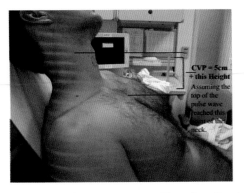

FIGURE 6-18 • **Determining the central venous pressure.** (Photo from *Practical Guide to Clinical Medicine: Cardiovascular Exam*. Available from: https://meded.ucsd.edu/clinicalmed/heart.html.)

Findings and Their Meaning: Elevated CVP

- Elevation in CVP reflects elevated right heart filling pressures and is most commonly due to left-sided heart failure.
- Isolated right-sided heart failure, pericardial disease, and other less common processes can also cause elevation in CVP.
- It is very helpful to be able to determine whether CVP is normal (making heart failure unlikely) or elevated.
- Clinicians also note changes in the height of CVP with the use of diuretics and other medications as a way of gauging the response of heart failure to treatments (ie, the height of the CVP goes down with effective treatment).

Heart failure (HF) is a clinical syndrome where cardiac dysfunction causes characteristic symptoms and findings as described in **Figure 6-19**. HF is broadly characterized based on ventricular function, including Heart Failure with Reduced Ejection Fraction (HFrEF) and Heart Failure with Preserved Ejection Fraction (HFpEF). The ejection fraction is typically determined by ultrasound.

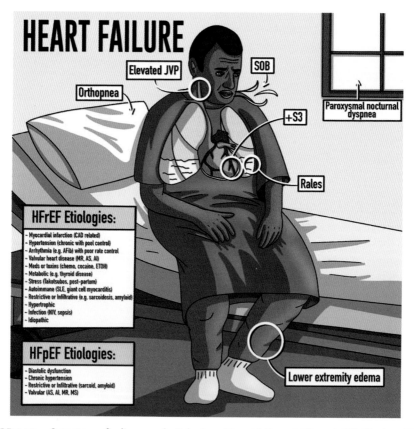

FIGURE 6-19 • Symptoms, findings, and etiologies of heart failure. A Fib, atrial fibrillation; AI, aortic insufficiency; JVP, jugular venous pressure; MR, mitral regurgitation; MS, mitral stenosis; SLE, systemic lupus erythematosus; SOB, shortness of breath. (Reproduced with permission from Cathy Cichon, MD.)

LOWER EXTREMITY EXAM

This area of the physical exam is included as part of a screening evaluation for asymptomatic disease in healthy or at-risk populations. It is also performed in the setting of specific presenting symptoms or findings (eg, leg pain, wound healing problems, shortness of breath, edema). The knee exam is covered in Chapter 14.

Arterial and Venous Anatomy

It is helpful to be familiar with the names of the main branches of the peripheral arterial system (**Figure 6-20**). Veins travel in parallel and often have the same names as arteries. Identifying named veins during the exam is not typically relevant.

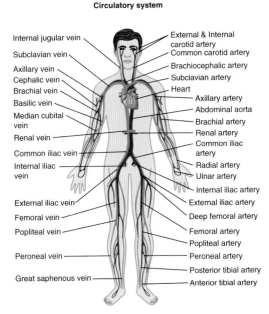

FIGURE 6-20 • **Vascular anatomy.** (Reproduced with permission from Hamm RL, ed. *Text and Atlas of Wound Diagnosis and Treatment.* 2nd ed. New York: McGraw Hill; 2019.)

Normal Function of Peripheral Vascular System

Normally functioning arteries carry blood to the peripheral tissues, meeting metabolic needs by delivering oxygen and other nutrients. Arterial pressure is generated by the heart and further regulated by the tone of the peripheral arterioles.

The venous and lymphatic systems provide the path for blood and interstitial fluid to return to the heart, removing carbon dioxide and other metabolic waste. The pressure generated in veins and lymphatics is low, and flow follows the pressure gradient from the periphery to the right atrium of the heart. Valves in the deep veins of the legs and lymphatics, as well as the pumping action of surrounding muscles, further enhances flow in the correct direction (**Figure 6-21**).

PEARL: Arterial disease (blood flow out to the periphery) causes problems with tissue perfusion (eg, ischemic pain, impaired wound healing). Venous disease (blood flow from periphery to the heart) most commonly causes pooling of blood and edema.

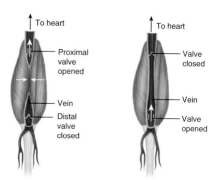

FIGURE 6-21 • **Venous valves and their function.** (Reproduced with permission from Hamm RL, ed. *Text and Atlas of Wound Diagnosis and Treatment.* 2nd ed. New York: McGraw Hill; 2019.)

The lymphatics (vessels and nodes) play an important role in the immune system, helping to fight off infection by removing pathogens, as well as identifying and destroying other abnormal cells and absorbing fat from the intestines. They transport protein-rich lymphatic fluid from the interstitial space to the heart. The lymphatic vessels are very thin and travel through lymph nodes en route to the heart. While the channels are not identifiable on exam, the nodes are often palpable and can provide some insights into the function and disorders affecting the lymph system.

THE PERIPHERAL VASCULAR EXAM

The Femoral Region

The patient should be lying down and the area to be examined thoughtfully exposed. All clothing should be removed, and the patient should be in a gown, with further exposure facilitated via the use of a sheet (**Figure 6-22**).

- Begin by simply looking at the area, which is on either side of the crease separating the leg from the groin region. Make note of any discrete swellings, which might represent adenopathy or a femoral hernia.
- Palpate the area, identifying the femoral pulse. It is typically easily palpable in the inguinal crease, located midway between the pubic bone and the anterior iliac crest. Use the tips of your second, third, and fourth fingers. If there is a lot of soft tissue, you will need to push firmly.
- Note if there is any inguinal/femoral adenopathy (lymph nodes that surround the femoral artery and vein). Lymph nodes up to 1 cm in size are typically nonpathologic.
- If you feel any lymph nodes, note if they are firm or soft, fixed in position or freely mobile, and painful or nontender.

PEARL: Palpating the large arteries (femoral, popliteal, dorsalis pedis, and posterior tibial) that perfuse the leg and foot can help identify the site(s) of obstruction to flow in the setting of arterial insufficiency.

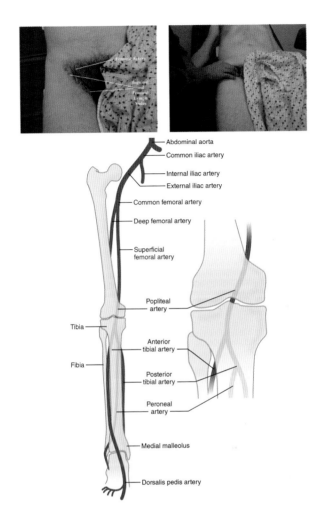

FIGURE 6-22 • **Examination of the femoral area and arterial anatomy.** (Photos [top] from *Practical Guide to Clinical Medicine: The Lower Extremities.* Available from: https://meded.ucsd.edu/clinicalmed/ extremities.html. Illustration [bottom] reproduced with permission from Tintinalli JE, Ma OJ, Yealy DM, et al, eds. *Tintinalli's Emergency Medicine: A Comprehensive Study Guide.* 9th ed. New York: McGraw Hill; 2020.)

Findings and Their Meaning: Femoral Area Abnormalities

- Palpable lymph nodes occur mostly commonly in the setting of infection, cancer, or selected autoimmune disorders.
  - In the setting of an infection (eg, cellulitis of the leg), the nodes can be acutely enlarged, tender, and warm.
  - In the setting of cancer (eg, melanoma of the distal leg), lymph nodes increase in size over time, are more firm and attached to each other and surrounding tissues.
  - Examination for distal cancer (eg, melanoma of leg, foot) as well as for systemic adenopathy (eg, as might occur with lymphoma) should also be performed.
  - Evidence for autoimmune disease should be explored during history taking and the rest of the exam, as these disorders can also cause adenopathy.

- A femoral hernia, if present, is visible on the anterior thigh, medial to the femoral artery, and may increase with Valsalva. These are much less common than inguinal hernias. See genital exam chapters (Chapters 9 and 11) for details.
- A nonpalpable or diminished pulse is suggestive of atherosclerotic disease in the femoral artery or more proximally.

The Popliteal Region

- Move down to the level of the knee. Ask the patient to slightly flex their lower leg.
- Place your hands around the knee and push the tips of your fingers into the popliteal fossa in an effort to feel the popliteal pulse (**Figure 6-23**). This artery is covered by a lot of tissue and can be difficult to identify, so you need to push pretty firmly.

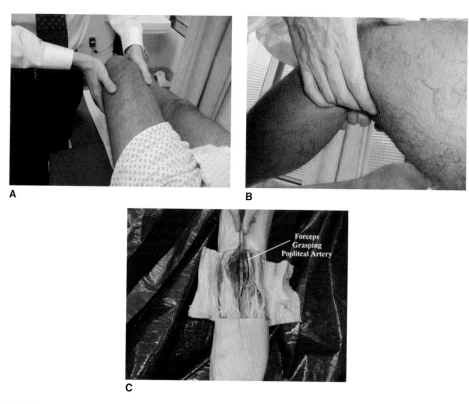

FIGURE 6-23 • **(A-C) Palpating popliteal artery.** (Photos from Practical *Guide to Clinical Medicine: The Lower Extremities.* Available from: https://meded.ucsd.edu/clinicalmed/extremities.html.)

Findings and Their Meaning: Popliteal Abnormalities

- Diminished pulses in the popliteal region can indicate atherosclerosis.
- Note whether the popliteal artery feels simply pulsatile (normal) or enlarged and aneurysmal (uncommon).

- Sometimes a fullness in the popliteal area can be from a Baker's cyst, which is a fluid collection that is typically asymptomatic (**Figure 6-24**). A Baker's cyst can become clinically relevant if it ruptures, causing acute lower leg swelling and raising concern about the possibility of a deep vein thrombosis (DVT).

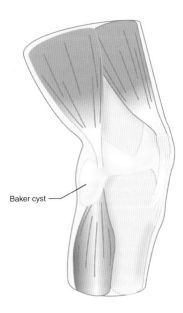

Baker cyst

FIGURE 6-24 • **Baker's cyst.** (Reproduced with permission from Simon RR, Sherman SC, Koenigsknecht SJ. *Emergency Orthopedics: The Extremities.* 5th ed. New York: McGraw-Hill; 2007.)

Observe and Inspect the Region Below the Knee

Turn your attention to the lower leg (ie, from the knee to the foot). Note the following:

- Skin color: Normal skin color should be consistent with the rest of the body.
- Note any obvious growths or skin changes.
- Check the bottom of the foot and between the toes: These are common places where infection can start, particularly in patients with diabetes who are predisposed as a result of sensory impairment, arterial insufficiency, or both.

Findings and Their Meaning: Observable Abnormalities

- A shiny, hairless appearance is sometimes seen with arterial insufficiency. Note any dilated or varicose superficial veins. Redness is associated with cellulitis, acute bacterial infection of the skin (**Figure 6-25**).
- Note any nail abnormalities including thickening, deformity, and slow growth. See Chapter 16, Dermatologic Exam, for additional information about nail pathology.

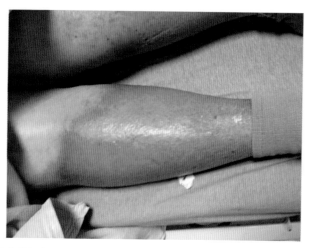

FIGURE 6-25 • **Cellulitis.** (From Knoop KJ, Stack LB, Storrow AB, Thurman RJ, eds. *The Atlas of Emergency Medicine.* 5th ed. New York, McGraw-Hill; 2021, Figure 12.2. Reproduced with permission from photo contributor: Robert Tubbs, MD.)

Assessing Temperature of the Skin

- Normal tissue is warm, although there is a range across patients.
- It is easiest to assess temperature using the back of your hand.
- Compare one side to the other, as well as distal and proximal.
- Arterial insufficiency can cause the skin to feel cool. This tends to be more pronounced distally (ie, toward the feet).
- Infection, on the other hand, causes increased flow and relative warmth.
- In cases where arterial insufficiency and infection occur simultaneously, impaired inflow of blood may generate less warmth (and also less redness) than might otherwise be expected.

Assessing for Edema

- In the normal state, hydrostatic (**Figure 6-26**) and oncotic (provided by proteins in the blood) forces favor retention of fluid within the vascular system.

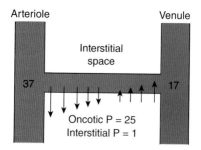

FIGURE 6-26 • **Pressure gradients across the interstitial space.** (Reproduced with permission from Elmoselhi A. *Cardiology: An Integrated Approach.* New York: McGraw Hill; 2018.)

- Normal pressures create a gradient (Figure 6-26) across the vascular system, which drives the blood in the correct direction (ie, heart → arteries → arterioles → capillaries → interstitial space → capillaries → venules → veins → back to the right atrium of the heart).

- The normally functioning vascular system allows:
  - Blood to reach the extremities through the arteries
  - Exchange of nutrients and waste products to occur between the capillaries and interstitial spaces
  - Return of the fluid through the venous and lymphatic systems

Normally, there is no edema (extravascular fluid) in the lower legs.
- The legs and feet should appear symmetric.
- The boney edges of the malleoli should appear sharp and distinct (**Figure 6-27**).
- The extensor tendons on the top of the foot should appear well defined.

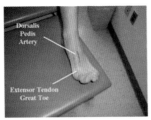
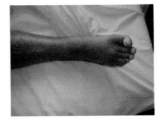
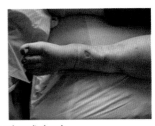

Normal	2+ edema (to above ankle)	4+ edema (to knee)	
1+	Minimal	Barely detectable impression	2 mm
2+	Mild	Slight indentation	4 mm
3+	Moderate	Deeper indentation	6 mm
4+	Severe	Very deep indentation	8 mm

*Tracking changes in weight is very useful when assessing and managing edema.

Average Marble
1 cm Diameter

FIGURE 6-27 • **Quantifying edema.** (Photos from *Practical Guide to Clinical Medicine: The Lower Extremities*. Available from: https://meded.ucsd.edu/clinicalmed/extremities.html.)

Findings and Their Meaning: Edema

- Edema occurs when the forces (hydrostatic and oncotic) which typically maintain fluid in blood vessels become altered such that there is accumulation within the interstitial space. The cause(s) (**Figure 6-28**) can typically be identified by history, exam, labs and imaging.
- Fluid tends to first "fill in" the spaces between the extensor tendons on the top of the foot, causing them to appear less defined. The edges of the malleoli will also become less distinct.
- If you are not sure whether fluid is present, push on the area for several seconds, release, and then gently rub your finger over that same spot, feeling for the presence of a "divot," referred to as pitting.
- As edema progresses, it tends to move up the leg (ie, from foot to ankle to calf to knee). Noting the proximal extent of the edema is one maker of severity. Systemic processes like heart failure typically cause symmetric edema.
- Inflammatory or other processes that increase capillary permeability can also contribute to edema.
- Chronic edema can lead to darkening of the skin of the lower extremity.

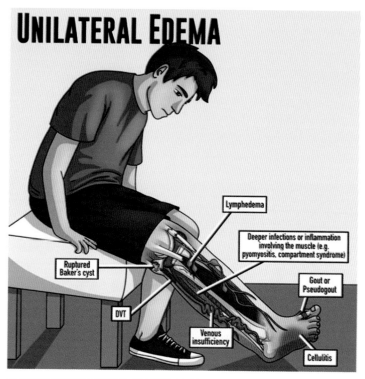

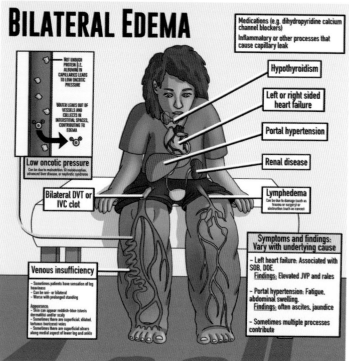

FIGURE 6-28 • Causes of unilateral versus bilateral edema. DVT, deep vein thrombosis; IVC, inferior vena cava. (Reproduced with permission from Cathy Cichon, MD.)

There is a subjective scale for rating edema, ranging from "trace at the ankles" to "4+ to the level of the knees." After examining many patients, you will develop a sense of what is a lot and what is not. Edema can also be quantified by estimating of the depth in millimeters of the "divot" left after applying steady pressure to the skin, best done over the tibial region. A comparison of the different ways of quantifying edema is shown in Figure 6-27.

You can consider edema and its etiologies based on whether it is unilateral or bilateral (Figure 6-28).

Lymphedema

This is a much less common cause of chronic leg swelling. It is related to impaired lymphatic drainage, which can occur secondary to an array of conditions including chronic infections, disrupted lymphatics, and obesity. It may also be idiopathic. There is wide range of severity. It feels somewhat doughy on palpation, with skin redundancy sometimes causing overlapping folds (**Figure 6-29**).

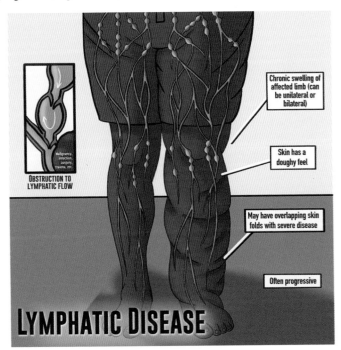

FIGURE 6-29 • **Lymphedema.** (Reproduced with permission from Cathy Cichon, MD.)

Capillary Refill

- Push on the tip of the great toe or the nail bed until blanching occurs.
- Then release and note how long it takes for the red color to return, a reflection of blood inflow to the distal aspect of the lower extremity. Normal is <2 to 3 seconds.

Findings and Their Meaning: Delayed Capillary Refill

- Capillary refill that takes longer than 2 to 3 seconds is abnormal and consistent with decreased perfusion (eg, from peripheral arterial disease).
- Refill may also be delayed in the setting of significant hypovolemia or hypotension, as decreased blood volume available for perfusion is shunted away from the extremities to feed more vital organs.

The Distal Pulses

- Pulses are assessed to identify the presence of arterial vascular disease. The less prominent the pulses, the greater is the chance that there is occlusive arterial disease.
- This is not a perfect correlation, however, as pulses may be palpable even when significant disease is present (eg, atherosclerosis may be affecting the smaller, microvascular system).
- A history of pain or cramps with activity is suggestive of arterial insufficiency and is important to ask about.
- The location of the blockage(s) will dictate the symptoms and findings. Aortoiliac disease, for example, will cause symptoms in the hips/buttocks and a loss of the femoral pulse, whereas disease affecting the more distal vessels will cause symptoms in the calves and feet.

The Dorsalis Pedis Artery

- Located just lateral to the extensor tendon of the big toe, the dorsalis pedis artery is identified by asking the patient to flex their toe while you provide resistance to this movement (**Figure 6-30**).
- Gently place the tips of your second, third, and fourth fingers adjacent to the tendon and feel the pulse.
- If you cannot identify it, try palpating more proximally (artery gets bigger as you move toward the heart) and/or more laterally.

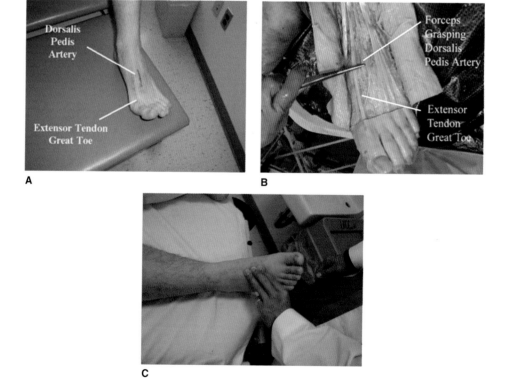

FIGURE 6-30 · (A-C) Palpating dorsalis pedis artery. (Photos from *Practical Guide to Clinical Medicine: The Lower Extremities.* Available from: https://meded.ucsd.edu/clinicalmed/extremities.html.)

- Common pitfalls include pushing too hard and/or mistaking your own pulse for that of the patient. Use your other hand to palpate the patient's radial artery or your own carotid simultaneously to help sort this out.

The Posterior Tibial Artery

- The posterior tibial artery is located just behind the medial malleolus (**Figure 6-31**).
- Palpate the area posterior to the medial malleolus, using the tips of your fingers.
- Pitfalls mentioned with the dorsalis pedis also apply here.
- If there is a lot of edema, you will have to push your way through the fluid-filled tissue to get down to the level of the artery.

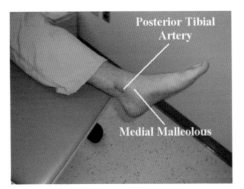
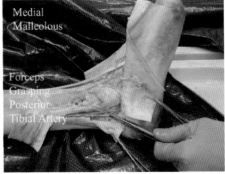

A   B

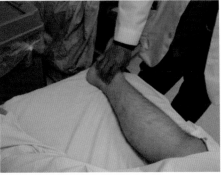

C

FIGURE 6-31 • **(A-C) Palpating posterior tibial artery.** (Photos from *Practical Guide to Clinical Medicine: The Lower Extremities*. Available from: https://meded.ucsd.edu/clinicalmed/extremities.html.)

- If you are unable to palpate a pulse, use Doppler (**Figure 6-32**) to identify the location of the artery. Mark the spot with a pen and then go back and again try to feel it with your fingers. In this way, you will be able to determine if the vessel was not palpable based on limited blood flow or if you are experiencing a problem with your technique.

Pulses are rated on a scale ranging from 0 (not palpable) to 2+ (normal). As with edema, this is subjective, and it will take you a while to develop a sense of relative values. In the event that the pulse is not palpable, the Doppler signal generated is also rated, ranging from 0 to 2+.

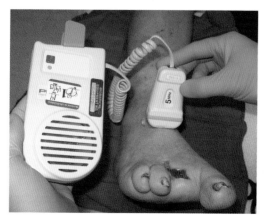

FIGURE 6-32 • Using Doppler to identify dorsalis pedis artery. Note loss of toes from prior amputations due to peripheral arterial disease. (Reproduced with permission from Hamm RL, ed. *Text and Atlas of Wound Diagnosis and Treatment*. 2nd ed. New York: McGraw Hill; 2019, Figure 4-17.)

Findings and Their Meaning: Diminished or Absent Pulses and Peripheral Arterial Disease

- As peripheral arterial disease (PAD) progresses, pulses often become harder to palpate, eventually becoming nonpalpable.
- The skin may become relatively pale as a result of underperfusion. Loss of hair can also occur.
- In severe cases, wounds may be slow to heal, ulcers can form, infections can occur, and it may even progress to gangrene (black discoloration, indicating tissue death).
- Symptoms and findings associated with PAD are described in **Figure 6-33**.

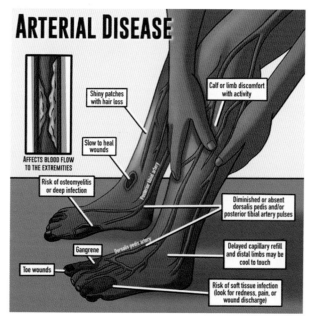

FIGURE 6-33 • Symptoms and findings of peripheral aterial disease. (Reproduced with permission from Cathy Cichon, MD.)

A comparison of venous, arterial, and lymphatic disease is presented in **Table 6-1**.

TABLE 6-1 • Diagnoses at a Glance: Comparison of Venous, Arterial, and Lymphatic Disease

Type of Vasculature Affected	Symptoms	Findings
Arterial disease • Affects blood flow to the extremities • Development is associated with atherosclerotic risk factors: smoking, hypertension, diabetes, hyperlipidemia, male > female, age > 50	• Ischemia results in progressive calf/limb discomfort with activity (claudication). As disease worsens, symptoms are provoked with less activity • Slow to heal wounds can develop. • Increased risk of infection in soft tissues • Persistent or deep ulcers, with risk of osteomyelitis • Acute ischemic symptoms can occur, often the result of embolic events (eg, atrial fibrillation)	• Distal extremity can feel cooler to touch • Diminished or absent distal pulses (dorsalis pedis and posterior tibial) • Delayed capillary refill • Sometimes shiny appearance of leg, hair loss • Wounds or ulcers can affect toes, feet, lateral > medial lower leg • With severe disease, higher risk for gangrene (dead, black tissue) • If there is coexistent diabetes (a common risk factor), there may be distal numbness (from neuropathy), predisposing to wounds at bottom of feet (cannot feel and hard to see) • Skin or bone infections can occur, causing redness, discharge, and sometimes sinus tracts that extend to level of bone **Distal toe ulcer in patient with peripheral arterial disease.** (Reproduced with permission from Hamm RL, ed. *Text and Atlas of Wound Diagnosis and Treatment.* 2nd ed. New York: McGraw Hill; 2019, Figure 4-14.)
Venous disease • A disorder affecting return of blood from the extremity • Associated with immobility, obesity, prior deep venous thrombosis (DVT), heart failure	• Leg swelling that worsens when in a dependent position (eg, prolonged sitting). Also worsened by immobility • Unilateral venous insufficiency results from local processes affecting that limb (eg, prior or acute DVT)	Edema • Sometimes brown/blue chronic discoloration from hemosiderin deposition • Sometimes ulcers develop, which tend to be superficial and along the medial aspect of the leg • If isolated venous disease, peripheral pulses normal • If related to elevated central venous pressure, should have elevated jugular venous pressure and rales (if left heart failure),

(Continued)

TABLE 6-1 • Diagnoses at a Glance: Comparison of Venous, Arterial, and Lymphatic Disease (Continued)		
Type of Vasculature Affected	Symptoms	Findings
	• Systemic problems like heart failure, advanced kidney disease or cirrhosis typically cause bilateral edema; often accompanied by generalized symptoms of shortness of breath and dyspnea on exertion (for heart failure) or ascites (for cirrhosis). • Sometimes patients experience a sensation of leg heaviness from edema • Chronic edema can lead to skin breakdown and ulcer formation.	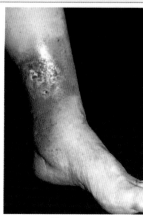 **Chronic venous insufficiency with ulcer.** (Reproduced with permission from Kang S, Amagai M, Bruckner AL, et al, eds. *Fitzpatrick's Dermatology.* 9th ed. New York: McGraw Hill; 2019, Figure 148-14.)
Lymphatic disease • Obstruction to or disruption in lymphatic flow at the level of the lymph vessels or nodes • Lymphatic disruption can occur from prior bacterial infections, filarial infections affecting the lymph system, trauma, surgery, cancer, obesity, or congenital causes • It can also be idiopathic	• Chronic swelling of affected limb (can be uni- or bilateral) • Worse when legs are dependent • Often progressive • Patients with lymphedema are predisposed to soft tissue infections, often from *Streptococcus*	• Edema that can be uni- or bilateral • Edema can have a doughy feel • Over time, skin thickens and loses normal texture • With severe disease, may develop overlapping skin folds • If primary process affects lymph nodes, they may be enlarged and/or feel abnormal (eg, firm, multiple) • If nodal abnormalities are related to malignancy, primary cancer might be apparent (eg, melanoma, lymphoma) 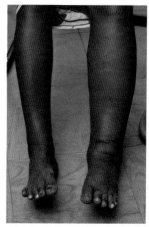 **Left leg lymphedema.** (From Knoop KJ, Stack LB, Storrow AB, Thurman RJ, eds. *The Atlas of Emergency Medicine.* 5th ed. New York: McGraw-Hill; 2021, Figure 21.24. Reproduced with permission from photo contributor: Lawrence B. Stack, MD.)

🖥 TELEHEALTH TIPS

- Historical information should be obtained in the usual fashion. Symptoms such as shortness of breath, chest pain, and edema can be further defined using your history-taking tools.
- Vital signs (VS) are always useful and easily obtained if the patient has an automatic measuring device at home. VS should include recent weights (if they have a scale) if they are being treated for heart failure.
- If someone is particularly short of breath, this might be evident by any of the following:
  - Limited ability to speak due to breathlessness
  - Obvious use of accessory muscles (those in the neck)
  - Pursed lip breathing
  - Rapid, shallow breathing, or general discomfort
- Those with chest pain of cardiovascular origin might appear uncomfortable, sweaty, or with their hand held to their chest. This type of appearance requires referral to an Emergency Department.
- The chest can be viewed if the patient takes off their shirt. Skin changes of herpes zoster or trauma (potential causes of chest pain) might be visualized. Cardiac problems do not typically cause surface abnormalities.
- If there is a focal area of pain on the chest wall, ask the patient to reveal the area on camera and point with one finger to identify where it hurts the most. They can be directed to push on or around it to see if this exacerbates the pain, as might occur with a process affecting the skin or soft tissues. It helps to have good lighting, with the source directed at the area of interest.
- Lower extremity edema can often be appreciated on camera. It helps to have the patient rest their feet on a chair to increase visibility and angle the camera to frame the lower extremities.
  - You can get a sense of fluid accumulation by noting whether you can see extensor tendons on the top of the foot and the distinct margins of the malleoli.
  - Look for sock indentation lines on the ankles and if present, ask the patient if they are new or worse.
  - If the patient applies gentle pressure to the edematous area with their fingertip and holds this pressure for 5 to 10 seconds, you may be able to see a small imprint (pitting) when the patient removes pressure.
  - The height of the edema (eg, ankle, mid-tibia) might also be noticeable.
- If there is edema, note if it is symmetric (as occurs with heart failure) versus asymmetric (raising the possibility of a DVT or other process restricted to one leg).
- Jugular venous pressure assessment may be feasible in some patients if they are able to recline to approximately 30 degrees and reveal the right side of their neck to the camera.
- The feet should be viewed with socks removed, looking for skin breaks, ulcers, redness, or other abnormalities.
- If the patient is able (or they have a caregiver who can hold the camera for them), have them display the bottom of their feet as well. For body parts that may be difficult to view by video even with the assistance of a caregiver, consider asking the patient to take a photograph and share it through a secure health portal.
- Those with concerning symptoms or findings usually need to be referred for in-person evaluation with appropriate urgency.

✓ SUMMARY OF SKILLS CHECKLIST

- ❏ Clean your hands
- ❏ Elevate head of table to approximately 30 degrees
- ❏ Gown and drape appropriately
- ❏ Inspect precordium
- ❏ Palpate left ventricle (LV); Identify PMI

Auscultation
- ❏ Identify S1 and S2 in 4 valvular areas with diaphragm
- ❏ Listen for physiologic splitting of S2
- ❏ Assess for murmurs
- ❏ Assess for extra heart sounds (S3, S4) with bell over LV

Carotid Artery
- ❏ Palpation (*special test)
- ❏ Auscultation (*special test)

Internal Jugular Vein
- ❏ Assess central venous pressure

Assess Femoral Area
- ❏ Palpate for nodes (*special test)
- ❏ Palpate femoral pulse (*special test)

Assess Knees (Nonmechanical Exam)
- ❏ Color, swelling
- ❏ Palpate popliteal artery pulse (*special test)

Assess Ankles and Feet
- ❏ Color, temperature, capillary refill
- ❏ Check for edema
- ❏ Observe for any skin breakdown or ulcerations (including between toes, soles)

Pulses
- ❏ Palpate dorsalis pedis artery
- ❏ Palpate posterior tibial artery
- ❏ Clean your hands

BIBLIOGRAPHY

Badgett R, Mulrow C, Lucey C. Can the clinical examination diagnoses left-sided heart failure in adults? In: Simel D, Drummond R, eds. *The Rational Clinical Exam*. New York: McGraw-Hill; 2009:183-193.

Bergan J, Schmid-Schönbein GW, Coleridge Smith PD, et al. Chronic venous disease. *N Engl J Med*. 2006;355:488-498.

Blankfield RP, Finkelhor RS, Alexander JJ, et al. Etiology and diagnosis of bilateral leg edema in primary care. *Am J Med*. 1998;105:192-197.

Boulton A, Kirsner RS, Vileikyte L. Neuropathic diabetic foot ulcers. *N Engl J Med*. 2004;351:48-55.

Carabello BA, Crawford FA. Valvular heart disease. *N Engl J Med*. 1997;337:32-41.

Chambers BR, Norris JW. Outcome in patients with asymptomatic neck bruits. *N Engl J Med*. 1986;315:860-865.

Choudhry N, Etchells E, Cescon D, Etchells E, Oddone E. Does this patient have aortic regurgitation? In: Simel D, Drummond R, eds. *The Rational Clinical Exam*. New York: McGraw-Hill; 2009:419-431.

Chun PKD, Dunn BE. Clinical clue of severe aortic stenosis: simultaneous palpation of the carotid and apical impulses. *Arch Intern Med*. 1982;142:2284-2288.

Conn DC, Cole JS. The cardiac apex impulse: clinical and angiographic correlation. *Ann Intern Med*. 1971;75:185-191.

Constant J. *Bedside Cardiology*. 4th ed. Boston: Little, Brown and Co.; 1993.

Cook D, Simel D. Does this patient have abnormal central venous pressure? In: Simel D, Drummond R, eds. *The Rational Clinical Exam*. New York: McGraw-Hill; 2009:125-135.

Creager M, Kaufman JA, Conte MS. Acute limb ischemia. *N Engl J Med*. 2012;366:2198-2206.

Ducas J, Magder S, McGregor M. Validity of the hepatojugular reflux as a clinical test of congestive heart failure. *Am J Cardiol*. 1983;52:1299-1303.

Etchells E, Bell C, Robb K., Cescon D, Etchells E, Oddone E. Does this patient have an abnormal systolic murmur? In: Simel D, Drummond R, eds. *The Rational Clinical Exam*. New York: McGraw-Hill; 2009:433-447.

Goldberg C. Digital DDx (cardiovascular symptoms or conditions). Accessed December 31, 2022. http://digitalddx.com/symptoms_list/5/.

Goldberg C. UCSD's practical guide to clinical medicine (exam of the lower extremities). Accessed December 31, 2022. https://meded.ucsd.edu/clinicalmed/extremities.html.

Goldberg C. UCSD's practical guide to clinical medicine (the cardiovascular exam). Accessed December 31, 2022. https://meded.ucsd.edu/clinicalmed/heart.html.

Hurst JW, Hopkins LC, Smith RB. Noises in the neck. *N Engl J Med*. 1980;302:362-363.

Lembro NJ, Dell'Italia LJ, Crawford MH, O'Rourke RA. Bedside diagnosis of systolic murmurs. *N Engl J Med*. 1988;318:1572-1578.

Lewinter M. Acute pericarditis. *N Engl J Med*. 2014;371:2410-2416.

Maisel A, Atwood E, Goldberger AL. Hepatojugular reflux: useful in the bedside diagnosis of tricuspid regurgitation. *Ann Intern Med*. 1984;101:781-782.

McGee S. *Evidence Based Physical Diagnosis* (Part 8: The heart). New York: Elsevier; 2022:295-415.

McMurray J. Systolic heart failure. *N Engl J Med*. 2010;362:228-238.

Nellen M, Gotsman MS, Vogelpoel L, Beck W, Schrire V. Effects of prompt squatting on the systolic murmur in idiopathic hypertrophic obstructive cardiomyopathy. *Br Med J*. 1967;3:140-143.

Nelzen O, Bergqvist D, Lindhagen A. Venous and non-venous ulcers: clinical history and appearance in a population study. *Br J Surg*. 1995;81:182-187.

Redfield M. Heart failure with preserved ejection fraction. *N Engl J Med*. 2016;375:1868-1877.

Roldan C, Shively BK, Crawford MH. Value of the cardiovascular physical examination for detecting valvular heart disease in asymptomatic subjects. *Am J Cardiol*. 1996;77:1327-1331.

Sauve J, Laupacis A, Ostbye T, et al. Does this patient have a clinically important carotid bruit? In: Simel D, Drummond R, eds. *The Rational Clinical Exam*. New York: McGraw-Hill; 2009:103-110.

Screening for asymptomatic carotid artery stenosis: US Preventive Services Task Force Recommendation Statement. *JAMA*. 2021;325(5):476-481.

Singer A, Tassiopoulos A, Kirsner RS. Evaluation and management of lower-extremity ulcers. *N Engl J Med*. 2017;377:1559-1567.

Sumpio BE. Foot ulcers. *N Engl J Med*. 2000;343:787-792.

Wang C, FitzGerald J, Schulzer M, Mak E, Ayas N. Does this dyspneic patient in the emergency department have congestive heart failure? In: Simel D, Drummond R, eds. *The Rational Clinical Exam*. New York: McGraw-Hill; 2009:195-213.

Wells P, Owen C, Doucette S, et al. Does this patient have a deep vein thrombosis? In: Simel D, Drummond R, eds. *The Rational Clinical Exam*. New York: McGraw-Hill; 2009:235-246.

White C. Intermittent claudication. *N Engl J Med*. 2007;356:1241-1250.

7

Pulmonary Exam

Rebecca E. Sell, MD

INTRODUCTION

The pulmonary exam is a standard part of the screening evaluation for routine patient visits and also performed when patients present with specific concerns or findings (eg, shortness of breath, wheezing) that may be caused by lung disease.

The 4 major components of the lung exam (inspection, palpation, percussion and auscultation) are also used to examine the heart and abdomen. Learning the appropriate techniques at this juncture will therefore enhance your ability to perform these other examinations as well. Vital signs, an important source of information, are discussed in Chapter 3.

For a discussion of gown management and tips for respectfully examining your patients, please see this section in Chapter 6, Cardiovascular exam.

REVIEW OF LUNG ANATOMY

Understanding the lung exam is enhanced by recognizing the relationship between surface structures, the skeleton, and the main lobes of the lung. Some surface markers (eg, nipples of the breast) do not always maintain their precise relationship to underlying structures, but they provide a rough guide to which lobe is beneath and can be quickly correlated with findings on chest x-ray or computed tomography (CT) scan. **Figure 7-1** demonstrates these relationships. Note how far up the back the lower lobes go and that the upper lobes are best heard anteriorly. The multicolored areas of the lung model identify precise anatomic segments of the various lobes, which cannot be appreciated on examination. Main lobes are outlined in black.

The lungs are contained within the visceral (lung side) and parietal (chest wall side) pleura, which normally contains a small amount of lubricating pleural fluid (**Figure 7-2**). In disease, excess fluid or air or a tumor can fill that space, contorting the normal anatomy of the lungs. This will be suggested by exam findings discussed in this chapter and confirmed with imaging studies.

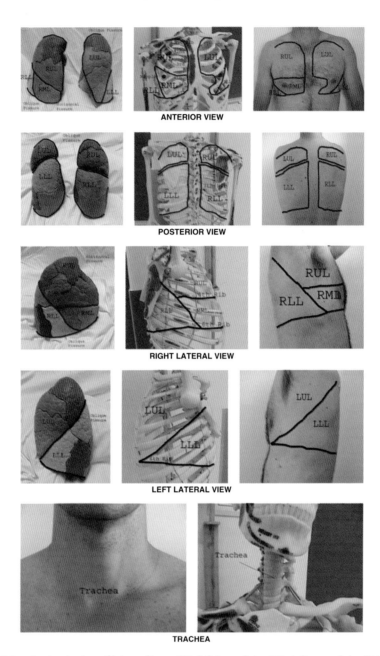

ANTERIOR VIEW

POSTERIOR VIEW

RIGHT LATERAL VIEW

LEFT LATERAL VIEW

TRACHEA

FIGURE 7-1 • Anatomic view of lobes of lung. LLL, left lower lobe; LUL, left upper lobe; RLL, right lower lobe; RML, right middle lobe; RUL, right upper lobe. (Photos from *Practical Guide to Clinical Medicine: Lung Exam*. Available from: https://meded.ucsd.edu/clinicalmed/lung.html.)

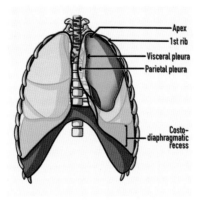

FIGURE 7-2 · **Lungs and pleural spaces.** (Reproduced with permission from Cathy Cichon, MD.)

NORMAL LUNG FUNCTION

The lung is responsible for bringing oxygen into the bloodstream and removing carbon dioxide. Breathing is driven by the respiratory center in the midbrain and pons and occurs without thought, responding to changes in oxygen and carbon dioxide levels in the blood. Key elements include the following:

- *Inhalation (inspiration)* is active and caused by shortening and downward contraction of the diaphragm and contraction of the intercostal muscles, drawing air into the lungs (**Figure 7-3**).
- *Exhalation (expiration)* is passive and occurs when the diaphragm and intercostal muscles relax, driving air out of the lungs (Figure 7-3).
- *Forced exhalation* is active and occurs with contraction of the abdominal and chest wall muscles inward and may be seen when coughing or in respiratory distress.
- The depth of inhalation and the rate increase in settings of physiologic stress (eg, exercise) to rid the body of excess carbon dioxide.

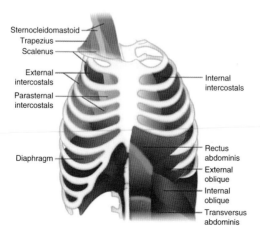

FIGURE 7-3 · **Inhalation and exhalation.** (Reproduced with permission from Michael A. Grippi et al. *Fishman's Pulmonary Diseases and Disorders*, 6e. New York: McGraw Hill LLC; 2023.)

- Air travels down through the branching airways (bronchi and bronchioles) until it reaches the alveolar sacs where gas exchange occurs (**Figure 7-4**).
- Pathology at any point along this path can affect lung function. The history and physical exam provide insight into the site(s) of pathology.

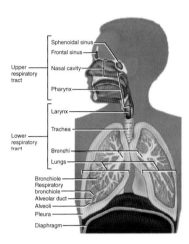

FIGURE 7-4 · **Airway anatomy.** (Reproduced with permission from Mescher AL. *Junqueira's Basic Histology Text and Atlas.* 16th ed. New York: McGraw Hill; 2021.)

OBSERVATION AND INSPECTION

It is remarkable how much information can be gained from watching a patient breathe. Pay close attention to:

- General comfort, position, and breathing pattern of the patient: Do they appear distressed, labored, or diaphoretic? Are they seated comfortably with regular deep breaths, or are they seated leaning forward with hands pressed down to straighten their posture and further optimize mechanics (eg, tripod position) (**Figure 7-5**)?

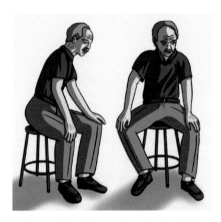

FIGURE 7-5 · **Patient with emphysema bending over in tripod position.** (Reproduced with permission from Cathy Cichon, MD.)

- Ability to speak: At times, respiratory rate may be too fast, or work of breathing so great, that patients may not be able to speak more than a few words before needing to take another breath. Inability to complete a full sentence (let alone several) is a bad sign!
- Use of accessory muscles of breathing (ie, muscles in the neck area including sternocleidomastoid and scalenes, which may be contracting and outlined with each effort): This suggests increased respiratory effort and distress (**Figure 7-6**).

> **PEARL:** Respiratory Rate x Tidal Volume (the amount of air moved with each breath) is referred to as the minute ventilation. Increases can result from lung disease, but also as the compensatory effort for a systemic metabolic acidosis, where the body tries to remove acid by breathing it out. Increased work of breathing is not always caused by the lungs!

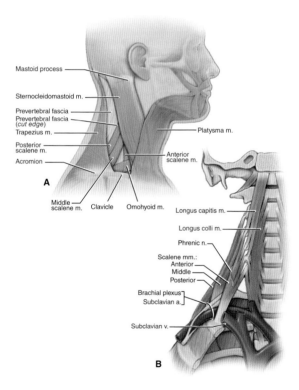

FIGURE 7-6 • **Neck muscles.** (Reproduced with permission from Morton DA, Foreman KB, Albertine KH. *The Big Picture: Gross Anatomy, Medical Course & Step 1 Review.* 2nd ed. New York: McGraw Hill; 2019.)

- Breathing through pursed lips (prolonged exhalation through lips making a whistle shape) (**Figure 7-7**): This may be seen in patients with severe obstructive lung disease who are often unable to fully exhale their entire breath, leading to air trapping and discomfort. By pursing their lips on exhalation, they may create additional positive airway pressure, stenting airways open and allowing more air to be exhaled.

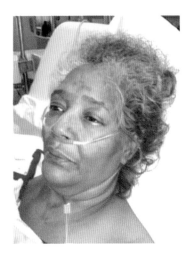

FIGURE 7-7 · **Breathing through pursed lips.** (Reproduced with permission from Tobin MJ, ed. *Principles and Practice of Mechanical Ventilation.* 3rd ed. New York: McGraw Hill; 2013, Figure 4-3 [upper right panel].)

- Mental status: Depressed mental status along with abnormal breathing is an emergency. This can be seen with either hypoxia or hypercapnia. The clinical history and an arterial blood gas can help you decide the cause. For example:
  - Worsening COVID-19 pneumonia and decreasing oxygen levels despite oxygen supplementation may lead to confusion and agitation on top of respiratory distress.
  - Anxiety followed by lethargy and decreased level of consciousness may occur with worsening hypercapnia from a chronic obstructive pulmonary disease (COPD) exacerbation or excess opiate use.

You can't always wait for the blood gas; sometimes these patients need emergent mechanical ventilation based on clinical appearance and inability to protect their airway

Any Audible Breathing Noises

- *Gurgling* may be heard when patients are unable to cough up secretions and mucus from the trachea and large airways.
- *Wheezing* on exhalation is the sound of air moving through narrowed airways and may occur in asthma exacerbations and may sometimes be heard without a stethoscope.
- *Stridor* is a high-pitched, harsh wheezing sound that may occur with upper airway and tracheal obstruction; this is an emergency and must be acted on right away!

Color of the Patient and Extremity Assessment

- Blue around the lips and nail beds suggests cyanosis (**Figure 7-8**). This can be acute, indicative of a severe problem with oxygen delivery. Or it can be chronic, as occurs in some patients with congenital heart disease or end-stage lung disease.
- Nicotine staining on thumb and first finger or around lips or mustache. This suggests significant smoking, which should be evident on history.

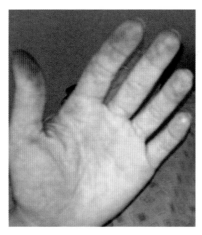

FIGURE 7-8 · Cyanosis of the finger-tips, also visible in nail beds. (Reproduced with permission from Loscalzo J, Fauci AS, Kasper DL, et al, eds. *Harrison's Principles of Internal Medicine*. 21st ed. New York: McGraw Hill; 2022, Figure 281-3C.)

● Clubbing: This is an uncommon flattening of the angle between the nail bed and adjacent skin occurring in some patients with congenital heart disease, malignancy, and some chronic lung diseases such as cystic fibrosis (**Figure 7-9**). The cause is debated and not simply due to hypoxia. Abnormal levels of platelet-derived growth factor and vascular endothelial growth factor are likely involved. A patient may have clubbing of fingers and/or toes, so be sure and look at the feet as well. The normal angle becomes obtuse, leading to a clubbed shape and loss of the "diamond-shaped window" you normally see when holding 2 fingers together nail-to-nail. New clubbing always merits an explanation.

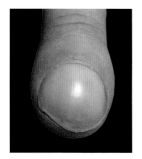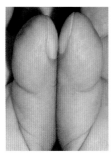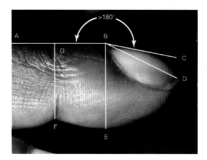

FIGURE 7-9 · Clubbing (left), loss of diamond window (middle), and obtuse angle (right). (From Usatine RP, Smith MA, Mayeaux EJ Jr, Chumley HS. *The Color Atlas and Synopsis of Family Medicine*. 3rd ed. New York: McGraw Hill; 2019, Figures 53-2 (left), 53-4 (middle), and 53-3 (right). Reproduced with permission from Richard P. Usatine, MD.)

● Edema: Swollen ankles (see Chapter 6, Cardiovascular Exam, for additional details) raises the possibility that the patient's shortness of breath could be related to pulmonary edema (**Figure 7-10**).

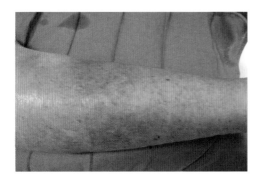

FIGURE 7-10 · **Lower extremity edema.** (Reproduced with permission from Hamm RL, ed. *Text and Atlas of Wound Diagnosis and Treatment.* 2nd ed. New York: McGraw Hill; 2019, Figure 3-52.)

Breathing Patterns

Normal and abnormal breathing patterns are described in **Table 7-1**.

TABLE 7-1 · Normal and Abnormal Breathing Patterns				
	Patients	Pattern	Etiology	Management
Normal breathing	Healthy patients at rest			
Cheyne-Stokes breathing	Heart failure, stroke, sedation, sleep or with acid-base disturbances		Delay between change in ventilation and sensation of new pCO2	Treat the underlying cause
Obstructive sleep apnea	Older adults (mostly men) who are more likely obese		Upper airway obstructs flow during sleep, leading to apnea and hypoxia and intermittent arousals	Continuous positive airway pressure (CPAP) machine while asleep, hypoglossal nerve stimulation, weight loss
Kussmaul's	A compensatory response to severe metabolic acidosis such as diabetic ketoacidosis		Increased minute ventilation (respiratory rate × tidal volume) to compensate for acidosis	Treat the underlying cause

Source: Table created by Rebecca E Sell, MD.

Special Testing: Noting the Direction of the Abdominal Wall Movement During Inspiration

Normal: The abdominal wall should move *out* and down on inspiration as the diaphragm contracts and pushes downward into the belly, drawing air in though the mouth and filling the lungs.

Abnormal: Abdominal wall moves *in* on inspiration. This occurs most commonly with diaphragmatic paralysis or severe diaphragmatic flattening (with air trapping from severe COPD) when the chest wall muscles take over as the primary inspiratory muscles. This pulls the abdominal wall contents up (cephalad) and in. This is referred to as paradoxical breathing. If you suspect this, place your hand on the patient's abdomen as they breathe, which should accentuate its movement.

Shape of Chest and Spine

The shape of the chest and spine can provide important information about pulmonary disease and function. The normal thorax has a shape that is optimized for breathing, allowing the diaphragm to shorten and chest to expand during inspiration (**Figure 7-11**). Assessing the shape of the chest is done by looking from the front, back, and sides.

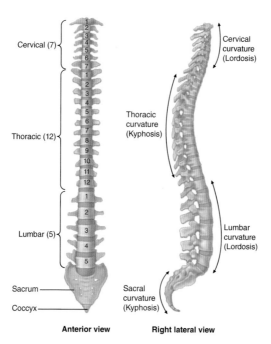

FIGURE 7-11 · **The shape of the spine.** (Reproduced with permission from Gauthier Cornuelle A, Gronefeld DH. *Radiographic Anatomy Positioning*. New York: McGraw-Hill; 1998.)

Findings and Their Meaning: Abnormal Shape of the Chest

Abnormalities in chest shape may be congenital, arise from trauma or surgery, or result from disorders or other degenerative process. Noting these findings will give insight into a patient's symptoms and underlying disease.

A few variants include the following:

• Pectus excavatum: This deformity of the anterior chest—inward and posterior displacement of the lower portion of the sternum—is congenital and more common in men (**Figure 7-12**). Its severity is measured by the Pectus Severity Index, which describes the ratio of the lateral diameter of the chest transverse (TR) to the sternum-to-spine distance Anterior-Posterior (AP) at the point of maximal depression.
• Barrell chest: Increased diameter of the chest wall from anterior to posterior, seen with hyperinflated lungs from COPD (Figure 7-12).

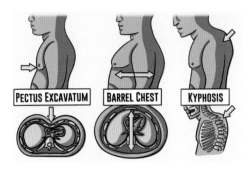

FIGURE 7-12 · **Pectus excavatum with inward displacement of the sternum; barrel chest with a large anterior-posterior diameter; and kyphosis with excessive thoracic curvature.** (Reproduced with permission from Cathy Cichon, MD.)

● Kyphosis: Abnormal excessive curvature of the thoracic spine often seen in older adults that effectively decreases total lung volume (Figure 7-12). It causes decreased vital capacity (the ability to take a deep breath) and reduced exercise tolerance.

PALPATION

Palpation is done when a patient has specific pulmonary complaints but is not necessary when a patient is asymptomatic.

Special Testing: Investigating Areas That Are Painful or Abnormal in Appearance

● If there is pain at a site, inspect for a rash or bruising, as the presence of vesicles could suggesting Zoster. Be sure to wear gloves when exploring a rash or exposed wound!
● If there is pain at a site and no superficial skin changes, it is important to carefully palpate the area, looking for a mass or cyst. If there is a discrete enlarged or inflamed area (suggestive of an abscess) or mass (suggestive of tumor), palpate carefully to determine size and character (eg, firm, fluctuant).
● Does the pain localize to a specific location like bone or muscle?

Special Testing: Chest Excursion

With complaints of shortness of breath, it is helpful to determine if both right and left lung are ventilating equally.

● After warming your hands, place them flat of the mid-third of the back (below the scapula) with a thumb on either side of the spinous process (**Figure 7-13**).
● When the patient takes a deep breath, your hands should lift symmetrically outward and your thumbs slightly separate.

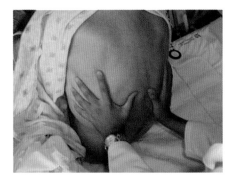

FIGURE 7-13 · **Testing pulmonary excursion.** (Photo from *Practical Guide to Clinical Medicine: Lung Exam*. Available from: https://meded.ucsd.edu/ clinicalmed/lung.html.)

- Processes that lead to asymmetric lung expansion (as when something fills the pleural space like fluid or air, or if a lung has been removed) will lead to the hand on that side moving less. This does not occur with small or subtle changes.
- Decreased excursion overall, where the hands move minimally when the patient inhales, may occur with hyperexpanded lungs like in COPD.

Special Testing: Tactile Fremitus

Lungs transmit sound as vibratory waves through the chest to the back, and this is known as fremitus.

- Fremitus can be detected by placing the ulnar aspect of each hand firmly on each side of the posterior chest wall between the rib spaces and having the patient say "Ninety-nine." This is repeated until the entire posterior chest is examined (**Figure 7-14**).

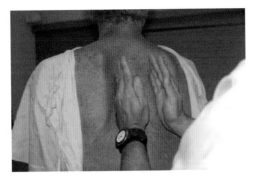

FIGURE 7-14 · **Testing for tactile fremitus.** (Photo from *Practical Guide to Clinical Medicine: Lung Exam.* Available from: https://meded.ucsd.edu/clinicalmed/lung.html.)

- Increased fremitus is heard when sound passes through consolidated lung (sound travels quicker through solids) and vibratory sensation is stronger. This may occur if there is a large pneumonia or tumor.
- Fremitus is decreased when there is a large pleural effusion.

PEARL: Fremitus is a subtle finding and most helpful to detect asymmetry (ie, increased fremitus on one side suggesting underlying pneumonia) rather than relative increase or decrease from normal (**Figure 7-15**).

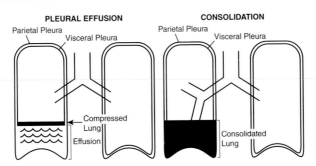

FIGURE 7-15 · **Fremitus is decreased with a pleural effusion and increased with a consolidated lung.** (Illustrations from Practical Guide to Clinical Medicine: Lung Exam. Available from: https://meded.ucsd.edu/clinicalmed/lung.html.)

PERCUSSION

This technique, similar to drumming, makes use of the fact that striking a surface covering an air-filled structure (eg, normal air-filled lung) will produce a resonant note. Percussing over areas of abnormal lung or the pleural space may alter the tone that is generated.

Percussion Technique

- If percussing with your right hand, stand to the left side of the patient's back.
- Ask the patient to cross their hands to opposite shoulders and pull forward, pulling apart the scapulae and opening up the back.
- Place the last 2 phalanges of your left middle finger firmly against the patient's back between the ribs. This will be the target for your percussing hand. Try to keep the rest of your hand off the patient to avoid dampening the sound (**Figure 7-16**).
- Allow the right (percussing) hand to swing freely from the wrist, hammering the soft part of the tip of the right middle finger against the distal interphalangeal joint (ie, the last joint) of your left middle finger. The impact should be crisp, so it helps to have short fingernails to avoid hurting yourself.

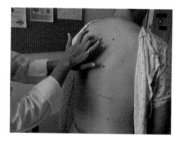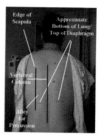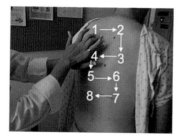

FIGURE 7-16 · Percussing the lung fields. (Photos from *Practical Guide to Clinical Medicine: Lung Exam.* Available from: https://meded.ucsd.edu/clinicalmed/lung.html.)

- 2 to 3 taps at each spot should be enough, noting the resonance of the sound. Then move your hand down a few interspaces and repeat. In general, percussion in about 5 locations should cover one of the posterior lung fields.
- Move your hands across to the opposite posterior lung to compare and contrast the sounds and work your way down the lung fields back and forth.
- With normal lungs, you will note that when you leave the thorax, percussion becomes duller. It is not particularly important to identify the exact location of the diaphragm, although if you are able to note a difference in level between maximum inspiration and expiration, all the better.

Special Testing: Identifying Paralysis of the Diaphragm

- Diaphragmatic weakness can occur with disorders of the right and/or left phrenic nerve (branch of the vagus that innervates the diaphragm) or with disorders that affect the muscle or neuromuscular junction (eg, amyotrophic lateral sclerosis).
- When the diaphragm is weak or paralyzed, it will not contract and descend normally, which causes shortness of breath.

- This shortness of breath is worse when lying flat (no help from gravity and abdominal contents pushing up into chest) or in a swimming pool (where the weight of the water makes it harder for the compensating chest wall muscles to expand the lung).
- To detect this on exam:
  - Ask the patient to exhale completely and identify the level of the diaphragm (bottom of lung) using percussion.
  - Then ask the patient to take a deep breath, hold it, and percuss again, noting if the diaphragm has descended. If the diaphragm is not working normally, the amount of change will be small or not appreciable.

Findings and Their Meaning: Abnormalities on Percussion

Percussion over normal lungs produces a resonant, drum-like sound.

Diminished resonance occurs if fluid accumulates in the pleural space (effusion) or within the lung (consolidation) or if the diaphragm is paralyzed and does not descend to normal levels. It is most notable when it is asymmetric.

- Effusions and infiltrates can be more easily understood using a sponge to represent the lung. In this model, an infiltrate is depicted by the blue coloration that has invaded the sponge itself (**Figure 7-17**, sponge on left). An effusion is depicted by the blue fluid upon which the lung is floating (sponge on right).

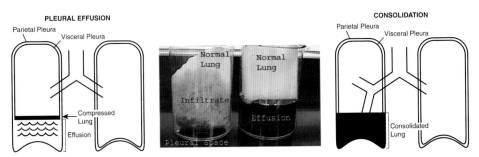

FIGURE 7-17 · **Effusion versus infiltrate.** (Photo and illustrations from *Practical Guide to Clinical Medicine: Lung Exam*. Available from: https://meded.ucsd.edu/clinicalmed/lung.html.)

Increased resonance occurs if there is extra air in the chest (**Figure 7-18**). As with diminished resonance, it is most notable when asymmetric.
- Chronic hyperinflation and air trapping from COPD (Figure 7-18)
- Acute air trapping in the pleural space such as from a pneumothorax

Hot tip: You can practice percussion on yourself! Try finding your own stomach bubble, which should be around the left costal margin. Note that due to the location of the heart, tapping over your left chest will produce a different sound than when performed over your right. Percuss your walls (if they are sheet rock) and try to locate the studs. Tap on containers filled with various amounts of water. This not only helps you develop a sense of the different tones that may be produced but also allows you to practice the technique.

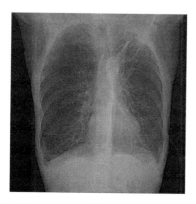
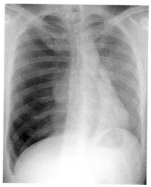

FIGURE 7-18 • **Hyperexpanded lung with air trapping in chronic obstructive pulmonary disease on the left and right-sided pneumothorax in image on right.** (Left photo: Reproduced with permission from Tintinalli JE, Ma OJ, Yealy DM, et al, eds. *Tintinalli's Emergency Medicine: A Comprehensive Study Guide.* 9th ed. New York: McGraw Hill; 2020, Figure 70-1. Right photo: Reproduced with permission from McKean SC, Ross JJ, Dressler DD, Scheurer DB, eds. *Principles and Practice of Hospital Medicine.* 2nd ed. New York: McGraw Hill; 2017, Figure 114-7.)

AUSCULTATION

Prior to listening over any one area of the chest, remind yourself which lobe of the lung is heard best in that region. This can be quite helpful in trying to pin down the location of pathologic processes that may be restricted by anatomic boundaries (eg, typical lobar pneumonia). Many disease processes (eg, pulmonary edema, bronchoconstriction) are diffuse, producing abnormal findings in multiple fields. Remember:

- Lower lobes occupy the majority of the posterior fields
- Right middle lobe heard in right axilla
- Lingula in left axilla
- Upper lobes in the anterior chest and at the top one-quarter of the posterior fields

Technique (**Figure 7-19**):

- Put on your stethoscope so that the earpieces are directed away from you and engage the diaphragm (for those stethoscopes with rotating heads); apply firm pressure for tunable scopes.

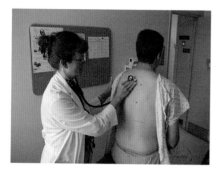
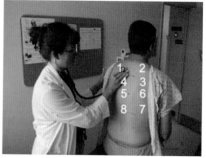

FIGURE 7-19 • **Auscultating the lung fields.** (Photos from *Practical Guide to Clinical Medicine: Lung Exam.* Available from: https://meded.ucsd.edu/clinicalmed/lung.html.)

- Stand to the patient's side; consider warming up the stethoscope head by rubbing it against the gown. Begin with the upper aspect of the posterior lung fields. Listen over one spot and then move the stethoscope to the same position on the opposite side and repeat. This again makes use of one lung as a source of comparison for the other.
- The entire posterior chest can be covered by listening in roughly 4 to 6 places on each side. If you hear something abnormal, you will need to listen in more places to fully characterize.
- The lingula and right middle lobes can be examined while you are standing behind the patient. This can be appreciated by listening to 1 or 2 spots over each area.
- Then, move around to the front and listen to the anterior fields in the same fashion. This is generally done while the patient is still sitting upright and listening in 1 to 2 spots on each side.
- Finally, listen over the trachea. This produces a different sound than when listening over the rest of the lung, as the trachea is large and proximal to the mouth, generating an unfiltered sound.

Additional Tips and Tricks

- Often when you ask a patient to "take a breath," they will inhale and hold it. Make sure you ask them to breathe in *and* out.
- Do not make your patient hyperventilate! Ask them to take slow deep breaths through an open mouth; this provides a large enough volume of air to detect more subtle abnormalities. Sometimes you might need to give them a break and take a pause between deep breaths.
- Asking a patient to cough a few times may clear airway secretions and open up small atelectatic (ie, collapsed) airways.
- If the patient is unable to sit up (eg, in cases of neuromuscular weakness, critical illness), auscultation can be performed while the patient is lying on their side. Do not be afraid to ask for help in positioning your patient. If this cannot be accomplished, a basic exam of anterior and lateral lung fields is still possible as the patient remains supine.

Findings and Their Meaning: Breath Sounds

- Vesicular breath sounds: This is the soft inspiratory sound as air rushes into the lungs in healthy individuals with normal tidal breathing and minimal sound on exhalation. This is normal.
- Wheezing: This is a high-pitched whistling type of noise usually produced on exhalation (rarely on inspiration) when air is forced through airways narrowed by bronchoconstriction, secretions, and/or associated mucosal edema.
  - Most common with a diffuse process affecting all lobes of the lung like asthma or COPD and can be heard in all lung fields.
  - When airway narrowing is severe and diffuse, the expiratory phase of respiration gets longer (relative to inspiration). Clinicians refer to this as a decreased inspiration-to-expiration ratio.
  - Wheezing can be subtle and is more obvious when exhaling at a fast rate. Ask the patient to take a breath and blow out hard and fast like they are blowing out a match or candle (with pursed lips), and you may hear expiratory wheezing.

PEARL: Focal wheezing (heard only in one location) suggests a local airway narrowing in a single anatomic airway like a foreign body obstruction or endobronchial tumor.

- Stridor: This is an audible and harsh inspiratory wheeze that signifies obstruction at the level of the vocal cords/trachea.
  - This can be a medical emergency if there is an obstructing lesion at that level of the trachea.
  - It can occur with vocal cord and laryngeal edema after a breathing tube is removed and may mean a patient needs urgent reintubation.
  - Stridor can also be heard with paradoxical vocal cord motion where the vocal cords come together on inspiration instead of opening. This can be a neurologic or functional disorder.
- Rales (ie, crackles): These soft scratchy sounds occur with processes that cause fluid to accumulate within the alveolar and interstitial spaces. It is similar to the sound produced when rubbing strands of hair together close to the ear.
  - Pulmonary edema is the most common cause, at least in the older adult population, and results in symmetric crackles. This tends to occur first in the most dependent portions of the lower lobes and extend from the bases toward the apices as more pulmonary edema accumulates.
  - Pneumonia, on the other hand, can result in discrete areas of alveolar filling and, therefore, produce crackles restricted to a specific region of the lung.
- Dry crackles: This sound is like that of Velcro pulling apart. It is heard most commonly with pulmonary fibrosis, a disease seen in older adults with progressive shortness of breath, and tends to be at the lung bases.
- Rhonchi: Secretions that roll around in larger airways, as might occur with bronchitis or other mucus-creating process, can produce a gurgling-type noise, similar to the sound produced when you suck the last bits of a milkshake through a straw.
- Tubular or bronchial breath sounds: Large airway noises (like those heard normally over the trachea) transmit through consolidated lung, as occurs with pneumonia. It is very similar to the sound of breathing through a snorkel.
  - Furthermore, if you direct the patient to say the letter "E," it is detected during auscultation over the involved lobe as a nasal-sounding "A." These "E" to "A" changes are referred to as egophony.
  - The first time you detect it, you will think that the patient is actually saying "A." Have them repeat it several times to assure yourself that they are really following your directions! This is an uncommon finding and only assessed if auscultation suggests consolidation.
- Very little noise: Auscultation of patients with severe, stable emphysema will produce very little sound. These patients suffer from significant lung destruction and air trapping, resulting in their breathing at small tidal volumes that generate almost no noise. Wheezing occurs when there is a superimposed acute inflammatory process (see above).

Findings and Their Meaning: Painting the Best Clinical Picture

Many of the above techniques are complimentary:

- Dullness detected on percussion, for example, may represent either lung consolidation or a pleural effusion.
- Auscultation over the same region should help to distinguish between these possibilities, as consolidation generates bronchial breath sounds, whereas an effusion is associated with a relative absence of sound.

- Similarly, fremitus will be increased over consolidation and decreased over an effusion. As such, it may be necessary to repeat certain aspects of the exam, using one finding to confirm the significance of another.
- Few findings are pathognomonic. They have their greatest meaning when used together to paint the most informative picture.

Examples of how these findings might be put together to paint the most accurate picture are described in **Table 7-2** and **Figure 7-20**.

TABLE 7-2 · Lung Exam Findings Suggestive of Effusion, Consolidation, or Pneumothorax				
	Auscultation (Breath Sounds)	Percussion	Fremitus	Egophony
Effusion	↓ or absent	Dull	↓	No
Consolidation	Bronchial	Dull	↓	Present
Pneumothorax	↓ or absent	Hyperresonant	Not applicable	No

Source: Table created by Rebecca E Sell, MD.

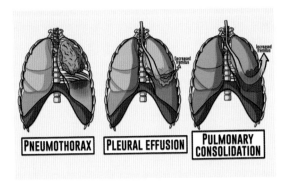

FIGURE 7-20 · **Pneumothorax, pleural effusion, and consolidated lung.** (Reproduced with permission from Cathy Cichon, MD.)

THE DYNAMIC LUNG EVALUATION

It is common for patients to only have symptoms when they are exerting or exercising, and they may have a normal exam seated at rest. In such cases, consider observed ambulation (with the use of a pulse oximeter) as a dynamic extension of the cardiac and pulmonary examinations.

- Quantifying a patient's exercise tolerance in terms of *distance* and/or *time* walked can provide objective information critical to the assessment of activity-induced symptoms.
- It may also help unmask illness that would be inapparent unless the patient was asked to perform a task that challenged their impaired reserves.
- Pay attention to the rate at which the patient walks, duration of activity, distance covered, development of dyspnea, changes in heart rate and oxygen saturation, ability to talk during exercise, and anything else that the patient identifies as limiting their activity.
- You can use this objective information to review changes over time at subsequent visits.

PEARL: Clinicians use a 6-minute walk test (6MWT) to examine functional capacity in patients with heart and lung disease. In addition to distance, baseline and 6-minute oxygen saturation, heart rate, and Borg dyspnea scale score are recorded.

TELEHEALTH TIPS

Investigating pulmonary concerns can be done in a telehealth visit.

- Historical information can be obtained in the usual fashion. Relatively common symptoms such as shortness of breath, cough, wheezing, and functional limitations can be further shaped by use of your history-taking tools.
- If someone is particularly short of breath, this might be evident during your discussion by any of the following:
  - Limited ability to speak due to breathlessness
  - Obvious use of accessory muscles (those in the neck)
  - Pursed lip breathing
  - Rapid, shallowing breathing or general comfort
- Consider asking the patient to walk across the room and come back as a limited way of assessing exercise tolerance.
- Occasionally, you may hear wheezing. To accentuate the wheeze, ask the patient to forcibly exhale while you listen. It helps if the environments on both patient and provider side are quiet.
- You might also get a sense of the frequency and/or severity of coughing by noting if it interferes with the interview. The quality of the cough (dry or wet sounding) might also be apparent.
- Lower extremity edema might be appreciated on camera. It helps to have the patient rest their feet on a chair to increase visibility and to angle the camera to frame the lower extremities. A few key areas include the following:
  - You can get a sense of fluid accumulation by noting whether you can see extensor tendons on the top of the foot and the distinct margins of the malleoli.
  - Look for sock indentation lines on the ankles and ask the patient if they are new or worse.
  - If the patient applies gentle pressure to the edematous area with their fingertip and holds this pressure for 5 to 10 seconds, you may be able to see a small imprint (pitting) when the patient removes pressure.
  - The height of the edema (eg, ankle, mid-tibia) might also be noticeable, as well as whether it is uni- or bilateral.
  - In patients with volume overload states, weight should be considered a vital sign.
- If there is a focal area of pain on the chest wall, you can ask the patient to reveal the area on camera and point with one finger to identify where it hurts the most. They can be directed to push on or around it to see if that exacerbates the pain, as might occur with a process affecting the skin or soft tissues. Skin changes of herpes zoster or trauma (potential causes of chest pain) might be visualized. It helps to have good lighting, with the source directed at the area of interest.
- Those with concerning symptoms or findings usually need to be referred for in-person evaluation with appropriate urgency.

SUMMARY OF SKILLS CHECKLIST

❑ Clean your hands
❑ Gown and drape appropriately
❑ Examine hands, fingers, and nails and lower legs (edema)

Observe and Inspect Chest

❑ General observation: note use of accessory muscles, general respiratory effort, ability to speak, audible noises, breathing pattern
❑ Shape of chest, spine

Palpation (*Special Test)
❏ Assess chest excursion (*if concern for asymmetric ventilation)
❏ Assess for fremitus (*if concern for effusion or consolidation)

Percussion
❏ Percuss posterior lung fields, top to bottom and comparing side to side
❏ Identify amount of diaphragmatic descent with inhalation (*special test: if concern for diaphragmatic paralysis)
❏ Percuss right anterolateral chest (middle lobe) and anterior lobes (bilateral)

Auscultation
❏ Listen with diaphragm to posterior lung fields, top to bottom and comparing side to side
❏ Listen to right middle lobe and then the lingula areas
❏ Listen to anterior lung fields
❏ Listen over trachea
❏ Assess for egophony (*special test: if concern for effusion or consolidation)
❏ Clean your hands

*Special test: Not done on routine exam; reserved for specific clinical situations.

BIBLIOGRAPHY

Acres JC, Kryger MH. Clinical significance of pulmonary function tests: upper airway obstruction. *Chest.* 1981;80:207-211.

Al-Qadi M, Artenstein AW, Braman SS. The "forgotten zone": acquired disorders of the trachea in adults. *Respir Med.* 2013;107(9):1301-1313.

Andrews JL, Badger TL. Lung sounds through the ages: from Hippocrates to Laennec to Osler. *JAMA.* 1979; 241: 2625-30.

Badgett RG, Tanaka DJ, Hunt DK, et al. Can moderate chronic obstructive pulmonary disease be diagnosed by historical and physical findings alone? *Am J Med.* 1993;94:188-196.

Bohadana A, Izbicki G, Kraman SS. Fundamentals of lung auscultation. *N Engl J Med.* 2014;370:744-751.

Enright P. The six-minute walk test. *Resp Care.* 2003;48(8):783-785.

Feller-Kopman D, Light R. Pleural disease. *N Engl J Med.* 2018;378:740-751.

Forgacs P. The functional basis of pulmonary sounds. *Chest.* 1978;73:399-405.

Forgacs P. Lung sounds. *Br J Dis Chest.* 1969;63:1-12.

Goldberg C. Digital DDx: pulmonary symptoms or conditions. Accessed January 1, 2023. http://digitalddx.com/symptoms_list/4/.

Goldberg C. UCSD's practical guide to clinical medicine (lung exam). Accessed January 1, 2023. https://meded.ucsd.edu/clinicalmed/lung.html.

Heckerling PS, Tape TG, Wigton RS, et al. Clinical prediction rule for pulmonary infiltrates. *Ann Intern Med.* 1990;113:664-670.

Holleman DR, Simel DL. Does the clinical examination predict airflow limitation? In: Simel D, Drummond R, eds. *The Rational Clinical Exam.* New York: McGraw-Hill; 2009:149-162.

King DK, Thompson T, Johnson DC. Wheezing on maximal forced exhalation in the diagnosis of atypical asthma: Lack of sensitivity and specificity. *Ann Intern Med.* 1989;110:451-455.

Light D. Pleural effusion. *N Engl J Med.* 2002;346(25):1971-1977.

Loudon R, Murphy RLH. Lung sounds. *Am Rev Respir Dis.* 1984;130:663-673.

Mannino DM, Etzel RA, Flanders D. Do the medical history and physical examination predict low lung function? *Arch Intern Med.* 1993;153:1892-1897.

Metlay J, Kapoor W, Fine M. Does this patient have community-acquired pneumonia? Diagnosing pneumonia by history and physical examination. In: Simel D, Drummond R, eds. *The Rational Clinical Exam.* New York: McGraw-Hill; 2009:527-537.

Myers K, Farquhar D. Does this patient have clubbing? In: Simel D, Drummond R, eds. *The Rational Clinical Exam.* New York: McGraw-Hill; 2009:163-172.

Osmer JC, Cole BK. The stethoscope and roentgenogram in acute pneumonia. *Southern Med J.* 1966;59:75-77.

Schapira JM, Schapira MM, Funahashi A, McAuliffe TL, Varkey B. The value of the forced expiratory time in the physical diagnosis of obstructive airways disease. *JAMA.* 1993;270:731-736.

Spiter MA, Cook DG, Clarke SW. Reliability of eliciting physical signs in examination of the chest. *Lancet.* 1988;1:873-875.

Stubbing DG Mathur PN, Roberts RS, Campbell EJM. Some physical signs in patients with chronic airflow obstruction. *Am Rev Respir Dis.* 1982;125:549-552.

Thacker RE, Kraman SS. The prevalence of auscultatory crackles in subjects without lung disease. *Chest.* 1982;6:672-674.

West JB. *Pulmonary Pathophysiology.* 4th ed. Baltimore: Williams and Wilkins; 1992.

West JB. *Respiratory Physiology.* 4th ed. Baltimore: Williams and Wilkins; 1990.

Wilkins RL, Dexter JR, Murphy RLH, DelBono EA. Lung sound nomenclature survey. *Chest.* 1990;98:886-889.

Wunderdink R. Community-acquired pneumonia. *N Engl J Med.* 2014;370:543-551.

8

Abdominal Exam

Charlie Goldberg, MD

INTRODUCTION

The major components of the abdominal exam include observation, percussion, and palpation. Pelvic, genital, and rectal exams, each of which can provide important insights about abdominal symptoms, are discussed in chapters dedicated to those areas.

When to Perform the Abdominal Exam

- The abdominal exam can be part of a screening exam, although it will have the greatest likelihood of identifying significant findings when patients have risk factors for disease; for example, assessing for signs of liver disease in patients with alcohol use disorder.
- The exam should be performed when a patient has symptoms suggestive of abdominal pathology (eg, pain, bloating).
- Sometimes, nonspecific symptoms (eg, weight loss, fevers without focal complaints) as well those in a seemingly distant part of the body might also have their root cause in the abdomen. A complete exam covering all organ systems is necessary in these settings.
- Early learners should perform as many exams as possible, with the goal of developing skills to become comfortable recognizing the range of normal.
- Correlating history and exam findings with definitive diagnoses (eg, made via imaging, endoscopy, labs, or laparoscopy/laparotomy) is a very helpful way of learning.

Think Anatomically

- When looking, feeling, and percussing, imagine what organs live in the area that you are examining.
- The abdomen can be divided into 4 quadrants: right upper, right lower, left upper, and left lower (**Figure 8-1**). By thinking in anatomic terms, you can remind yourself of what resides in a particular quadrant and therefore what might be identifiable during both normal and pathologic states (**Figure 8-2**).

As with all aspects of the exam, it is useful to develop a systematic approach, such that you perform it the same way each time. This develops patterns and muscle memory, helping you to avoid inadvertently skipping any key elements.

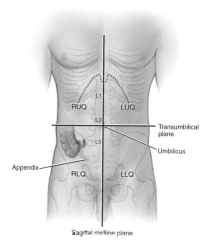

FIGURE 8-1 · Quadrants of the abdomen. (Reproduced with permission from Morton DA, Foreman KB, Albertine KH. *The Big Picture: Gross Anatomy, Medical Course & Step 1 Review*. 2nd ed. New York: McGraw Hill; 2019.)

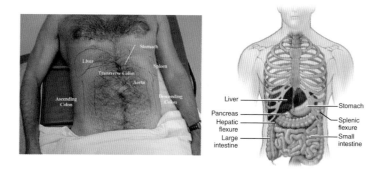

FIGURE 8-2 · Superficial and subsurface anatomy of the abdomen. (Left photo: *From Practical Guide to Clinical Medicine: Exam of the Abdomen*. Available from: https://meded.ucsd.edu/clinicalmed/ abdomen.html. Right illustration: Reproduced with permission from Morton DA, Foreman KB, Albertine KH. *The Big Picture: Gross Anatomy, Medical Course & Step 1 Review*. 2nd ed. New York: McGraw Hill; 2019.)

OBSERVATION

Important information can be gathered from watching the patient and looking at the abdomen. This requires complete exposure of the region.

- Ask the patient to lie on the examination table, bed, or gurney. Having them dressed in a gown and underwear facilitates optimal exposure.
- Take a sheet and drape it over their lower body such that it just covers the upper edge of their underwear or so that it crosses the top of the pubic region if they are completely undressed (**Figure 8-3**).

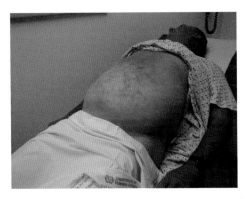

FIGURE 8-3 • **Draping the abdomen to achieve appropriate exposure.** (Photo from *Practical Guide to Clinical Medicine: Exam of the Abdomen.* Available from: https://meded.ucsd.edu/clinicalmed/abdomen.html.)

- This allows full exposure while at the same time permitting the patient to remain reasonably covered.
- The gown can then be withdrawn so that the area extending from just below the breasts to the pelvic brim is uncovered, remembering that the superior margin of the abdomen extends beneath the rib cage.
- The patient's hands should remain at their sides with their head resting on a pillow.
- Having the patient bend their knees so that the soles of their feet rest on the table can further relax the abdomen.
- Make sure that the lighting is adequate. Paying attention to small details creates an environment that gives you the best chance of performing an accurate exam.
- By convention, the abdominal exam is performed with the provider standing on the patient's right side.

> PEARL: Thoughtful exposure of the entire abdomen is critical in order to identify observable abnormalities.

Findings and Their Meaning: Abdominal Shape and Appearance

- Pay particular attention to the shape and size of the abdomen, noting scars, asymmetries, or protrusions.
- Key scars to note include port marks from a range of laparoscopic procedures; a right upper quadrant scar consistent with cholecystectomy; a right lower quadrant scar consistent with appendectomy; or a lower abdominal mid-line scar in a woman consistent with prior cesarean section. Noticing scars on patients who have not mentioned prior surgeries should prompt additional history taking.
- The contours of the abdomen can be best appreciated by standing at the foot of the table and looking up toward the patient's head. Is the abdomen flat? Distended? If enlarged, does this appear symmetric, or are there focal protrusions, perhaps linked to underlying masses, hernias, or other structural pathology?
- Global abdominal enlargement is usually caused by air, fluid, or fat (**Table 8-1**).

TABLE 8-1 • Diagnoses at a Glance: Common Causes of Abdominal Protrusions or Enlargement

Cause of Enlargement	Symptoms	Appearance
Abdominal obesity • From intra-abdominal and subcutaneous fat	• No acute symptoms • Typically develops over years	• Generalized obesity, elevated body mass index • See Figure 8-3
Ascites (fluid within abdominal cavity) • Typical cause is cirrhosis, resulting in portal hypertension	• Sometimes discomfort if significant accumulation • Tense ascites can make it difficult to take a deep breath • Smaller amounts of fluid can be asymptomatic or cause mild sense of fullness • Often accompanied by other symptoms and findings associated with liver disease (see Table 8-2).	 (From Knoop KJ, Stack LB, Storrow AB, Thurman RJ, eds. *The Atlas of Emergency Medicine.* 5th ed. New York: McGraw-Hill; 2021, Figure 7.71. Reproduced with permission from photo contributor: Lawrence B. Stack, MD.)
Incisional hernia • Protrusion at site of prior surgery, secondary to failure of fascia to keep contents within the abdominal cavity	• Range from small to large • Can increase over time • Can sometimes get bigger with Valsalva or if patient is asked to raise head, chest, or legs off of the exam table • Can be asymptomatic • Pain, nausea, and vomiting often occur when bowel is incarcerated or strangulated within the hernia	 (From Knoop KJ, Stack LB, Storrow AB, Thurman RJ, eds. *The Atlas of Emergency Medicine.* 5th ed. New York: McGraw-Hill; 2021, Figure 7.52A. Reproduced with permission from photo contributor: Lawrence B. Stack, MD.)
Umbilical hernia • Failure of fascia beneath the umbilicus • Often congenital; can also develop associated with obesity and/or ascites	• Protrusion at umbilicus • Can sometimes get bigger with Valsalva or if patient is asked to raise head, chest, or legs off of the exam table • Range from small to large • Often asymptomatic • Pain, nausea, and vomiting often occur when bowel is incarcerated or strangulated within the hernia	 (From Knoop KJ, Stack LB, Storrow AB, Thurman RJ, eds. *The Atlas of Emergency Medicine.* 5th ed. New York: McGraw-Hill; 2021, Figure 7.59. Reproduced with permission from photo contributor: Lawrence B. Stack, MD.)

AUSCULTATION

Special Testing: Auscultation for Bowel Sounds

As food and liquid course through the intestines via peristalsis, noise, referred to as bowel sounds or borborygmi, is generated. There is a wide range of normal in terms of the frequency with which these sounds are generated. The assessment of bowel sounds has been taught as a "standard" component of the physical exam. However, in the asymptomatic patient, bowel sound assessment does not offer useful clinical information because whatever pattern the patient has will be normal for them and is not in and of itself pathognomonic for any particular process.

The presence or absence of bowel sounds has particular value in the setting of concerns about bowel obstruction. Listening for bowel sounds is presented here as an adjuvant test to be used in that setting.

When there is concern for bowel obstruction, patients will typically have symptoms (eg, nausea, vomiting, decreased flatus) and findings (eg, abdominal distention, generalized or focal pain). Bowel sounds may also be abnormal.

- Gently place the diaphragm of the stethoscope on the abdomen and listen for approximately 10 seconds (**Figure 8-4**).
- The stethoscope can be placed over any area of the abdomen because there is no true compartmentalization and sounds produced in one area can generally be heard throughout.
- Note whether any sounds are present as well their frequency. Absent, infrequent, or increased sounds (ie, anything different than normal) may add supporting evidence that an obstruction is present.
- Although listening to bowel sounds in asymptomatic patients does not offer important clinical insights, it can help learners develop a sense of the range of normal.

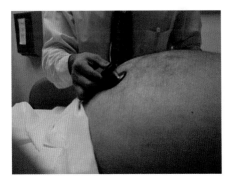

FIGURE 8-4 · **Abdominal auscultation.** (Photo from *Practical Guide to Clinical Medicine: Exam of the Abdomen.* Available from: https://meded.ucsd.edu/clinicalmed/abdomen.html.)

Special Testing: Auscultation for Bruits

Assessing for bruits can be done in specific situations where there is clinical concern that narrowed vessels (most commonly the result of atherosclerosis) are contributing to symptoms or organ dysfunction.

Bruits are high-pitched sounds caused by turbulent blood flow through a vessel narrowed by atherosclerosis (most common), inflammation (eg, vasculitis), or fibrosis (eg, fibromuscular dysplasia). This causes a soft "shshhing" sound that occurs with each contraction of the heart (ie, simultaneous with the pulse).

Assessing for bruits should be done in specific situations where there is clinical concern that narrowed vessels are causing pathology. These include the following:

- Concern for renal artery stenosis, when a patient has some combination of impaired renal function, difficult-to-control hypertension, and known vascular disease or risk factors. The presence of a bruit lends supporting evidence for the existence of renal artery stenosis.
- Concern for mesenteric atherosclerosis (eg, narrowing of celiac, superior mesenteric, or inferior mesenteric arteries). Symptoms associated with chronic mesenteric ischemia include postprandial abdominal pain, food avoidance, and weight loss. This typically occurs in patients with risk factors for atherosclerosis or known disease.
- Unusual conditions such as vasculitis, where inflammation causes vessel narrowing. This is often accompanied by additional symptoms (eg, weight loss, joint pain, fever, abdominal pain).

Assessing for abdominal bruits:

- To listen for renal artery bruits, place the diaphragm of your stethoscope a few centimeters above the umbilicus, along the lateral edges of either rectus muscle.
- Auscultate centrally above and below the umbilicus in order to assess for bruits in the mesenteric arteries (**Figure 8-5**).

> PEARL: Auscultation plays a minor supporting role in the abdominal exam. Listening should be pursued if there is clinical suspicion for disease.

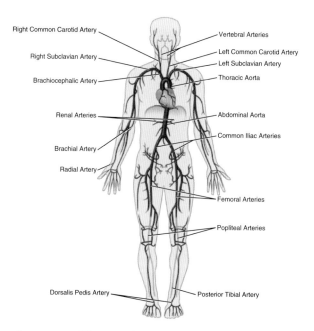

FIGURE 8-5 · **Vascular anatomy.** (Illustration from *Practical Guide to Clinical Medicine: Exam of the Abdomen.* Available from: https://meded.ucsd.edu/clinicalmed/abdomen.html.)

PERCUSSION

Percussion plays a supporting role in helping to assess for intra-abdominal pathology. It provides some insights into whether an area of the abdomen contains a solid organ, gas, or liquid.

- The technique for percussion is the same as that used for the lung exam.
- Place the middle finger of your nondominant hand firmly against the abdomen (**Figure 8-6**).
- Strike the distal interphalangeal joint of the middle finger 2 or 3 times with the tip of the middle finger of your dominant hand.
- Use a floppy wrist action (see section on percussion in Chapter 7, Pulmonary exam) to create the correct percussive note.
- There are 2 basic sounds that can be elicited:
  - Tympanic (drum-like) sounds produced by percussing over air-filled structures.
  - Dull sounds that occur when a solid structure (eg, liver) or fluid (eg, ascites) lies beneath the region being examined.

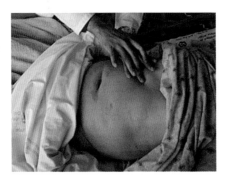

FIGURE 8-6 · **Abdominal percussion.** (Photo from *Practical Guide to Clinical Medicine: Exam of the Abdomen.* Available from: https://meded.ucsd.edu/clinicalmed/abdomen.html.)

Percussing the liver area:

- Start just below the right breast in line with the middle of the clavicle, at a point that you are reasonably certain is over the lungs. Percussion in this area should produce a relatively resonant note.
- Move your hand a few centimeters toward the liver and repeat. After doing this several times, you will be over the liver, which will produce a duller-sounding tone.
- Continue moving your hand and percussing, until the sound changes once again to resonant. At this point, you will have reached the inferior margin of the liver.
- The total span of the normal liver is variable, depending on the size of the patient (between 6 and 12 cm), and the liver is usually fully covered by the ribs.
- If the liver seems enlarged, this can be further explored during palpation (ie, the liver should be palpable).
- Do not get discouraged if you have a hard time picking up the different sounds because the changes can be quite subtle, particularly if there is a lot of subcutaneous fat.

Percussing the rest of the abdomen:

- The normal abdomen is filled with the small and large intestines.
- Percussing each of the 4 quadrants will generate mostly tympanic tones.

- Occasional dullness is encountered if you are on top of intestines that are filled with liquid.
- The stomach should produce a tympanic sound, identified with percussion over the left lower rib cage, close to the sternum.
- Performing percussion on asymptomatic patients early in your training allows you to hone your technique and develop an appreciation for the range of normal.

Findings and Their Meaning: Unexpected Tympany or Dullness

- In the setting of distention of unclear etiology, percussion can provide insights about whether the underlying cause is gas (eg, within the intestines), organomegaly (eg, liver or spleen), a mass (eg, primary or metastatic cancer), or fluid (ascites).
- Dullness in the left upper quadrant and over the left lower ribs may suggest splenomegaly, which can be further explored during palpation.
- Percussion can also help to correlate symptoms with objective findings. For example, in a patient complaining of bloating, finding an abdomen that has distension and tympany on percussion would suggest that the bloating is related to gas retention, and this could help to narrow the differential diagnosis (eg, small bowel bacterial overgrowth, mechanical obstruction).

PALPATION

Palpation plays a vital role in identifying intra-abdominal pathology. When palpating, it is important to move slowly, thinking about which organs live in each area that is being explored. Keys to examining the patient with abdominal pain are described in a later section dedicated to this topic.

- Warm your hands by rubbing them together before placing them on the patient.
- The pads and tips (the most sensitive areas) of the index, middle, and ring fingers are used to locate the edges of organs as well as deeper structures. You can use either your dominant hand alone or both hands, with the nondominant hand resting on top of the other (**Figure 8-7**).
- Apply slow, steady pressure, avoiding any rapid/sharp movements that are likely to startle the patient or cause discomfort.
- Examine each quadrant separately, imagining what structures lie beneath your hands and what you might expect to feel.
- Start by palpation at a superficial level, examining each of the 4 quadrants. Then move to deeper palpation. In order to be systematic, start in the right lower quadrant.

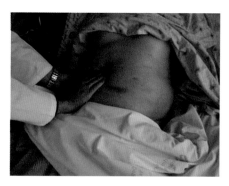

FIGURE 8-7 · **Abdominal palpation.** (Photo from *Practical Guide to Clinical Medicine: Exam of the Abdomen.* Available from: https://meded.ucsd.edu/clinicalmed/abdomen.html.)

- Gently push down (posterior) and then toward the patient's head, with your hand angled as shown in Figure 8-7. Advance your hands a few centimeters cephalad and repeat until ultimately you are at the bottom margin of the ribs.
- Push posterior and then toward the head while the patient takes a deep breath. This makes it easier to feel the liver edge, as the downward movement of the diaphragm will bring the liver toward your hand. If you detect the edge, note its character (firm vs soft) and determine if you can feel a consistent edge as you move your palpating hand medially and laterally.
- You can also try to "hook" the edge of the liver with your fingers (**Figure 8-8**). Flex the tips of the fingers of your right hand (claw-like). Then push down in the right upper quadrant and pull upward (toward the patient's head) as you try to catch the edge of the liver. This is a nice way of confirming the presence of a palpable liver edge felt during initial palpation.

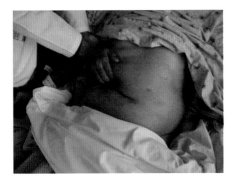

FIGURE 8-8 · **Hooking edge of the liver.** (Photo from Practical Guide to Clinical Medicine: Exam of the Abdomen. Available from: https://meded.ucsd.edu/clinicalmed/abdomen.html.)

- The tip of the xyphoid process, the bony structure at the bottom of the sternum, may be directed outward or inward and can be mistaken for an abdominal mass (**Figure 8-9**). You should be able to distinguish it by noting its location relative to the rib cage and sternum.
- Now move toward the left upper quadrant. The normal spleen is not palpable. When enlarged, it tends to grow toward the pelvis and the umbilicus (ie, down and across). Move your hand toward the left upper quadrant, palpating deeply. You can use your other hand to push in from the patient's left flank, directing an enlarged spleen (an unusual finding) toward your right hand.

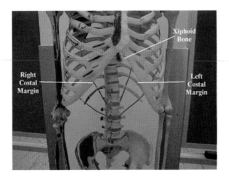

FIGURE 8-9 · **Location of xiphoid process.** (Photo from Practical Guide to Clinical Medicine: Exam of the Abdomen. Available from: https://meded.ucsd.edu/clinicalmed/abdomen.html.)

- Splenomegaly is usually more difficult to appreciate than hepatomegaly. The edge of the spleen, when palpable, tends to be soft and rounded – varying based on the cause of splenomegaly.
  - If you identify the spleen, repeat the exam with the patient turned onto their right side, which causes the spleen to move toward your examining hand.
- Then move to the left lower quadrant, the area of the sigmoid colon. It does not typically generate a characteristic palpable sensation.
- Then palpate across the suprapubic area. You will not typically feel any discrete masses or structures.
- Then try to identify the abdominal aorta. First push down with a single hand in the area just above the umbilicus. If you are able to identify the pulsating aorta with one hand, try to determine if it is enlarged, as occurs with an abdominal aortic aneurysm (AAA). Orient your hands so that the thumbs are pointed toward the patient's head. Then push deeply and try to position them so that they are on either side of the blood vessel. This is a crude technique and provides a general sense of size (normal width is <3 cm).
  - Recall that the aorta is a retroperitoneal structure and can be very hard to appreciate in obese patients.
  - Based on US Preventive Services Taskforce guidelines, one-time screening for AAAs should be offered to men older than 64 years who have a smoking history. This is typically accomplished with ultrasound.

What Can You Expect to Feel?

In general, do not be discouraged if you are unable to identify anything discrete during palpation of healthy, asymptomatic patients.

- The body has evolved to protect critically important organs (eg, liver and spleen beneath the ribs; kidneys and pancreas deep in the retroperitoneum).
- It is, for the most part, during pathologic states that these organs become identifiable to the careful examiner.
- However, you will not be able to recognize abnormal until you become comfortable identifying variants of normal, a theme common to the examination of any part of the body. It is therefore important to practice on as many patients as possible early in your training.
- It is also quite easy to miss abnormalities if you rush or push too vigorously, so take your time and focus on the tips/pads of your fingers.

Findings and Their Meaning: Abdominal Mases

- If you identify a mass in the abdomen, determine its size, shape, and whether it appears to arise from a known structure found in that area.
- Note if it appears to be connected to other structures or independent.
- Identify if it is superficial (eg, in the subcutaneous tissue of the abdominal wall) or deeper and within the abdominal cavity. Also identify whether it is isolated or accompanied by other masses.
- Characterize the consistency of the mass (eg. firm vs soft). Firm is often concerning for cancer.
- Note also if it is painful or painless.

PEARL: If you identify a mass, think pathoanatomically as you consider possible etiologies. Consider what normally lives in that area, as these are the structures that might become palpable if enlarged.

Special Testing: Assessing for Costovertebral Angle Tenderness

- Assessing for kidney area pain should be done when patients have symptoms of pyelo-nephritis (kidney infection). Patients typically will have some combination of acute low back/flank pain, nausea, vomiting, fever, urinary frequency, urgency, and dysuria.
- As the kidneys lie in the retroperitoneum, place one hand over the costovertebral angle (ie, where the bottom-most ribs articulate with the vertebral column) as this is the region of the kidney (**Figure 8-10**).
- Firmly strike that hand with the bottom of your other fist. This will often cause pain (ie, costovertebral angle tenderness) if the underlying kidney is inflamed (Figure 8-10).

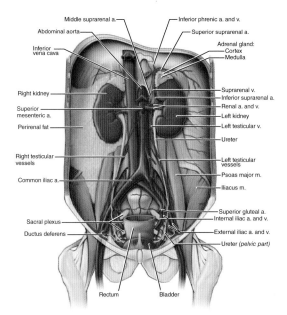

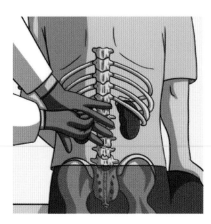

FIGURE 8-10 · **Location of the kidneys (posterior view) and assessing for costovertebral angle tenderness.** (Top illustration: Reproduced with permission from Morton DA, Foreman KB, Albertine KH. *The Big Picture: Gross Anatomy, Medical Course & Step 1 Review.* 2nd ed. New York: McGraw Hill; 2019, Figure 11-4. Bottom illustration: Reproduced with permission from Cathy Cichon, MD.)

Special Testing: Examination of the Patient With Abdominal Pain

- Note whether the patient moves around or prefers to lie still.
  - Those with peritonitis (eg, appendicitis) tend to avoid movement, as any motion causes further peritoneal irritation and pain.
  - By comparison, patients with kidney stones will appear very uncomfortable, moving frequently or walking around, searching for a position that might offer relief from the colicky pain caused by ureteral contraction around an obstructing stone.
- In the event that a patient presents complaining of pain in any region of the abdomen, have them first try to localize the area with a single finger.
- Examine each of the other abdominal quadrants first before turning your attention to the area of pain. This should help to keep the patient as relaxed as possible and limit voluntary and involuntary guarding (ie, superficial muscle tightening that protects intra-abdominal organs from being poked), allowing you to gather the greatest amount of clinical data.

> PEARL: In the setting of abdominal pain, ask the patient to localize the most intense area of symptoms with a single finger. Examine painful regions last.

- As you examine, think about what might be causing the pain based on your knowledge of anatomy. Some processes cause localized (somatic) pain. Others cause generalized symptoms (visceral pain) or pain that is referred to more distant regions of the body (**Figure 8-11**). A few examples include the following:
  - Early appendicitis causes central discomfort (visceral pain), which then moves to the right lower quadrant (somatic pain) as the peritoneum becomes inflamed.
  - Splenic or hepatobiliary inflammatory processes (including cholecystitis) can cause referred discomfort to the left and right shoulders, respectively.
  - Processes affecting retroperitoneal structures (eg, AAAs, pancreatitis, kidney infection or stone) often generate pain that is referred to the back.

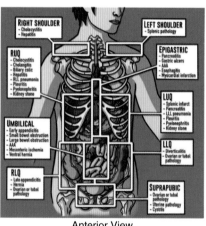
Anterior View

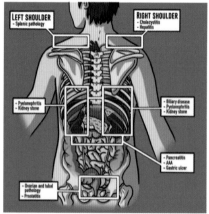
Posterior View

FIGURE 8-11 • **Anatomy of acute abdominal pain.** Location of pain and common causes (anterior and posterior views). AAA, abdominal aortic aneurysm; LLL, left lower lobe; LLQ, left lower quadrant; LUQ, left upper quadrant; RLL, right lower lobe; RLQ, right lower quadrant; RUQ, right upper quadrante. (Reproduced with permission from Cathy Cichon, MD.)

- Processes in the chest (eg, a heart attack affecting the inferior wall of the heart, pneumonia of the lower lobes of the lung, pleural processes) can cause epigastric or upper abdominal symptoms.
- The key to making any of these diagnoses is an awareness about the types of pain caused by various pathologic processes, obtaining the relevant history, and performing an appropriate exam. This allows you to begin the localization process. Labs and imaging are also critical in making these diagnoses, ordered based on the history and exam.
- Make sure to glance at the patient's face while examining a tender area. This can be particularly revealing when evaluating otherwise stoic individuals. Most patients will grimace when painful areas are examined.
- The goal is to obtain relevant information while generating the minimum amount of discomfort.
- Note that certain coexisting conditions (eg. spinal cord injury with impaired sensation) may allow pathologic processes to exist without causing pain. Altered immune systems (eg. from the use of steroids, immune modulating agents, or underlying disorders) may limit the normal inflammatory response, resulting in fewer symptoms. Patients on either end of the age spectrum may also have fewer or atypical symptoms. Finally, those with cognitive issues or challenges expressing themselves (eg. caused by mental illness, intoxication, or other acute or chronic processes) may have a difficult time describing symptoms.

Special Testing: Assessing for Peritoneal Signs (peritonitis)

- Inflammation of the peritoneum often generates specific findings, and patients usually feel sick, with abnormal vital signs and other indicators of significant illness. Several exam techniques can be revealing, noting that it is best to get the necessary information with the fewest maneuvers possible in order to minimize patient discomfort.
  - Shake tenderness: If you put your hands on either side of the patients hips and gently rock them from side to side, the patient will report increased pain in the affected area.
  - Cough tenderness: Similar localization of pain when the patient coughs.
  - Palpating over the affected area (eg, right lower quadrant in setting of acute appendicitis) reproduces the pain.
  - Guarding: The abdominal muscles contract due to severe underlying inflammation, protecting the area when it is examined. With advanced peritonitis, the entire abdominal wall may become rigid.
  - Rebound pain: Pushing down in the area and then letting go makes the pain worse.

Special Testing: Assessing for Ascites

This is done in the setting of abdominal distention, peripheral edema, and risk factors or other findings suggestive of underlying liver disease. The most common cause of ascites is portal hypertension, which in turn is often the result of cirrhosis. The presence of risk factors for cirrhosis should be sought, including: chronic hepatitis C or B, alcohol use disorder, obesity with resultant nonalcoholic steatohepatitis, or combinations of these processes. Note that there needs to be a lot of fluid (eg, 1 L or more, in particular if the patient is obese) before it is detectable on exam. None of these special tests can definitively rule in or out ascites. They can raise or lower the suspicion that there is fluid in the abdomen. Following the history and exam, if there is clinical concern for ascites, ultrasound is typically the next step in defining its presence. Any fluid identified is then typically sampled and tested in order to determine its cause.

Identifying Bulging Flanks
- In the setting of large amounts of ascites, the flanks can bulge (**Figure 8-12**).
- Percussion over the flanks should generate a dull tone if there is fluid.
- The absence of dullness and bulging flanks suggests that large volume ascites is not present.

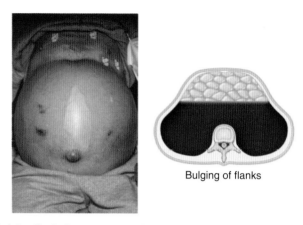

Bulging of flanks

FIGURE 8-12 · **Bulging flanks from ascites.** (Left photo: From Knoop KJ, Stack LB, Storrow AB, Thurman RJ, eds. *The Atlas of Emergency Medicine*. 5th ed. New York: McGraw-Hill; 2021, Figure 7.71. Reproduced with permission from photo contributor: Lawrence B. Stack, MD. Right illustration: Reproduced with permission from Suneja M, Szot JF, LeBlond RF, Brown DD. *DeGowin's Diagnostic Examination*. 11th ed. New York: McGraw Hill; 2020.)

Identifying a Fluid Wave When observation and/or percussion are suggestive of ascites, assess for a fluid wave:
- Ask the patient or an observer to place their hand so that it is oriented longitudinally over the center of the abdomen. They should press firmly so that subcutaneous tissue and fat do not jiggle.
- Place your right hand on the left side of the abdomen and your left hand opposite, so that both are equidistant from the umbilicus.
- Firmly tap on the abdomen with one hand while the other hand remains against the abdominal wall (**Figure 8-13**).

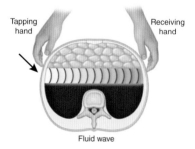

Tapping hand

Receiving hand

Fluid wave

FIGURE 8-13 · **Assessing for a fluid wave.** (Reproduced with permission from Suneja M, Szot JF, LeBlond RF, Brown DD. *DeGowin's Diagnostic Examination*. 11th ed. New York: McGraw Hill; 2020.)

- If there is a lot of ascites present, you may be able to feel a fluid wave (generated within the ascites by the tapping maneuver) strike against the abdominal wall under your receiving hand.
- You will typically need to examine multiple patients with ascites before being able to confidently identify the wave-like impulse.

Identifying Shifting Dullness

- In the presence of a large volume of ascites, the fluid will collect along the posterior aspect of the abdomen and the intestines will "float" to the surface. Using percussion, you can approximate the fluid-intestine interface (**Figure 8-14**).
- Start by percussing near the umbilicus. This will generate a tympanic tone, as gas-filled bowel is underneath this area. Then slide your hand down the side of the abdomen a few centimeters and repeat percussion. Keep moving your hand downward and repeating percussion until you reach the point where it generates a dull note. This is the place where your hand is over the ascites. Mark the location on the skin with ink or a small impression.
- Then have the patient turn on their side. Due to gravity, the fluid will now collect along the part of the abdomen that is closest to the bed and the intestines will float to the top, which is now toward the side that's turned upward. Repeat the process described above, noting the new location of the fluid-intestine interface. Mark this location on the skin (Figure 8-14).
- Compare the mark made when the patient was supine with that made when they were on their side. The location of the intestine-fluid interface will have shifted upward, toward the umbilicus.
- This is referred to as shifting dullness and, when present, is suggestive of significant ascites.

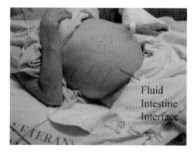 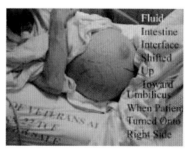

FIGURE 8-14 · **Fluid-intestine interface marked with patient supine (image on left).** When resting on their right side (image on right), the location of the intestine-fluid interface shifts upward, as the fluid collects in the newly dependent portion of the abdomen. (From Usatine RP, Smith MA, Mayeaux EJ Jr, Chumley HS. *The Color Atlas and Synopsis of Family Medicine*. 3rd ed. New York, McGraw Hill; 2019, Figures 63-6 and 63-7. Reproduced with permission from Charlie Goldberg, MD, copyright University of California, San Diego.)

Findings Associated with Advanced Liver Disease

Liver disease typically results from years of hepatic inflammation, ultimately leading to fibrosis and decline in normal liver function. Histologically, this is referred to as cirrhosis. This can be driven by a number of different processes, most commonly chronic alcohol use, fatty liver, viral hepatitis (B or C), hepatotoxic medications, or combinations of these processes. There are many other less common causes of acute and chronic liver disease not described here. It is important to realize that a cirrhotic liver can be markedly enlarged (in which case, it is often palpable) or shrunken and nonpalpable.

Ultimately, the liver may become unable to perform some or all of its normal functions. There are multiple clinical manifestations of this, none of which are pathognomonic for liver disease. Given that patients with liver disease are frequently encountered in hospitals and clinics, some of the most common findings are described in **Table 8-2**. Non-hepatic causes would need to be excluded based on history, exam, and appropriate studies.

TABLE 8-2 • Diagnoses at a Glance: Findings Commonly Associated with Advanced Liver Disease

Condition and Etiology	Symptoms	Findings
Hyperbilirubinemia • Most commonly secondary to cirrhosis or other disorders affecting the liver and/or the biliary drainage system (eg, obstruction of the bile ducts which connect the liver to the small intestines). • Also from hemolysis of red blood cells, a prehepatic cause of hyperbilirubinemia. • Detectable when the total bilirubin (combination of direct and indirect fractions of bilirubin) exceeds approximately 3 mg/dL • Becomes increasingly noticeable as levels rise (eg, approaching 10 mg/dL or higher) • Good lighting and contrast make jaundice and icterus more apparent	• Yellowed sclera (icterus) • No other eye symptoms • Yellowing of skin (jaundice) • Often accompanied by itching • In patients with dark skin, jaundice can be harder to appreciate	(From Knoop KJ, Stack LB, Storrow AB, Thurman RJ, eds. *The Atlas of Emergency Medicine.* 5th ed. New York: McGraw-Hill; 2021, Figure 27.21. Reproduced with permission from photo contributor: Lawrence B. Stack, MD.)
Bilirubinuria (elevated levels of bilirubin in urine) • Associated with elevated direct bilirubin (ie conjugated bilirubin – which has been processed by the liver). • Caused by processes that damage the liver or obstruct the pathways that allow bile to drain into the intestines.	• Dark yellow/orange, foamy urine • Sometimes described as tea or cola colored. • May have jaundice and icterus; also itching • No other urinary symptoms	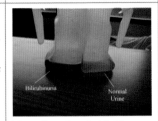 (Photo from *Practical Guide to Clinical Medicine: Exam of the Abdomen.* Available from: https://meded.ucsd.edu/clinicalmed/abdomen.html.)

(Continued)

TABLE 8-2 • Diagnoses at a Glance: Findings Commonly Associated with Advanced Liver Disease (Continued)		
Condition and Etiology	Symptoms	Findings
Ascites • Typically secondary to portal hypertension, which is most commonly the result of cirrhosis • Large volume (eg, >1 L) has to be present in order to identify on exam	• Generalized abdominal discomfort and fullness, varying with the amount of fluid present. • Sometimes weight gain. • Tense ascites can cause shortness of breath (ascites pushes up diaphragms, limiting ability to breathe deeply). • History may indicate presence of risk factors for cirrhosis (eg, Hepatitis C, alcohol use disorder). • If ascites becomes infected (known as spontaneous bacterial peritonitis), patients develop a range of symptoms and findings including: abdominal pain, fever, confusion, gastrointestinal bleeding, and other signs of acute illness.	• Presence of bulging flanks, fluid wave, shifting dullness and peripheral edema are suggestive of ascites (See Figures 8-12, 8-13 and 8-14).
Breast development (gynecomastia) • Results from elevation in estrogen-to-testosterone levels in patients with cirrhosis.	• Painless bilateral breast development	(From Usatine RP, Smith MA, Mayeaux EJ Jr, Chumley HS. *The Color Atlas and Synopsis of Family Medicine.* 3rd ed. New York, McGraw Hill; 2019, Figure 63-8. Reproduced with permission from Richard P. Usatine, MD.)
Spider angioma • Dilated arterioles in skin • Often easiest to see on upper chest • Due to hormonal changes as above	• No symptoms related to the arterioles	(Reproduced with permission from Soutor C, Hordinsky MK. *Clinical Dermatology: Diagnosis and Management of Common Disorders.* 2nd ed. New York: McGraw Hill; 2022, Figure 20-16.)

(Continued)

TABLE 8-2 • Diagnoses at a Glance: Findings Commonly Associated with Advanced Liver Disease (Continued)		
Condition and Etiology	Symptoms	Findings
Testicular atrophy • Due to hormonal changes as above	• Can contribute to decreased energy/fatigue and impaired libido.	• Symmetric decrease in size of testes
Palmar erythema • Due to hormonal changes as above	• No hand related symptoms.	 (From Usatine RP, Smith MA, Mayeaux EJ Jr, Chumley HS. *The Color Atlas and Synopsis of Family Medicine.* 3rd ed. New York, McGraw Hill; 2019, Figure 63-3. Reproduced with permission from Richard P. Usatine, MD.)
Lower extremity edema • Related to portal hypertension and fluid retention. • For patients with concern for liver disease, it is the finding most commonly associated with ascites.	• Sometimes sensation of heaviness in legs from fluid (painless). • May report weight gain.	 (Reproduced with permission from Kemp WL, Burns DK, Brown TG. *Pathology: The Big Picture.* New York: McGraw Hill; 2008, Figure 8-3B.)
Coffee ground emesis • Caused by upper gastrointestinal tract bleeding, which could be from portal hypertension and esophageal varices or portal gastropathy • Can also bleed from non–liver-related processes (eg, ulcers, esophagitis) • Sometimes vomited blood can appear bright red	• Dark vomitus • Severe illness (hypotension, tachycardia) if significant blood loss, as often occurs with varices (bleeding into the open esophageal space). • Other manifestations of portal hypertension (eg, ascites, edema, melena, confusion) may be present	 (Photo from *Practical Guide to Clinical Medicine: Exam of the Abdomen.* Available from: https://meded.ucsd.edu/clinicalmed/abdomen.html.)

(Continued)

TABLE 8-2 • Diagnoses at a Glance: Findings Commonly Associated with Advanced Liver Disease (Continued)

Condition and Etiology	Symptoms	Findings
Melena • Blood in stool from upper gastrointestinal bleeding • Can be caused by portal hypertension and esophageal varices or portal gastropathy - or from processes unrelated to portal hypertension	• Black, tarry/sticky stool • Severe illness if significant blood loss • Sometimes confusion • Other manifestations of portal hypertension (eg, ascites, edema, hematemesis, confusion) may be present	 (From Knoop KJ, Stack LB, Storrow AB, Thurman RJ, eds. *The Atlas of Emergency Medicine.* 5th ed. New York: McGraw-Hill; 2021, Figure 25.37. Reproduced with permission from photo contributor: Alan B. Storrow, MD.)
Encephalopathy (confusion) • Related to portal hypertension and inability of liver to metabolize toxins absorbed from the gastrointestinal tract. • Often precipitated by an acute event (eg, gastrointestinal bleed, spontaneous bacterial peritonitis)	• Can be anywhere on spectrum from somnolence, slower processing, irritability, confusion to agitation.	• Often other findings of portal hypertension (eg, ascites, edema, gastrointestinal bleeding) and liver disease are present. • May have asterixis: Repetitive, involuntary flexion of hands when the patient is directed to hold them up in hyperextension.

TELEHEALTH TIPS

- Effective history taking can be performed in the telehealth environment.
- Overall comfort of the patient can be noted on camera. Also, it is possible to note whether movement causes pain. Vital signs are typically helpful in identifying acute illness or decompensation.
- Visualizing the abdomen in the seated patient is challenging. A few things that you may be able to accomplish include the following:
  - Patients can expose their abdomen to give you a general sense of the size, shape, and/or superficial abnormalities, as well as skin findings such as herpes zoster. The camera has to be pointed at this area, which can be difficult for a patient who is alone.
  - Having the patient lie down and asking a caregiver to orient the camera to the abdominal area can help with visualization.
- Localizing symptoms may be enhanced by asking the patient to point with a single finger to the place that is causing their discomfort. Remember that abdominal processes can cause pain that is referred elsewhere. And pathologic processes in other parts of the body (eg, chest) can cause symptoms in the abdomen.
- Visualization of a hernia may be apparent if the patient is instructed to Valsalva (ie, "bear down").
- Yellow discoloration of skin or eyes might be visible.

- Lower extremity edema can be appreciated on camera. It helps to have the patient rest their feet on a chair to increase visibility and angle the camera to frame the lower extremities.
  - You can get a sense of fluid accumulation by noting whether you can see extensor tendons on the top of the foot and the distinct margins of the malleoli (socks off).
  - Look for sock indentation lines on the ankles and ask the patient if they are new or worse.
  - If the patient applies gentle pressure to the edematous area with their fingertip, you may be able to see a small imprint (pitting) when the patient releases their finger.
  - The height of the edema (eg, ankle, mid-tibia) might also be noticeable as well as whether it is uni- or bilateral.
  - In patients with volume overload states (eg, portal hypertension from cirrhosis), their weight should be considered a vital sign.
- Clear plans for follow-up, additional testing, and when to seek emergency department evaluations should be described.
- Those with concerning symptoms or findings usually need to be referred for in-person evaluation with appropriate urgency.

✅ SUMMARY OF SKILLS CHECKLIST

❑ Clean your hands

Observation
❑ Gown and drape appropriately, allowing full exposure
❑ Exam done from right-hand side of the patient's body
❑ Observe and inspect abdomen
❑ Shape, scars, color, symmetry, unusual protrusions

Auscultation
❑ Listen with diaphragm (*special test—relevant if abdominal pain and symptoms suggestive of bowel obstruction)
❑ Listen for bruits (*special test—relevant if hypertension in young patients, resistant or accelerated hypertension, otherwise unexplained kidney disease)

Percussion
❑ Percuss all quadrants
❑ Percuss liver span
❑ Percuss area of spleen, stomach

Palpation
❑ Palpate all quadrants superficially
❑ Palpate all quadrants deeply; think about what "lives" in each area
❑ Assess for liver edge (with inspiration)
❑ Palpate region of spleen
❑ Palpate area of aorta (*special test—if risk factors for AAA)
❑ Assess costovertebral angle for tenderness (*special test—if concern for pyelonephritis)
❑ Clean your hands

BIBLIOGRAPHY

Baudendistel T, Carcamo-Molina D. Chapter 37. Jaundice. In: Henderson M, et al, eds. *The Patient History*. 2nd ed. New York: McGraw Hill; 2012.

Benal W, Wendon J. Acute liver failure. *N Engl J Med*. 2013;369:2525-2534.

Birger M, Rud B, Kirkegaard T, et al. Accuracy of abdominal auscultation for bowel obstruction. *World J Gastroenterol.* 2015;21(34):1018-1024.

Clair D, Beach J. Mesenteric ischemia. *N Engl J Med.* 2016;374:959-968.

Felder S, Margel D, Murrell Z, et al. Usefulness of bowel sound auscultation: a prospective evaluation. *J Surg Educ.* 2014;71(5):768-773.

Fitzgibbons R, Forse R. Groin hernias in adults. *N Engl J Med.* 2015;372:756-763.

Ford A, Talley NJ, Veldhuyzen van Zanten S, et al. Will the history and physical examination help establish that irritable bowel syndrome is causing this patient's lower gastrointestinal tract symptoms? *JAMA.* 2008;300(15):1793-1805.

Forsmark C, Vege SS, Wilcox CM. Acute pancreatitis. *N Engl J Med.* 2016;375:1972-1981.

Friedman L, Gee MS, Misdraji J. A 19-year-old woman with nausea, jaundice and pruritus (jaundice/autoimmune hepatitis). *N Engl J Med.* 2010;363:2548-2555.

Harrison's Principles of Internal Medicine. 18th ed. New York, NY: McGraw-Hill; 2012.

Goldberg C. Digital Ddx: gastrointestinal symptoms or conditions. Accessed January 1, 2023. http://digitalddx.com/symptoms_list/6/.

Goldberg C. UCSD's practical guide to clinical medicine: exam of the abdomen. Accessed January 1, 2023. https://meded.ucsd.edu/clinicalmed/abdomen.html.

Jacobs D. Diverticulitis. *N Engl J Med.* 2007;357:2057-2066.

Jacobs D. Hemorrhoids. *N Engl J Med.* 2014;371:944-951.

Kahrilas P. Gastroesophageal reflux disease. *N Engl J Med.* 2008;359:1700-1707.

Kerlin M, Tokar J. Acute gastrointestinal bleeding. *Ann Intern Med.* 2013;159(3):ITC2-1.

Lederle F. Abdominal aortic aneurysm. *Ann Intern Med.* 2009;150(9):ITC5-1.

McGee S. *Evidence Based Physical Diagnosis (the Abdomen).* Philadelphia: Elsevier; 2022:417-446.

Park AE, Targarona E, Weltz A. The Spleen. In: Brunicardi F, et al, eds. *Schwartz's Principles of Surgery.* 11th ed. New York: McGraw-Hill, 2019.

Schubert M, Sridhar S, Schade RR, et al. What every gastroenterologist needs to know about common ano-rectal disorders. *World J Gastroenterol.* 2009;15(26):3201-3209.

Silen W. *Cope's Early Diagnosis of the Acute Abdomen.* 22nd ed. New York: Oxford University Press; 2010.

Talley N. How to do and interpret a rectal exam in GI. *Am J Gastroenterol.* 2008;103:820-822.

Trowbridge R, Rutkowski N, Shojania K. Does this patient have acute cholecystitis? In: Simel D, Drummond R. eds. *The Rational Clinical Exam.* New York: McGraw-Hill; 2009:137-147.

9

Male Genital and Rectal Exams

Charlie Goldberg, MD

INTRODUCTION

Because the male genital and rectal exams involve examining sensitive areas of the body, you need to communicate well with your patients, clearly explaining each aspect of the exam and why it is important prior to beginning. Obtain verbal consent and have a chaperone in the room to assist and observe.

Trauma-Informed Care

- Many patients have experienced physical or sexual trauma in their lifetime, which they may or may not disclose.
- Providers can create a safer space for trauma-informed care if they explain carefully, ask permission, take their time, move slowly, and empower the patient to opt out or stop the exam at any time. Apply the same principles discussed in Chapter 11, the Gynecologic exam.

THE GENITAL EXAM

Indications for Performing the Male Genital Exam

- To explore genital area symptoms (eg, testicular mass or pain, penile discharge).
- To assess for genital area findings in patients with systemic disorders or risk factors that can manifest in this region of the body.

Preparing and Positioning the Patient

- If they have not already done so, ask the patient to remove their underwear and put on a gown.
- It is easier to examine the penis and testicles with the patient standing and the examiner seated or standing in front of them. If that is not possible, the exam can also be performed with the patient supine on the table.

Observation and Examination of the Penis and Scrotum

- Expose the area to be examined. If the patient is standing, have them lift up their gown. If supine, ask them to pull their gown up so that the area is exposed, using a sheet to cover the rest of the body.
- Put on a pair of non-sterile gloves.
- Make note of the main anatomic structures as identified in **Figure 9-1**: glans and shaft of the penis, urethral opening, testicles, and scrotum.
- Note any obvious skin abnormalities on the penis, scrotum, or surrounding areas.

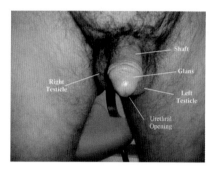
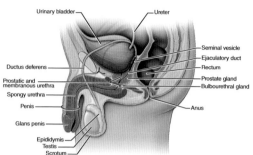

FIGURE 9-1 · Male genital anatomy. (Left photo: From Practical *Guide to Clinical Medicine: Male Genital and Rectal Exam.* Available from: https://meded.ucsd.edu/clinicalmed/genital.html. Right illustration: Reproduced with permission from Morton DA, Foreman KB, Albertine KH. *The Big Picture: Gross Anatomy, Medical Course & Step 1 Review.* 2nd ed. New York: McGraw Hill; 2019.)

- Examine the glans (ie, the head of the penis).
- If the patient is uncircumcised, draw back the foreskin so that you can look at the glans in its entirety.
  - Make sure that you return the foreskin to its normal position.
- Examine the shaft and the base of the penis for any skin abnormalities (eg, pigmented areas, ulcers, vesicles), in particular if the patient complains of seeing or feeling something in that region.
- Observe the scrotum. You will need to gently move the penis in order to thoroughly evaluate this area.
- Palpate any abnormal-appearing area to further characterize it (eg, to determine if it is a process within the scrotal wall vs deeper structures).

PEARL: Adequate exposure of the genital area is critical in order to identify external abnormalities.

Findings and Their Meaning: Genital Area Skin Findings

Common skin findings in the genital region are described in **Table 9-1**.

TABLE 9-1 · Diagnoses at a Glance: Skin Findings in the Genital Region

Condition	Etiology and Symptoms	Findings
Herpes simplex virus (HSV)	• Spread through sexual contact • Can occur in men or women; in the perirectal, oral, and genital areas • There is sometimes a burning discomfort days prior to appearance of clear vesicle(s) on a red base • Vesicle(s) resolve(s) spontaneously in 1-3 weeks • Recurs in 70%-90% of cases	(Reproduced with permission from Taylor SC, Kelly AP, Lim HW, Serrano AMA, eds. *Taylor and Kelly's Dermatology for Skin of Color.* 2nd ed. New York: McGraw Hill; 2016, Figure 58-7.)

(Continued)

TABLE 9-1 • Diagnoses at a Glance: Skin Findings in the Genital Region (Continued)

Condition	Etiology and Symptoms	Findings
Syphilis-related ulcer	• Spread through sexual contact • First manifestation of syphilis; can later have systemic symptoms and findings (secondary, tertiary, neurologic) • Occurs on average 3 weeks after sexual encounter • Can occur in men or women; in the perirectal, oral, and genital areas; may go unrecognized • Painless and resolves spontaneously	 (Reproduced with permission from Kang S, Amagai M, Bruckner AL, et al, eds. *Fitzpatrick's Dermatology*. 9th ed. New York: McGraw Hill; 2019, Figure 170-3.)
Human papillomavirus (HPV)–associated condyloma	• Spread through sexual contact • Can occur in men or women; in the perirectal, oral, and genital areas • Painless warts, occurring singly or in clusters • Can regress spontaneously or persist	 (Reproduced with permission from Wolff K, Johnson RA, Saavedra AP, Roh EK. *Fitzpatrick's Color Atlas and Synopsis of Clinical Dermatology*. 8th ed. New York: McGraw Hill; 2017, Figure 30-1.)
Pearly penile papules	• Small (1-2 mm) papules, on edge of glans • Asymptomatic and unchanging with time • Normal and common (19% incidence) • Have no clinical significance, although it can cause concern for patients if mistaken for warts	 (Reproduced with permission from Wolff K, Johnson RA, Saavedra AP, Roh EK. *Fitzpatrick's Color Atlas and Synopsis of Clinical Dermatology*. 8th ed. New York: McGraw Hill; 2017, Figure 34-1.)
Balanitis (inflammation of the glans)	• Red, itchy, sometimes painful eruption on head of penis; sometimes discharge also present • Typically from *Candida*, related to moist environments (uncircumcised); can also result from bacteria, contact • Predisposed if patient has poorly controlled diabetes	 (From Usatine RP, Smith MA, Mayeaux EJ Jr, Chumley HS. *The Color Atlas and Synopsis of Family Medicine*. 3rd ed. New York: McGraw Hill; 2019, Figure 142-1. Reproduced with permission from Richard P. Usatine, MD.)

Findings and their Meaning: Disorders Associated With the Foreskin—Paraphimosis and Phimosis

- If the foreskin is not replaced so that it covers the head of the penis, it can cause paraphimosis. This is when the foreskin is trapped behind the glans, leading to venous and arterial obstruction (**Figure 9-2**, left). This in turn can cause necrosis of the head of the penis.
  - Returning the foreskin over the glans prevents this from occurring.
- Phimosis, by contrast, occurs when foreskin cannot be retracted from its position covering the glans (Figure 9-2, right). This is a chronic condition, resulting from adhesions between the glans and foreskin. It can interfere with hygiene of the glans and obstruct urination.

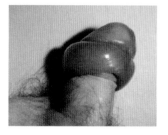 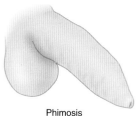

Phimosis

FIGURE 9-2 · **Paraphimosis and phimosis.** (Left photo: From Knoop KJ, Stack LB, Storrow AB, Thurman RJ, eds. *The Atlas of Emergency Medicine.* 5th ed. New York: McGraw-Hill; 2021, Figure 8.22. Reproduced with permission from photo contributor: Lawrence B. Stack, MD. Right illustration: Reproduced with permission from Tintinalli JE, Ma OJ, Yealy DM, et al, eds. *Tintinalli's Emergency Medicine: A Comprehensive Study Guide.* 9th ed. New York: McGraw Hill; 2020.)

Examining the Testes and Cord Structures

- The testes produce sperm and testosterone and are located in the scrotum. The coiled, sperm-producing tubules within the testis are connected to the epididymis, located at the top of each testicle. During ejaculation, the vas deferens carries sperm from the epididymis, through the prostate, to the penis (**Figures** 9-1 and **9-3**).
- The testes should appear as 2 discrete swellings, although if the room is particularly cold, they may retract toward the inguinal canal (see Figure 9-8).

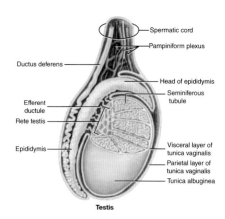

Testis

FIGURE 9-3 · **Anatomy of testicles.** (Reproduced with permission from Hoffman BL, Schorge JO, Halvorson LM, et al, eds. *Williams Gynecology.* 4th ed. New York: McGraw Hill; 2020.)

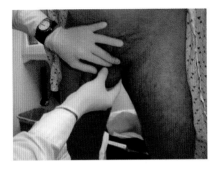

FIGURE 9-4 · **Examining the testes.** (Photo from *Practical Guide to Clinical Medicine: Male Genital and Rectal Exam.* Available from: https://meded.ucsd.edu/clinicalmed/genital.html.)

- Gently examine each testicle separately. Palpate using your thumb and next 2 fingers of your examining hand (**Figure 9-4**).
- Each testicle should be of the same consistency and size. If there is a significant difference in size (or absence of one of the testes), ask the patient if this has always been the case. They may have had one surgically removed or perhaps suffer from a congenitally undescended testis.
- Identify the epididymis, a discrete structure that lies toward the top of each testis.
- The vas deferens, testicular artery/vein, ilioinguinal nerve, lymphatics, and fatty tissue make up the spermatic cord, which runs from the epididymis up through the inguinal canal. The vas can sometimes be distinguished from the rest of these structures as it feels firm and wire-like.

Findings and Their Meaning: Testicular Mass or Enlargement

- The presence of a firm, discrete nodule in the testis raises the possibility of testicular cancer. This is typically slow growing and painless, requiring additional evaluation (ultrasound and referral to a urologist).
- Occasionally, the entire testis feels enlarged. This is most commonly caused by a hydrocele, which is a collection of fluid that fills a potential space surrounding the testis (**Figure 9-5**).

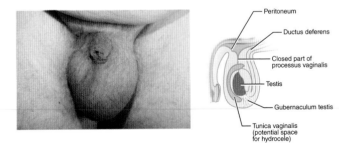

FIGURE 9-5 · **Anatomy and appearance of a hydrocele (left testicle in photo).** (Left photo: From Knoop KJ, Stack LB, Storrow AB, Thurman RJ, eds. *The Atlas of Emergency Medicine.* 5th ed. New York: McGraw-Hill; 2021, Figure 8.13A. Reproduced with permission from photo contributor: David Bryson. Reproduced from Bryson D. Transillumination of testicular hydrocele. *Clin Med Img Lib.* 2017;3(3):075. Right illustration: Reproduced with permission from Tintinalli JE, Ma OJ, Yealy DM, et al, eds. *Tintinalli's Emergency Medicine: A Comprehensive Study Guide.* 9th ed. New York: McGraw Hill; 2020.)

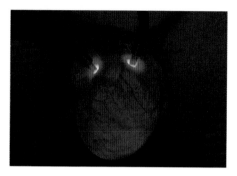

FIGURE 9-6 · **Transillumination of hydrocele, left testicle.** (From Knoop KJ, Stack LB, Storrow AB, Thurman RJ, eds. *The Atlas of Emergency Medicine.* 5th ed. New York: McGraw-Hill; 2021, Figure 8.13B. Reproduced with permission from photo contributor: David Bryson. Reproduced from Bryson D. *Transillumination of testicular hydrocele. Clin Med Img Lib.* 2017;3(3):075.)

- Hydroceles have a characteristic texture that is different from that of testicular tissue.
- You can also distinguish them from the body of the testis by transillumination (**Figure 9-6**). To assess, shut off the lights in the exam room and place a light on the scrotum, directly over the area in question.
- The fluid in a hydrocele allows the transmission of light, whereas testicular tissue will not.
- Acute testicular enlargement can be caused by infection within the body of the testis (orchitis).
- This is typically the result of infection that has spread from the bladder/prostate (urinary tract) or urethra (urethritis from sexually transmitted infection).
- The entire testicle, typically including the epididymis, becomes enlarged. The inflammation can spread from the testis to the skin of the scrotum, with resulting edema and erythema (**Figure 9-7**).
- There is no transillumination, as the inflamed testis does not allow the passage of light.
- Associated symptoms may include testicular pain, fevers/chills, malaise, urinary urgency, frequency, and dysuria.

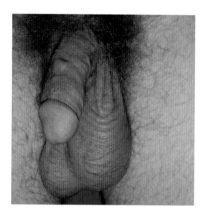

FIGURE 9-7 · Orchitis of left testicle. The left side of scrotum appears larger, with overlying redness and decreased wrinkles due to edema. (From Knoop KJ, Stack LB, Storrow AB, Thurman RJ, eds. *The Atlas of Emergency Medicine.* 5th ed. New York: McGraw-Hill; 2021, Figure 8.10. Reproduced with permission from photo contributor: Lawrence B. Stack, MD.)

- Testicular torsion is an acute process caused by spontaneous twisting of the testicle.
  - This compromises blood flow through the cord structures, causing acute ischemia and testicular demise if not addressed emergently.
  - It's associated with acute, severe, pain – most commonly occurring age <6 m and 10-20 yo.
  - The affected testicle may appear to be higher in the scrotum than normal, horizontally oriented, enlarged and tender (See Chapter 21, Adolescent Exam, Figure 21-3).
  - This is an emergency, requiring prompt evaluation by a urologist.

Findings and Their Meaning: Varicocele and Epididymal Cysts

- Dilated veins within the cord are referred to as a varicocele. They are discrete structures and are sometimes described as feeling like a bag of worms.
- Varicoceles are typically nontender on exam. Usually there are no external findings, although larger varicoceles may cause visible bulges through the scrotal skin. They are usually idiopathic and sometimes associated with infertility.
- Epididymal cysts are small, firm, nontender nodules within the epididymis. They are usually asymptomatic and do not have clinical significance.

EVALUATION FOR INGUINAL HERNIAS

- Hernias are a protrusion of intra-abdominal contents through a weakening of the structures that typically keep them contained within the abdominal cavity. In the inguinal region, these hernias are referred to as direct or indirect (most common) based on the path that they take (**Figure 9-8**).
- The exam may be notable for a bulge in the inguinal canal area on observation if the hernia is large (**Figure 9-9**).

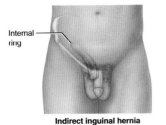
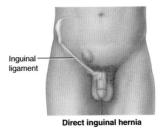

Internal ring

Inguinal ligament

Indirect inguinal hernia

Direct inguinal hernia

FIGURE 9-8 · **Inguinal area hernias.** (Reproduced with permission from Knoop KJ, Stack LB, Storrow AB, Thurman RJ, eds. *The Atlas of Emergency Medicine.* 5th ed. New York: McGraw-Hill; 2021.)

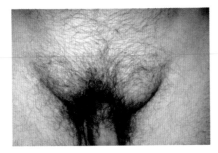

FIGURE 9-9 · **Left inguinal bulge.** (From Knoop KJ, Stack LB, Storrow AB, Thurman RJ, eds. *The Atlas of Emergency Medicine.* 5th ed. New York: McGraw-Hill; 2021, Figure 7.54. Reproduced with permission from photo contributor: Lawrence B. Stack, MD.)

- Before palpating this region, have the patient bear down (ie, Valsalva) or cough (ask them to turn their head so they do not cough on top of you) while you look at the inguinal region. Both of these maneuvers increase intra-abdominal pressure, making a hernia more apparent.
- If you are examining the right inguinal region, place the index finger of your right hand along the spermatic cord, inverting the scrotal skin as you trace the cord to where it emerges from the external ring of the inguinal canal. Place your other hand over the canal (**Figure 9-10**).
- Have the patient repeat the above maneuvers that increase intra-abdominal pressure and note if you can feel, with either hand, any bulging tissue that would be consistent with a hernia.

> **PEARL:** Subtle inguinal hernias can be appreciated when you ask the patient to Valsalva or cough while one hand is positioned over the inguinal canal and the finger of the other is placed along the cord.

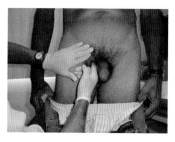 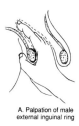

A. Palpation of male
external inguinal ring

FIGURE 9-10 · **Inguinal hernia exam.** (Left photo: From *Practical Guide to Clinical Medicine: Male Genital and Rectal Exam*. Available from: https://meded.ucsd.edu/clinicalmed/genital.html. Right illustration: Reproduced with permission from Suneja M, Szot JF, LeBlond RF, Brown DD. *DeGowin's Diagnostic Examination*. 11th ed. New York: McGraw Hill; 2020.)

- Exam of the left inguinal area is done in the same way, although hand positioning is reversed.
- Auscultation on top of a hernia may allow the detection of bowel sounds, which can be useful information if you are unsure as to the nature of an inguinal bulge.
- In the event that the patient is unable to stand, the examination can be performed as described, but with the patient supine.
- Inguinal hernias come in all sizes; they are sometimes restricted to the inguinal canal but, at other times, can extend into the scrotum.
- Distinguishing direct from indirect hernias based on exam is not clinically important as both should generally be repaired (to reduce the risk of incarceration or strangulation, the most feared complications).
- Hernias are generally nontender, although they may cause a general discomfort or sense of fullness as they enlarge. Acute pain and inflammation suggest incarceration or strangulation of the entrapped contents, which is a surgical emergency.

RECTAL AND PROSTATE EXAMS

Indications for Performing Male Rectal and Prostate Exams

- Assessment of perirectal symptoms (eg, rectal pain, discharge, mass).
- To provide insights about gastrointestinal bleeding (eg, stool color), neurologic function (eg, rectal tone, perirectal sensation), and prostate pathology (see Table 9-3).
- Assessment of those at high risk for perirectal disease (eg, anal cancer in patient with history human papillomavirus).

Preparing and Positioning the Patient

- If they have not already done so, ask the patient to remove their underwear.
- Rectal and prostate evaluations can be performed with the patient either standing or lying on their side on the exam table (**Figure 9-11**).
- The approach to trauma-informed care was described previously.

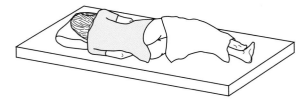
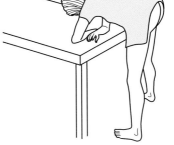

FIGURE 9-11 · **Positioning the patient for rectal and prostate exams.** (Reproduced with permission from Suneja M, Szot JF, LeBlond RF, Brown DD. *DeGowin's Diagnostic Examination*. 11th ed. New York: McGraw Hill; 2020.)

Examination of the Perirectal Area

- Make sure to explain everything that you are doing ahead of time to the patient (and why). If the patient is lying on an exam table, the remainder of their body should be covered. Ask them to turn onto their side and slide close to the edge of the table. Their knees should be tucked up tightly toward their chest. You may either sit or stand.
- For the standing exam, ask the patient to turn around and rest their chest on the exam table. This gives you an opportunity to perform the exam while providing the patient with something to lean against for support. The examiner may sit or stand.
- Separate the cheeks of the buttocks and look at the perirectal area. It is important to have adequate lighting.
- Make note of any abnormalities (common ones are described in **Table 9-2**).

TABLE 9-2 • Diagnoses at a Glance: Common Perirectal Disorders		
Condition	Etiology and Symptoms	Findings
External hemorrhoids (nonthrombosed)	· Visible on exam · Symptoms can be itching and painless bleeding · Caused by chronic straining during bowel movements	(Reproduced with permission from Suneja M, Szot JF, LeBlond RF, Brown DD. *DeGowin's Diagnostic Examination*. 11th ed. New York: McGraw Hill; 2020, Figure 9-29.)

(Continued)

TABLE 9-2 • Diagnoses at a Glance: Common Perirectal Disorders (Continued)		
Condition	Etiology and Symptoms	Findings
External hemorrhoids (thrombosed)	• Acute perirectal pain • Visible on exam • May have a history of nonthrombosed external hemorrhoids, with painless bleeding • Painful on palpation and vary in size	 (From Knoop KJ, Stack LB, Storrow AB, Thurman RJ, eds. *The Atlas of Emergency Medicine*. 5th ed. New York: McGraw-Hill; 2021, Figure 9.49. Reproduced with permission from photo contributor: Lawrence B. Stack, MD.)
Internal hemorrhoids	• Typically painless and not visible on external exam • Produce painless bleeding • When large, they may prolapse (protrude) to variable degrees • Typically caused by chronic straining with bowel movements	 Internal hemorrhoids (Reproduced with permission from Tintinalli JE, Ma OJ, Yealy DM, et al, eds. *Tintinalli's Emergency Medicine: A Comprehensive Study Guide*. 9th ed. New York: McGraw Hill; 2020.)
Anal fissure	• An acute tear of the external mucosa • Acute, significant pain when attempting bowel movement • Sometimes with small amounts of bleeding • Associated with constipation and chronic straining	 Rectal fissure and skin tag. (Photo from *Practical Guide to Clinical Medicine: Male Genital and Rectal Exam*. Available from: https://meded.ucsd.edu/clinicalmed/genital.html.)

(Continued)

TABLE 9-2 • Diagnoses at a Glance: Common Perirectal Disorders (Continued)		
Condition	Etiology and Symptoms	Findings
Perirectal condyloma	• Usually subacute and painless growths • Result from human papillomavirus (HPV) infection, spread through sexual contact • HPV is risk factor for squamous cancer of the anus	 (From Knoop KJ, Stack LB, Storrow AB, Thurman RJ, eds. *The Atlas of Emergency Medicine.* 5th ed. New York: McGraw-Hill; 2021. Reproduced with permission from photo contributor: Lawrence B. Stack, MD.) • Appear as single or multiple growths • Can increase in size and number • Can have similar findings in the genital area
Perirectal abscess	• Acute pain and swelling in perirectal area • May be associated with systemic symptoms of fevers, chills, and sweats if large	 (From Usatine RP, Smith MA, Mayeaux EJ Jr, Chumley HS. *The Color Atlas and Synopsis of Family Medicine.* 3rd ed. New York, McGraw Hill; 2019, Figure 68-5. Reproduced with permission from Charlie Goldberg, MD, copyright University of California, San Diego.) • On exam, there is a tender, often fluctuant area extending from the anal area to buttocks

Findings and Their Meaning: Perirectal Pathology

Common perirectal pathology is described in Table 9-2. Review of the normal anatomy of the colon, rectum, and anus helps to understand potential structural abnormalities (**Figure 9-12**).

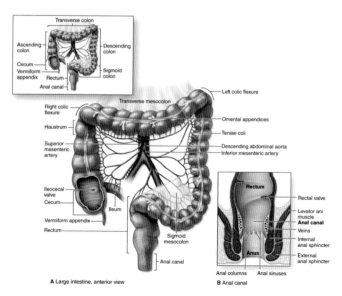

FIGURE 9-12 · **Normal anatomy of rectum and anus.** (Reproduced with permission from McKinley M, O'Loughlin VD. *Human Anatomy*. 2nd ed. New York: McGraw-Hill; 2021.)

The Digital Rectal Exam

- Place lubricant on the index finger of the examining hand.
- Place the well-lubricated index finger against the patient's anus, but do not yet place it into the rectum.
- Ask the patient to bear down as if they are trying to have a bowel movement. This helps to relax their external sphincter and should decrease discomfort. As they bear down, gently push forward until you have placed the entire finger within the anal canal.
- Rarely, there can be stenosis of the anus from an infiltrating process (eg, cancer) or scarring from prior inflammatory processes. If there is pain or your finger does not easily enter, stop and limit your exam to external palpation. Further exploration of stenosis typically requires referral to someone with appropriate expertise.
- As your finger enters, make note if it encounters any resistance. It may run into stool, which should easily move out of the way. A mass (eg, a rectal tumor) will not move. If this occurs, do not force your finger forward.
- Gently rotate your hand. Use the pad of your index finger to feel to the left, right, and then directly posterior (ie, toward yourself) and along the sacrum. Make note of any irregularities or masses.
- Orient your finger so that it is directed anteriorly (ie, toward the patient's umbilicus). It should now be resting on the prostate gland, which is palpated through the wall of the rectum (**Figure 9-13**).
- The prostate has 2 lobes with a cleft running between them. The lobes should feel symmetric. Firm nodules (or areas of diffuse firmness) are concerning for malignancy.
- Prostatic tenderness and induration can indicate infection.

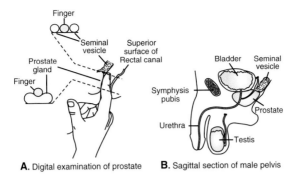

A. Digital examination of prostate   **B.** Sagittal section of male pelvis

FIGURE 9-13 • **Position of finger during digital rectal exam relative to prostate.** (Reproduced with permission from Suneja M, Szot JF, LeBlond RF, Brown DD. *DeGowin's Diagnostic Examination.* 11th ed. New York: McGraw Hill; 2020.)

- Note the size of the prostate. As you perform more exams, you'll develop an informed sense of what is normal versus enlarged. In general, you should be able to get your finger over the top of the gland. This may be difficult if:
  - The patient is obese and/or has large gluteal cheeks
  - You have small fingers
  - They have a big prostate
- Symptoms and findings associated with common conditions affecting the prostate are presented in **Table 9-3**.

TABLE 9-3 • Diagnoses at a Glance: Common Disorders Affecting the Prostate Gland		
Pathologic Process Affecting the Prostate	Symptoms	Findings
Benign prostatic hypertrophy (BPH) • A disorder related to the normal process of prostate gland enlargement, typically beginning at age >50 • As it enlarges, the prostate can mechanically interfere with (obstruct) the flow of urine from the bladder • The prostate can also cause irritative symptoms related to its growth	• Typically chronic and progressive • Obstructive symptoms: decreased force of stream, longer time required to void, hesitancy, difficulty starting/stopping stream • Irritative symptoms: urgency, frequency, nocturia, need to void again soon after urinating • Can cause acute or chronic kidney injury related to obstruction and subsequent hydronephrosis • Can also predispose to lower urinary tract infections if there is a high post void residual volume (urine remaining in bladder after urination).	• The prostate gland feels symmetrically large on digital rectal exam (DRE). • The consistency of the prostate should be uniform • There should not be any focal nodules or other areas of firmness that might suggest cancer • Rarely this is associated with a palpable bladder, which occurs if there is a significant amount of urinary retention leading to very high postvoid residual volumes over time

(Continued)

TABLE 9-3 • Diagnoses at a Glance: Common Disorders Affecting the Prostate Gland (Continued)

Pathologic Process Affecting the Prostate	Symptoms	Findings
Prostate cancer • A disorder that occurs in some men, typically age >50 • Other risk factors include family history, black patients	• Early in the course, it is asymptomatic • Notable that cancer can coexist with BPH because they have similar risk factors • Cancer can cause urgency, frequency, delayed emptying, and hematuria, none of which are specific • Metastatic disease causes bone pain. A common site is the spine, although it can spread to any bones	• Focal, firm nodules on DRE; with early disease, smaller areas, in 1 lobe of prostate • As cancer spreads within the prostate, it causes diffuse firmness and can be in 1 or both lobes; it can also spread to the seminal vesicles, which are at the top of the prostate • Bone pain that is progressive, otherwise unexplained, or associated with systemic symptoms is concerning for metastatic disease (prostate vs other)
Prostate infection (prostatitis) • Infection within the prostate • Typically spread from bladder, backward through the vas deferens into prostate • Typically gram-negative rods (same as other urinary tract infections); can also be related to urethritis from sexually transmitted infection (gonorrhea, chlamydia) • Can be acute or chronic (recurrent or persistent); similar organisms for both	• Acute: urinary frequency, urgency, dysuria, lower abdominal/pelvic pain • Can have fever, chills, systemic symptoms if severe • Chronic prostatitis typically causes persistent or recurrent urinary symptoms (urgency, frequency, dysuria, lower abdominal pain)	• Sometimes abnormal vital signs if acute, severe infection • Prostate tender on exam (pain elicited when the examining finger pushes on prostate) • Prostate itself may feel diffusely edematous; need to examine many prostates to develop an accurate sense of normal versus pathologic • Exam may be relatively normal, depending on magnitude of infection

- One helpful way of trying to feel the full extent of the prostate is to ask the patient to lean over the exam table (if standing), which has the effect of directing the prostate out toward you. If you still cannot adequately palpate the prostate, place your nonexamining hand on their anterior hip and draw the patient toward you as you push with your examining finger (**Figure 9-14**). Always inform the patient about what you are going to do and why. If the patient is lying on their side, direct them to pull their knees tightly toward their chest.

PEARL: Optimal positioning for the prostate exam is with the patient standing and leaning over the table, with the examiner seated or standing behind them.

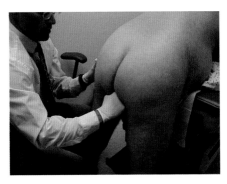

FIGURE 9-14 · **Positioning when examining the prostate with patient standing.** (Photo from *Practical Guide to Clinical Medicine: Male Genital and Rectal Exam.* Available from: https://meded.ucsd. edu/clinicalmed/genital.html.)

Assessment of Rectal Tone

- This can be done either at the beginning or the end of the examination, if there is concern for neurologic dysfunction (eg, if the patient has suggestive symptoms, such as fecal incontinence).
- In certain diseases of the central or peripheral nervous system, innervation of the sphincters that help maintain rectal continence may be affected (eg, in the setting of cauda equina syndrome, where there is sacral nerve root compression from a tumor or other mass), causing muscular tone to be diminished or absent.
- There is a certain subjective tightness that you will notice when your finger enters the rectum.
- You can further assess external sphincter tone by asking the patient to hold on to or squeeze your finger with their anus (explain why, as this is an unusual ask), allowing you to feel the contraction of this muscle.

> PEARL: Rectal tone can be appreciated by the general sense of pressure around the finger as it enters the anus. Asking the patient to "squeeze down" can make the tone more apparent.

Examination of the Stool

- There is often stool in the rectal vault that will coat your finger at the end of the exam. Inspect it after you withdraw your hand, in particular noting the color.

Findings and Their Meaning: Stool Color (**Figure 9-15**)

- Normal-appearing stool is brown.
- If there is bright red blood (ie, looks like typical blood), it implies that there is a bleeding source close to the anus.
  - This can be from hemorrhoids, colonic diverticula, polyps, inflammation (inflammatory bowel disease), cancer, arteriovenous malformation, or other causes.
  - Some of these processes are identifiable on exam (eg, external hemorrhoids), whereas others are internal and neither visible nor palpable.
  - Historical information can help, although definitive identification requires endoscopy.

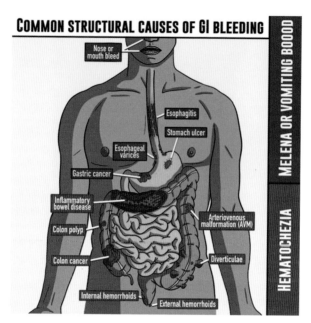

FIGURE 9-15 · Clinical connections: stool color and gastrointestinal bleeding. (Reproduced with permission from Cathy Cichon, MD.)

- When bleeding is from a more proximal source, the stool tends to appear darker (eg, maroon).
  - Rarely, bleeding from an upper gastrointestinal (GI) source (eg, esophagus, stomach, duodenum) can be of such large volume and so acute that it appears relatively red. More commonly, upper GI bleeding causes stool to have a darker color.
- Black, tarry (sticky) stool is referred to as melena (**Figure 9-16**). It occurs when blood released from the upper GI tract (esophagus, stomach, or duodenum) traverses the entire alimentary canal. It also has a characteristic odor. This can occur with any upper GI cause of bleeding (eg, gastric ulcers, varices, gastric or esophageal cancer). Black stools can also result from benign causes, such as ingestion of iron supplements or bismuth containing products (eg, Pepto Bismol).

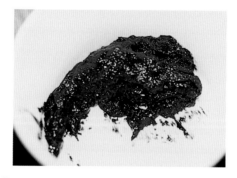

FIGURE 9-16 · **Melena.** (From Knoop KJ, Stack LB, Storrow AB, Thurman RJ, eds. *The Atlas of Emergency Medicine*. 5th ed. New York: McGraw-Hill; 2021. Reproduced with permission from photo contributor: Alan B. Storrow, MD.)

- Stool can be tested with a special agent designed to detect hemoglobin. This is referred to as assessing for occult blood (ie, blood that would not otherwise be identifiable). It is done if you are searching for objective evidence of GI blood loss when the stool appearance is equivocal or normal.

> **PEARL:** If there's concern for GI bleeding, looking at the color of the stool (either from a bowel movement or during physical exam) can provide important insights as to the anatomic source of the problem

Concluding the Exam

- Allow the patient to wipe themselves off with tissues. Provide them with privacy while they clean up and dress.
- To remove your stool-covered glove, take the index finger of your nonexamining hand (which should still be clean) and place it under the cuff of the other glove. Then pull that glove down toward your fingers, inverting it in the process.

TELEHEALTH TIPS

- Due to the sensitive nature of this exam, telehealth evaluation of this region is typically limited to history and counseling.
- Check with the patient to ensure they have privacy before continuing with sensitive history taking.
- Observation of sensitive organs may be completed following oral consent of the patient and agreement of the provider that use of the telehealth modality is clinically appropriate. Additionally, a chaperone is recommended for both patient and provider.
- Those with concerning symptoms or findings usually need to be referred for in-person evaluation with appropriate urgency.

SUMMARY OF SKILLS CHECKLIST

- ❏ Clean your hands and put on gloves
- ❏ Have chaperone present, discuss rational for exam with patient, obtain consent
- ❏ Position patient and yourself to perform genital exam
- ❏ Examine penis, testicles, epididymis, spermatic cord, and scrotum
- ❏ Examine inguinal area
- ❏ Position patient and yourself to perform rectal exam
- ❏ Examine perirectal area
- ❏ Perform digital rectal exam
- ❏ Allow patient opportunity to clean themselves
- ❏ Clean your hands

BIBLIOGRAPHY

Brock A, Cook JL, Nathaniel Ranney N, et al. A not-so-obscure cause of gastrointestinal bleeding (vascular ectasia). *N Engl J Med*. 2015;372:556-561.

Curhan GC. Chapter 318. Nephrolithiasis. In: Longo DL, et al, eds. *Harrison's Principles of Internal Medicine*. 21e. New York: McGraw-Hill; 2022.

Dixon JM, Elton RA, Rainey JB, Macleod DAD. Rectal examination in patients with pain in the right lower quadrant of the abdomen. *BMJ*. 1991;302:386-388.

Fitzgibbons R, Forse RA. Groin hernias in adults. *N Engl J Med*. 2015;372:756-763.

Goldberg C. UCSD's Practical Guide to clinical medicine: Male genital and rectal exam. Accessed December 30, 2022. https://meded.ucsd.edu/clinicalmed/genital.html.

Goldberg C. Digital DDx: Genitourinary and renal symptoms or conditions. Accessed December 31, 2022. http://digitalddx.com/symptoms_list/s&d_list/7/.

Gupta K, Trautner B. Urinary tract infection. *Ann Intern Med*. 2012;156(5):ITC3-1.

Hooton T. Uncomplicated urinary tract infection. *N Engl J Med*. 2012;366:1028-1037.

Rockey D. Occult gastrointestinal bleeding. *N Engl J Med*. 1999;341:38-46.

Rockey D, Cello JP. Evaluation of the gastrointestinal tract in patients with iron-deficiency anemia. *N Engl J Med*. 1993;329:1691-1695.

Schubert M, Sridhar S, Schade RR, et al. What every gastroenterologist needs to know about common ano-rectal disorders. *World J Gastroenterol*. 2009;15(26):3201-3209.

Sharma A, Wei JT. Benign prostatic hyperplasia and lower urinary tract symptoms. *N Engl J Med*. 2012;367:248-255.

Sharp VJ, Kieran K, Arlen AM. Testicular torsion: diagnosis, evaluation, and management. *Am Fam Phys*. 2013;88(12):835-840.

Sharp V, Takacs EB, Powell CR. Prostatitis: diagnosis and treatment. *Am Fam Phys*. 2010;82(4):397-406.

Talley N. How to do and interpret a rectal exam in GI. *Am J Gastroenterol*. 2008;103:820-822.

Trojian T, Lishnak TS, Heiman D. Epididymitis and orchitis: an overview. *Am Fam Phys*. 2009;79(7):583-587.

US Preventive Services Task Force. Recommendations for prostate cancer screening. Accessed December 30, 2022. https://www.uspreventiveservicestaskforce.org/uspstf/recommendation/prostate-cancer-screening.

Worcester E, Coe FL. Calcium kidney stones. *N Engl J Med*. 2010;363:954-963.

10

Breast Exam

Simerjot K. Jassal, MD

INTRODUCTION

Breast symptoms, including palpable mass, breast pain, and nipple discharge, are common. While most breast symptoms are due to a benign cause, breast cancer is one of the most common malignancies worldwide. It is the most common cancer in women (excluding nonmelanoma skin cancer) and the second most common cause of cancer death. 1 in 8 women in the United States will develop breast cancer in their lifetime. Evaluation should include a thorough medical and family history to assess risk and a clinical breast examination and breast imaging.

Most breast cancers are diagnosed by mammography, but approximately 25% of breast cancers are initially identified as a self-palpated mass. Less-frequent symptoms are breast pain; nipple discharge; erosion, retraction, enlargement, or itching of the nipple; and redness, generalized hardness, enlargement, or retraction of the breast. The breast-related history should include the following:

- When the mass or abnormality was first noticed
- Changes in size over time
- Associated pain and symptoms such as skin changes or nipple discharge
- Risk factors for breast cancer: age, deleterious *BRCA1/BRCA2* genes, history of chest radiation, history of atypical hyperplasia on biopsy, mother or sister with breast cancer, nulliparity, first-term pregnancy at or after age 30 years, menarche before age 12, menopause after age 55, dense breast, history of benign breast biopsy, alcohol use (>2 drinks per day), and postmenopausal combination hormonal therapy
- Ancestry: 1 in 40 people of Ashkenazi Jewish ancestry may carry a germline *BRCA* pathogenic mutation

Self-examination is not recommended for average-risk women by the American Cancer Society (ACS), American College of Obstetricians and Gynecologists (ACOG), or U.S. Preventive Services Task Force (USPSTF) due to lack of efficacy in the literature. ACOG recommends breast self-awareness for average-risk women, emphasizing patient education about breast changes.

INDICATIONS FOR PERFORMING THE BREAST EXAM

In the Asymptomatic Patient

The current guidelines for asymptomatic clinical breast examinations (CBEs) are controversial. Some guidelines (ACS and USPSTF) do not recommend CBEs for average-risk women because of conflicting efficacy in the literature. No studies demonstrate that it improves clinical outcomes (ie, detects cancer at an earlier stage, demonstrating positive impact on cancer-related morbidity or mortality) when performed as a stand-alone examination. Other guidelines (ACOG) advise CBEs may be offered to women at average risk with shared decision making.

In the Symptomatic Patient

The goal of the examination in the setting of symptoms is to better characterize the abnormality, identify underlying etiology, and direct additional evaluation and treatment. Breast symptoms in any patient merit careful history taking and, if indicated, evaluation of other organ systems. Breast symptoms may be caused by diseases elsewhere in the body. For example, inappropriate milk production may be due to a prolactin-secreting pituitary tumor, or breast enlargement in men may signify underlying liver disease.

Breast-related symptoms may include any of the following:

- *Discrete masses* detected by the patient, which may be benign or malignant
- *Pain*, which can be associated with benign hormonal changes in premenopausal women or, less commonly, malignancies
- *Unusual nipple discharge*, including blood or milk in a nonlactating woman
- *Discoloration or change in the quality of the skin*

ANATOMY AND FUNCTION

The breast is made up of milk-producing glands that are arranged into units known as lobules (**Figure 10-1**). These glands are connected via a series of ducts that join to form a common drainage path, terminating at the nipple. The nipple is surrounded by a ring of pigmented tissue known as the areola. Fibroelastic and fatty tissue provide support. The breast lies over the pectoralis muscle, on the thoracic cage. Each breast contains a network of lymphatic tissue, approximately 90% of which drains into a lymph node group in the ipsilateral axilla. The remaining 10% drains into the internal thoracic nodes, which are located beneath the sternum (not accessible by exam).

Boundaries of the breast are as follows:

- Superiorly by the clavicle
- Inferiorly by the inframammary crease
- Medially by the sternum
- Laterally by the latissimus dorsi

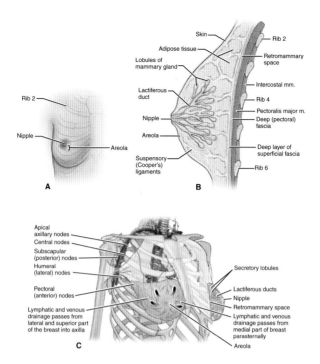

FIGURE 10-1 · Breast anatomy. (Reproduced with permission from Morton DA, Foreman KB, Albertine KH. *The Big Picture: Gross Anatomy, Medical Course & Step 1 Review.* 2nd ed. New York: McGraw Hill; 2019.)

PREPARATION

- Breast exams are sensitive and require discussion with the patient prior to beginning. This should include the reason the exam is recommended, the steps involved, and obtaining your patient's verbal consent prior to proceeding. Empower the patient to opt out or end the exam at any time if needed. Apply the same principles of trauma informed care discussed in Chapter 11, the Gynecologic Exam.
- Always have a chaperone with you when conducting a breast exam, to observe and assist, regardless of provider gender; document that you have done so.
- Give the patient privacy to undress from the waist up (including removing undergarments) and change into a gown.
- Have the patient put on the gown so that it opens in the front, which may make uncovering one breast at a time easier.

> **PEARL:** Explain in general terms what you are doing at each step: *"I'm looking on the outside first. Everything appears healthy and normal."*

Observation

- Visually examine both breasts initially in the upright position; have the patient uncover both breasts so that you can compare for differences or asymmetry.
- Observe with the arms hanging to the sides and with the arms overhead (**Figure 10-2**).

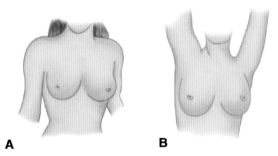

A   **B**

FIGURE 10-2 · **Breast observation.** (Reproduced with permission from Brunicardi FC, Andersen DK, Billiar TR, et al, eds. *Schwartz's Principles of Surgery.* 11th ed. New York: McGraw Hill; 2019.)

- Abnormal variations in breast size and contour, nipple retraction, edema, redness, or retraction of the skin can be identified.
- Asymmetry of the breasts and retraction or dimpling of the skin can often be accentuated by having the patient raise their arms overhead or press their hands on their hips to contract the pectoralis muscles.

> PEARL: Visually examine the breast and palpate the axillae with the patient seated. This improves your ability to identify visible abnormalities and palpate abnormal axillary nodes.

Findings and Their Meaning: Visible Abnormalities (Figure 10-3)

- Skin or nipple dimpling or retraction may result from a cancer growing underneath that area.
- Discoloration
  - Redness suggests infection or inflammation; in the postpartum patient, this is often due to mastitis, a diffuse inflammatory condition caused by congestion from inadequately expressed milk.
  - In a nonlactating patient, redness can represent inflammatory breast cancer. The skin may have a "peau d'orange" (orange peel) texture, caused by an uncommon, aggressive inflammatory malignancy.

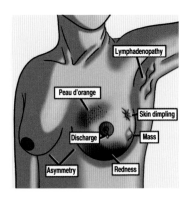

FIGURE 10-3 · **Visible abnormalities of the breast.** (Reproduced with permission from Cathy Cichon, MD.)

- Obvious masses: These may represent a benign finding or malignancy.
- Asymmetry between the 2 breasts: Although it is normal for there to be some asymmetry in size between the breasts, asymmetry can also be a sign of malignancy.

PALPATION OF THE AXILLA

- Evaluate the axillary lymph nodes with the patient seated because this improves the sensitivity of the axillary lymph node exam. The axillary lymph nodes are usually the first site of spread in the setting of breast cancer. Include the axilla in all of your breast exams.
- Have the patient rest their hand on your arm or shoulder, or support their arm with your nonexamining hand. This allows the arm and supporting structures to relax, which facilitates palpation. Use your left hand when examining the right axilla and your right hand when examining the left axilla. Direct the fingertips of the examining hand toward the apex of the axilla, anteriorly against the pectoralis muscle, posteriorly against the latissimus dorsi, and superiorly along the upper, inner aspect of the patient's arm. Then push the palmar aspect of the hand toward the chest wall. Identify any abnormal nodules or lumps that could represent axillary adenopathy (**Figure 10-4**).
- The axillary exam can be repeated when the patient is lying down.
- Most patients will not have palpable axillary lymph nodes. If you do feel discrete masses, make note of their number, firmness, and mobility. In general, malignancy is associated with firmness and adherence to each other and/or the chest wall.
- Adenopathy can be due to nonbreast pathology, including infections of the hand or systemic diseases. The rest of the history and exam will support these causes.

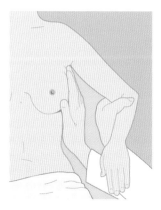

FIGURE 10-4 · **Palpating the axilla.** (Reproduced with permission from Papadakis MA, McPhee SJ, Rabow MW, McQuaid KR, eds. *Current Diagnosis & Treatment 2022.* New York: McGraw Hill; 2022.)

PALPATION OF THE BREAST

- The breasts should be palpated starting with the uninvolved breast first (if there is an area of concern).
- Have the patient lie flat on the table, and ask them to place the hand on the side to be examined behind their head, allowing easier access to breast and axilla (**Figure 10-5**).

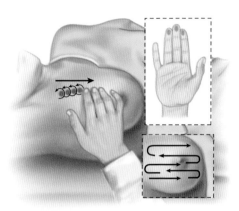

FIGURE 10-5 · Patient positioning and breast exam technique. (Reproduced with permission from Hoffman BL, Schorge JO, Halvorson LM, et al, eds. *Williams Gynecology*. 4th ed. New York: McGraw Hill; 2020.)

- Uncover only the breast that you are going to examine.
- All components of the exam should be done gently, with clear explanations provided about what to expect prior to each step.
- Examine the breast in a systematic fashion, ensuring all the tissue is palpated. The accuracy of the exam is increased by allowing adequate time. Time varies based on breast size. It can be technically challenging to assure that you have done a thorough examination of all the tissue in larger breasts. It may take 3 or more minutes to examine each breast.
- Use the pads of the middle 3 fingers of one hand (Figure 10-5).
- Press downward using a circular motion.
- Apply steady pressure to palpate to 3 levels of depth: first light, then medium, and then deep/to the level of the chest wall.
- Palpate the nipple and areolar regions.

While there are different methods of approaching the breast examination, the most important aspect is to palpate all of the tissue, including the axilla.

Three Methods for Systematic Examination of the Breast

Method 1: Vertical Strips Pattern

- Divide the breast into a series of overlapping vertical strips, evaluate each sequentially (Figure 10-5).
- Start at the clavicle, adjacent to the axilla.
- Move your hand down in a vertical line until you have reached the area below the breast.
- Then move a few centimeters medially and examine while moving up toward the top of the breast.
- When you reach the clavicle, move your fingers medially and repeat until you have evaluated the entire breast.
- There is a "tail" of breast tissue that extends from the lateral aspect of the structure toward the axilla; palpate this region as well.

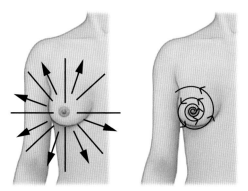

FIGURE 10-6 · Radial spoke and circular pattern techniques for systematic examination of the breast. (Drawing used from the UC San Diego School of Medicine. *Practical Guide to Clinical Medicine: Breast Exam.* Available from: https://meded.ucsd.edu/clinicalmed/breast.html.)

Method 2: Radial Spoke Pattern

- Divide the breast into a series of pie-type slices, with the nipple at the center (**Figure 10-6**).
- Start at the nipple, working outward toward the periphery of the slice that you are examining. Move your hands a few centimeters along each time.
- When you are clearly no longer over the breast, move to the next slice.
- Palpate the "tail" of the breast as described above.

Method 3: Concentric Circles Pattern

- Start at the nipple (Figure 10-6).
- Work along in circular fashion, moving in a spiral toward the periphery.
- Palpate the "tail" of the breast as described above.

After completing examination of the first breast, cover it and then uncover and examine the other breast. If space in the exam room allows, move to the other side of the table when examining the other breast.

> **PEARL:** No matter which technique you use, ensure that all of the breast tissue is palpated and that sufficient time is spent to thoroughly do so.

Findings and Their Meaning: Palpable Abnormalities

- Normal breasts have a lumpy consistency, created by the mix of lobular, ductal, and supporting tissue.
- Lobular tissue is replaced by fat with age; it is easier to identify masses in older patients.
- Masses:
  - Most masses are benign (**Table 10-1**).
  - Masses of concern tend to feel different from the rest of breast tissue (ie, "dominant mass") and firm, have irregular or hard-to-define borders, be fixed or stuck to adjacent tissue, and increase in size over time. Physical examination findings cannot reliably distinguish between a benign mass and a malignancy.
- If a mass or other abnormality is identified, it is important to clearly document the area of concern to allow accurate reidentification of the affected area for radiologic evaluation and for future clinical exams.

TABLE 10-1 • Differential Diagnosis of Breast Mass	
Type of Mass	Characteristics
Benign	
Fibroadenoma	Solid mass usually seen in young women; firm and often mobile; may be solid, multiple, or bilateral
Simple cyst	Fluid-filled mass; discrete, compressible, or ballotable; may be found in women of any age
Fibrocystic changes	Nodularity or diffuse thickening rather than a well-defined mass; may be bilateral, unilateral, or focal; common in premeno-pausal woman; may increase in size prior to onset of menses; associated tenderness may be cyclic
Galactocele	Milk retention cyst common in breastfeeding women
Fat necrosis	Breast mass that can develop after blunt trauma to the breast, or after injection of substances such as fat, paraffin, or silicone; an operative procedure; or radiation
Abscess	Localized collection of inflammatory exudate. Tender, often with inflamed overlying skin; fluctuance on palpation.
Malignant	
Infiltrating ductal carcinoma	Can be detected as a palpable mass; accounts for 70%-80% of invasive breast cancers
Infiltrating lobular carcinoma	Often presents as a prominent diffuse thickening of breast rather than as a discrete mass
Ductal carcinoma in situ	Rarely, noninvasive cancers with or without microinvasion can present as a palpable breast mass

- Although the quadrant system has been used in the past, a more precise way to document location of a mass is using the clock face system (**Figure 10-7**). Imagine that a clock face is superimposed on the breast. Use the numbers as a reference to describe the location of the abnormality. For example: "1 cm mobile, nontender, well-circumscribed mass at the 2 o'clock position of the left breast 6 cm from the edge of the areola."

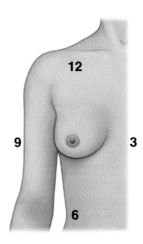

FIGURE 10-7 • **Describing location of an abnormality using the clock face system.** (Drawing used from the UC San Diego School of Medicine. *Practical Guide to Clinical Medicine: Breast Exam.* Available from: https://meded.ucsd.edu/clinicalmed/breast.html.)

- Describe the nature of the mass, including size, texture, mobility, well-circumscribed versus ill-defined borders, tender versus nontender to palpation, fluctuant, and with or without associated skin changes.

> PEARL: Thorough documentation of location and characteristics of a palpated abnormality will ensure that you or other clinicians (eg. a radiologist or surgeon) can identify the area on subsequent evaluation.

Tips to Consider and Pitfalls to Avoid

- Carefully evaluate any mass that the patient brings to your attention. Patients are often familiar with their bodies and can sometimes detect subtle or early changes concerning for malignancy that an examiner may not identify.
- Breast cancer can occur in young women (risk of invasive breast cancer is 1 in 2000 by age 30 and 1 in 233 by age 40). Masses should be appropriately evaluated regardless of age.
- While uncommon, breast cancer can occur in men (1 in 100 breast cancers are diagnosed in men). Any mass should be appropriately evaluated.
- Although not all masses represent malignancy, if you identify a discrete mass, it should be fully evaluated through examination, imaging, and, often, biopsy. A breast mass that does not have a corresponding abnormality on mammogram should still be evaluated for biopsy through referral to a breast surgeon. Exam and imaging alone cannot accurately distinguish a solid lesion as benign or malignant.

> PEARL: All palpated masses should be evaluated using clinical examination, imaging, and, if not definitely due to benign cause (eg, simple cyst), biopsy.

TELEHEALTH TIPS

- Due to the sensitive nature of this exam, telehealth evaluation of this region Is typically limited to history and counseling.
- Physical exam of sensitive organs may be completed following oral consent of the patient and agreement of the provider that use of the telehealth modality is clinically appropriate. Additionally, a chaperone is recommended for both patient and provider during the exam.
- Check with the patient to ensure they have privacy before continuing with sensitive history taking.

SUMMARY OF SKILLS CHECKLIST

- ❑ Explain rationale for exam and obtain verbal consent
- ❑ Give privacy while patient changes into gown
- ❑ Have chaperone present
- ❑ Clean your hands
- ❑ Guide patient verbally
- ❑ Examine the breasts visually with the patient seated
- ❑ Examine the axillae for lymph nodes with the patient seated
- ❑ Examine each breast thoroughly with the patient lying down
- ❑ Clean your hands
- ❑ Give patient privacy and time to dress
- ❑ Return to discuss findings and plan

BIBLIOGRAPHY

Goldberg C. Digital DDx (obstetric, gynecologic and breast symptoms or conditions). http://digitalddx.com/symptoms_list/9/. Accessed December 31, 2022.

Goldberg C. UCSD's practical guide to the clinical exam (breast exam section). Accessed November 11, 2022. https://meded.ucsd.edu/clinicalmed/breast.html.

Mango V, Bryce Y, Morris EA, Gianotti E, Pinker K. Commentary ACOG Practice Bulletin July 2017: Breast cancer risk assessment and screening in average-risk women. *Br J Radiol.* 2018;91(1090):20170907.

Nelson HD, Tyne K, Naik A, et al. Screening for breast cancer: an update for the U.S. Preventive Services Task Force. *Ann Intern Med.* 2009;151(10):727-737, W237-W242.

Oeffinger KC, Fontham ET, Etzioni R, et al. Breast cancer screening for women at average risk: 2015 guideline update from the American Cancer Society. *JAMA.* 2015;314(15):1599-1614. Erratum in: *JAMA.* 2016;315(13):1406.

Pleasant V. Management of breast complaints and high-risk lesions. *Best Pract Res Clin Obstet Gynaecol.* 2022;83:46-59.

Portnow LH, D'Alessio D, Morris EA, Bernard-Davila B, Mango V. Palpable breast findings in high-risk patients: are self- and clinical breast exams worthwhile? *J Breast Imaging.* 2021;3(2):190-195.

Practice Bulletin Number 179: breast cancer risk assessment and screening in average-risk women. *Obstet Gynecol.* 2017;130(1):e1-e16.

Siu AL; US Preventive Services Task Force. Screening for breast cancer: U.S. Preventive Services Task Force recommendation statement. *Ann Intern Med.* 2016;164(4):279-296. Erratum in: *Ann Intern Med.* 2016;164(6):448.

11

Gynecologic and Obstetric Pelvic Exam

Julia Cormano, MD

INTRODUCTION

A successful pelvic exam requires a conducive environment and good communication with your patient, as well as a gentle, trauma-informed care approach.

Let's Talk About Pronouns

The pronouns used in this chapter are she/hers and refer to a patient who identifies as female. However, it is important to remember to check with your patient about preferred pronouns. While anyone with gynecologic organs may need the examinations described in this chapter, it should not be assumed that your patient identifies as female. Be familiar with gender-neutral pronouns such as they, them, their, zie, ze, and hir.

Trauma-Informed Care

It is important to recognize the high prevalence and significant impact that a prior traumatic experience may have for your patient. Many patients have experienced physical or sexual trauma in their lifetime, which they may or may not disclose. Your patient's prior experience may impact your ability to conduct the exam and may mean your exam feels threatening or retraumatizing for them without your realizing it. Key aspects of trauma-informed care include the following:

- Creation of a physically and psychologically safe patient-provider relationship is critical to avoiding further psychological injury for your patient.
- Fostering your patient's sense of resiliency and control during your interactions improves overall health outcomes.
- Clearly explaining how the exam can help direct her care and asking her permission to proceed keeps the patient in a position of power during the exam. You can often still provide good care without a pelvic exam, if the patient declines.
- Providers can create a safer space for trauma-informed care if they take their time, move slowly, and empower the patient to stop the exam at any time.

Indications for Performing a Pelvic Exam

The decision to perform a pelvic examination should be collaborative between the patient and her provider. A pelvic exam should be performed when indicated by medical history or symptoms, typically for the following reasons:

- As part of preventative care for asymptomatic women to screen for gynecologic cancer and infection (eg, cervical cancer screening, sexually transmitted infection screening)
- Evaluation of a patient complaint of lower abdominal pain or vaginal symptoms (eg, abnormal vaginal bleeding or discharge, lower abdominal pain, vaginal mass or lesion, pelvic organ prolapse, urinary incontinence)
- As part of a routine full evaluation at the beginning of pregnancy
- Prior to a gynecologic procedure or surgery, to identify the size and shape of the uterus (eg, prior to intrauterine device placement)

GETTING STARTED

- Pelvic exams are invasive and require discussion with the patient prior to beginning. This should include the reason the exam is recommended, the steps involved, and obtaining your patient's verbal consent prior to proceeding. Empower the patient to opt out or end the exam at any time if needed.
- A chaperone should be present to observe and assist, regardless of provider gender.
- All necessary equipment should be readily available.
- The exam table should have footrests and be adjustable to maximize patient comfort, with an adjustable light source available. A goose-neck light or a lighted speculum works the best.
- Ideally, position your patient's bed so she is directed away from the door entry. Alternatively, ensure there is a curtain pulled around the table.
- Provide the patient with privacy so that they can put on a gown, drape, and remove undergarments.
- Keep the drape over her lower half for the entirety of the examination. Once she is positioned on the bed and you are seated, ask if she is ready to begin before lifting the drape to start your exam.
- All maneuvers should be done gently, with clear explanations provided about what to expect prior to each step.

Positioning

- The patient should be supine. Elevating the head of the table to 30 degrees usually makes the exam more comfortable and allows for eye contact (**Figure 11-1**).

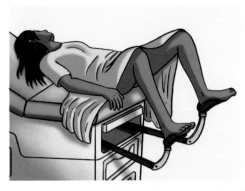

FIGURE 11-1 · **Pelvic exam positioning.** (Reproduced with permission from Cathy Cichon, MD.)

- Extend the footrests and ask the patient to place their feet in them. Encourage the patient to scoot toward the end of the table so that their sacrum is supported by the bottom edge, allowing the gluteal muscles to hang slightly over the edge. If the patient is not close enough to the edge of the table, speculum insertion will be difficult.
- Arrange the sheet so that that it covers up to their knees.
- Avoid unexpected or sudden movements. Monitor the comfort of the patient by watching their face.
- Ask the patient to position their legs so that there is space for you to sit and perform the exam. Use gentle verbal cues to assist them in positioning their legs such as, "Please relax your knees to the sides." Do not push the patient's legs open with your hands.

Examining Patients in the Emergency Department

Sometimes having your patient in a gynecology exam bed with footrests is not an option. This is particularly true in busy emergency departments or if a patient admitted to the hospital needs a gynecologic exam in a regular hospital bed. Get creative. You can use a bedpan! Place the bedpan upside down under the patient's sacrum, with a blanket or sheet covering it to make it less cold. Use a headlamp, flashlight, or a lighted speculum for visualization. Insist on appropriate privacy for your patient, usually with curtains.

EXTERNAL EXAM

Observation and Visual Inspection of Vulvar Area

Identify the following external structures (**Figure 11-2**):
- Mons pubis
- Labia majora
- Labia minora (has no hair)
- Prepuce (clitoral hood)
- Clitoris
- Urethral meatus (opening)

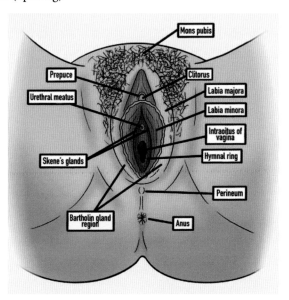

FIGURE 11-2 · External anatomy. (Reproduced with permission from Cathy Cichon, MD.)

- Skene's glands
- Hymenal ring (external to introitus)
- Vaginal opening (introitus)
- Bartholin glands areas
- Perineum
- Anus

> **PEARL:** Explain in general terms what you are doing at each step: *"I'm checking externally first. Everything appears healthy and normal."*

Palpation of discrete structures can be done as indicated by the presence of observed abnormalities or symptoms.

> **PEARL:** If palpation of a structure is indicated, let your patient know: *"You'll feel my touch as I look more carefully at your labia minora."*

Findings and Their Meaning: External Exam

What Is Normal to See?

- Physiologic discharge: Thin, white discharge without odor is often physiologic. During pregnancy and the luteal phase, the quantity of this discharge increases.
- Postmenopausal atrophy: Thinning of the tissues, especially vaginal mucosa, and less lubrication and discharge are normal after menopause.

Descriptions and images of common external exam pathologies are provided in **Table 11-1.**

TABLE 11-1 • Diagnosis at a Glance: Common Pathologic Findings Visible on the External Exam		
Structure	Findings	Pathology
Mons, labia majora, labia minora	Pustule and abscess	Plugged sebaceous gland cyst (sometimes called epidermoid cysts): White, typically <1 cm, may be multiple Abscess: Painful, fluctuant mass, red base, usually isolated
	Pedunculated lesions	Skin tags: Soft piece(s) of hanging skin, more common in patients with higher body mass index Condyloma acuminata (genital warts): Isolated or clusters of bumps, which often have a cauliflower-like appearance and may be itchy
	 Condyloma acuminata	(Reproduced with permission from Soutor C, Hordinsky MK. *Clinical Dermatology: Diagnosis and Management of Common Disorders.* 2nd ed. New York: McGraw Hill; 2022, Figure 32-15B.)

(Continued)

TABLE 11-1 • Diagnosis at a Glance: Common Pathologic Findings Visible on the External Exam (Continued)		
Structure	Findings	Pathology
	Irritated bumps	Molluscum: Multiple, round, painless, white or flesh-colored, dome-shaped papules 1-5 mm with central indentation
		Molluscum lesions (Reproduced with permission from Hoffman BL, Schorge JO, Halvorson LM, et al, eds. *Williams Gynecology*. 4th ed. New York: McGraw Hill; 2020, Figure 3-10.)
		Herpes: Clusters of vesicles on a red base, painful with burning and itching; can come and go spontaneously
		Herpes lesions (From Knoop KJ, Stack LB, Storrow AB, Thurman RJ, eds. *The Atlas of Emergency Medicine*. 5th ed. New York: McGraw-Hill; 2021, Figure 9.21. Reproduced with permission from photo contributor: Lawrence B. Stack, MD.)
	Skin discoloration	Lichen sclerosis: Chronic inflammatory disorder with itching, burning, and tearing; skin is thinned, whitened, and has a crinkled "cellophane appearance"; genital mucosa typically spared
		Lichen sclerosis (Reproduced with permission from Kang S, Amagai M, Bruckner AL, et al, eds. *Fitzpatrick's Dermatology*. 9th ed. New York: McGraw Hill; 2019, Figure 64-9E.)

(Continued)

TABLE 11-1 • Diagnosis at a Glance: Common Pathologic Findings Visible on the External Exam (Continued)

Structure	Findings	Pathology
		Carcinoma: Most common is squamous cell due to human papillomavirus infection. Palpation of mass is firm and irregular. Any vulvar discoloration should be biopsied. **Vulvar carcinoma** (Reproduced with permission from Hoffman BL, Schorge JO, Halvorson LM, et al, eds. *Williams Gynecology.* 4th ed. New York: McGraw Hill; 2020, Figure 31-4.)
Vaginal opening, Bartholin gland	Discrete swelling	Bartholin cyst: Unilateral, palpable, 2- to 4-cm swelling located at 5 or 7 o'clock position around vaginal opening. **Bartholin cyst** (Reproduced with permission from Hoffman BL, Schorge JO, Halvorson LM, et al, eds. *Williams Gynecology.* 4th ed. New York: McGraw Hill; 2020, Figure 4-12.)
		When a Bartholin gland cyst becomes infected, it forms a Bartholin abscess, leading to enlargement and worsening pain **Bartholin abscess** (Reproduced with permission from Hoffman BL, Schorge JO, Halvorson LM, et al, eds. *Williams Gynecology.* 4th ed. New York: McGraw Hill; 2020, Figure 3-18.)
Obstetrics lacerations (can occur during vaginal births)	Healed or healing laceration	First-degree laceration: tear through the vaginal mucosa Second-degree laceration: tear through the vaginal mucosa and perineal body (most common) Third-degree laceration: tear through the vaginal mucosa, perineal body, and rectal sphincter

(Continued)

TABLE 11-1 • Diagnosis at a Glance: Common Pathologic Findings Visible on the External Exam (Continued)		
Structure	Findings	Pathology
		Fourth-degree laceration: complete tear from vagina into rectum

(Reproduced with permission from Cathy Cichon, MD.) |
| Vaginal tissue visible externally | Bulge of vaginal tissue to the introitus or externally; worsens if patient coughs or Valsalva | Pelvic organ prolapse: A benign, common condition that can cause a vaginal bulge, voiding dysfunction, or sexual dysfunction. There may be prolapse of the uterus, prolapse of the bladder (cystocele), or prolapse of the rectum (rectocele). Risk factors include age, postmenopausal status, obesity, constipation, and history of vaginal deliveries.

(Reproduced with permission from Cathy Cichon, MD.) |

(Continued)

TABLE 11-1 • Diagnosis at a Glance: Common Pathologic Findings Visible on the External Exam (Continued)		
Structure	Findings	Pathology
		Progressive degrees of pelvic organ prolapse. This is not dangerous and only needs treatment if the patient is symptomatic or unable to void. ![A B C images] **A** **B** **C** Progressive degrees of pelvic organ prolapse. A: Stage 2, B: Stage 3, C: Stage 4. (Reproduced with permission from Hoffman BL, Schorge JO, Halvorson LM, et al, eds. *Williams Gynecology*. 4th ed. New York: McGraw Hill; 2020, Figure 24-8.)

INTERNAL EXAM

Speculum Exam

- Gain comfort with the speculum prior to using it during an exam (**Figure 11-3**). Practice opening and closing the blades, as well as widening the distance between the bills for improved visualization.
- If this is a patient's first exam, briefly show them the speculum and describe what you are going to do prior to starting.

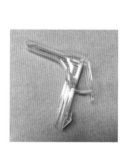 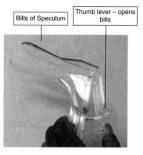

Bills of Speculum

Thumb lever – opens bills

FIGURE 11-3 • **Speculum.** (Photo from *Practical Guide to Clinical Medicine: The Pelvic Examination*. Available from: https://meded.ucsd.edu/clinicalmed/pelvic.html.)

> PEARL: Explain in general terms what you are doing at each step: *"Next, I'll use a speculum to examine your vagina and cervix. It's normal to feel pressure, but if anything hurts or pinches, please let me know."*

- The light sourced attached to the plastic version should make for easy visualization (**Figure 11-4**).

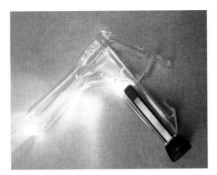

FIGURE 11-4 · **Speculum with light.** (Photo from *Practical Guide to Clinical Medicine: The Pelvic Examination.* Available from: https://meded.ucsd.edu/clinicalmed/pelvic.html.)

- For metal specula, use an external light (typically on a goose neck) to visualize the inside of the vagina and cervix.
- Note that specula come in various lengths and widths, allowing a range of sizes to fit the anatomy of your patient. A Graves speculum will fit most adult patients.
- Prior to starting the exam, lubricate the speculum with a water-soluble agent or warm water.
- Make sure that you have fully explained the process to the patient and continue to explain the steps prior to initiating each one.

> **PEARL:** While the patient is positioned on her back with her legs in lithotomy, let her know before you touch her: *"Next, you'll feel my touch."* Gently place the back of your hand against the inside of her upper thigh. *"I'll proceed with placing the speculum now."*

- Use the fingers of your nondominant hand to gently expose the introitus. You can use 2 fingers of that hand to apply downward pressure on the vaginal floor, and then gently place the speculum over those fingers and into the vagina. Especially if your patient is nonparous, insert the speculum partially sideways at first, and then rotate it upright (**Figure 11-5**).

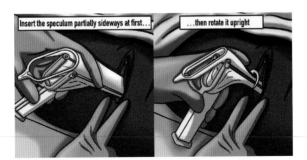

FIGURE 11-5 · **Insertion and rotation of speculum.** (Reproduced with permission from Cathy Cichon, MD.)

- Apply steady pressure in a downward angle until the speculum is fully inserted. Avoid touching the clitoris and urethra, which are highly innervated. Avoid accidentally pulling on pubic hair or pinching the labia. You can gently move the labia out of the way if pubic hair is catching in the speculum. Remove your nondominant hand from the introitus once the speculum is fully inserted.

- **Do not open the bills until the speculum is fully inserted.** Once fully inserted, use the thumb lever to open the bills while looking for the cervix through the opening of the speculum. The cervix should pop into view once the bills are sufficiently widened (**Figures 11-6** and **11-7**).

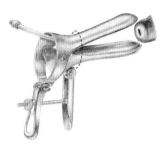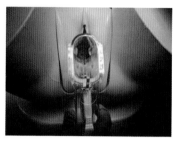

FIGURE 11-6 · **Opening of speculum and view through speculum.** (Left illustration: Reproduced with permission from Rishi Bhatnagar, MD. Right photo: Photo from *Practical Guide to Clinical Medicine: The Pelvic Examination.* Available from: https://meded.ucsd.edu/clinicalmed/pelvic.html.)

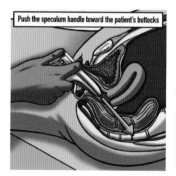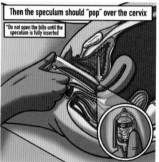

FIGURE 11-7 · **Position of speculum in relation to cervix.** (Reproduced with permission from Cathy Cichon, MD.)

- Once the cervix is visible, a plastic speculum will maintain that position. For a metal speculum, you will need to tighten the thumb screw to keep the bills of the speculum open while you complete your exam.
- If the cervix is not visible, you are either off to one side or not inserted deeply enough. To address this situation, close the bills, withdraw the speculum slightly and reposition, and then fully insert and open them again.

Pearls for When There Is Difficulty Visualizing the Cervix

- Close the blades of the speculum and reinsert fully into the posterior fornix. As you reopen the blades, gentle rock the speculum handle downward, allowing for the superior blade of the speculum to open to the other side of the cervix.
- If your patients has a larger body habitus or is multiparous with redundant vaginal tissue, consider a larger speculum if available.
- If finding the cervix still remains challenging, consider performing the bimanual exam first (described later in this chapter), which will allow you to feel the position of the cervix. Then go back and perform the speculum exam, using the information gained from the bimanual exam to assist in locating the cervix.

Findings and Their Meaning: Internal Exam

What Is Normal to See?

- Nulliparous os: If the patient has never delivered vaginally, the external os will have a round appearance.
- Multiparous os: If the patient has given birth vaginally, the os may appear more open and slit-like (**Figure 11-8**).

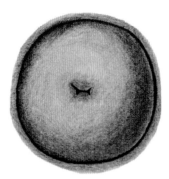

FIGURE 11-8 · **Appearance of cervical os after vaginal birth.** (Reproduced with permission from Rishi Bhatnagar, MD.)

- Squamocolumnar junction: The squamous epithelium of the external cervix meets the internal columnar epithelium, forming the endocervical canal at the squamocolumnar junction. This will be visible in most women and is the area for Pap smear collection (**Figure 11-9**).

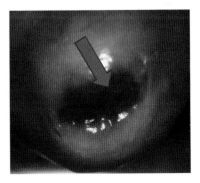

FIGURE 11-9 · **Squamocolumnar junction of cervix.** (From Usatine RP, Smith MA, Mayeaux EJ Jr, Chumley HS. *The Color Atlas and Synopsis of Family Medicine.* 3rd ed. New York: McGraw Hill; 2019, Figure 90-1. Reproduced with permission from E.J. Mayeaux, Jr., MD.)

- Physiologic discharge: Thin, odorless, mucous discharge is normal.
- Bleeding coming from the os is normal during a patient's menses. You can gently wipe this blood with a long cotton-tipped swab for better visualization and more accurate Pap collection.
- During pregnancy, the cervix may appear bluish due to hypervascularity and will be more friable, sometimes bleeding slightly during palpation on exam.

Descriptions and images of some commonly occurring pathologic findings visible on internal exam are provided in **Table 11-2.**

TABLE 11-2 • Diagnosis at a Glance: Common Pathologic Findings Visible on the Internal Exam		
Structure	**Findings**	**Pathology**
Vagina	Blood	Bleeding from the uterus, cervix, or vagina may collect in the vagina. Wiping the blood to identify the source will allow for appropriate differential diagnosis.
	Discharge	Trichomonal vaginitis: Yellowish/green, frothy, malodorous discharge. Can cause itching and pain with intercourse. Candida vaginitis: White, cottage cheese consistency. Causes itching, soreness, and sometimes pain with intercourse. Bacterial vaginosis: Thin, grayish, malodorous discharge. Can cause pain with intercourse.
	Vaginal atrophy	For women experiencing low-estrogen states (eg, breastfeeding, masculinizing therapy, postmenopausal), the vaginal tissue is thin and dry and can be more sensitive to exam and intercourse.
	Cervical growths	If smooth appearing and on squamous epithelium, most likely: Nabothian cysts (retention cysts)

Nabothian cyst

(Reproduced with permission from Hoffman BL, Schorge JO, Halvorson LM, et al, eds. *Williams Gynecology.* 4th ed. New York: McGraw Hill; 2020, Figure 4-15.)

Pedunculated or sessile polyps will also appear smooth. They may vary in size and often bleed slightly when touched.

Cervical polyp

(From Knoop KJ, Stack LB, Storrow AB, Thurman RJ, eds. *The Atlas of Emergency Medicine.* 5th ed. New York: McGraw-Hill; 2021, Figure 10.6. Reproduced with permission from photo contributor: Kevin J. Knoop, MD, MS.)

(Continued)

TABLE 11-2 • Diagnosis at a Glance: Common Pathologic Findings Visible on the Internal Exam (Continued)

Structure	Findings	Pathology
		If the mass is friable or irregular and originates in the columnar epithelium, there is concern for cervical carcinoma, and a biopsy should be obtained. **Cervical carcinoma** (Public Health Image Library, Centers for Disease Control and Prevention.)
Cervix	Cervical discharge	Pelvic inflammatory disease (PID): Yellowish discharge. Cervix may appear red/inflamed. Pain on manipulation of cervix (cervical motion tenderness) may also be present. PID can be a sequela of an initial chlamydia or gonorrhea infection, but PID cultures are often polymicrobial. **Purulent cervical discharge** (From Usatine RP, Smith MA, Mayeaux EJ Jr, Chumley HS. *The Color Atlas and Synopsis of Family Medicine.* 3rd ed. New York: McGraw Hill; 2019, Figure 87-3. Reproduced with permission from E.J. Mayeaux, Jr., MD.)
	Prolapsing fibroid	Smooth, ranging in size from 1-10 cm, palpable stalk connecting the fibroid to the cervix or up into the uterus. Typically smooth, firm, and nonfriable (see Table 11-3 for illustration).

Removing the Speculum

- This step should be done with care so as not to cause discomfort.
- First, pull the speculum back slightly so that the cervix is no longer between the bills. This will prevent you from pinching the cervix.
- Once you have cleared the cervix, close the speculum halfway.
- Observe the walls of the vagina as you withdraw the speculum, noting the appearance of the mucosa and any abnormalities such as growths or ulcers suggestive of cancer.
- Before you fully remove the speculum, close the bills and take pressure off the thumb piece so that it will not snap open when it exits the vagina. Avoid touching the urethra or clitoral areas.

PEARL: Ask permission while explaining the next step: *"Next, I'll place 2 fingers in your vagina to examine your uterus and ovaries. Is it okay to proceed?"*

BIMANUAL EXAM: PALPATING THE UTERUS AND ADNEXA/OVARIES

- Ask permission to examine the patient's uterus and ovaries. Explain that it will require you to place 2 fingers into her vagina.
- Place a small amount of lubricant on the middle and first fingers of your dominant hand.
- Separate the introitus and introduce the lubricated fingers of the dominant hand into the vagina. Be aware of your thumb and tilt your hand downward to keep your fingers away from the urethra and clitoral areas.
- Fully insert your 2 fingers inside the vaginal vault.
- Place your fingers under the cervix and gently push it up a few times. Mild patient discomfort is normal, but if it causes extreme pain or is intolerable to the patient, this may be consistent with cervical motion tenderness (concerning for pelvic inflammatory disease).
- Note the general consistency of the cervix and whether it is closed or open, firm or soft, and positioned posteriorly or anteriorly in the vagina.
- Then, with your fingers beneath the cervix (in the posterior fornix), again gently lift up (**Figure 11-10**). At the same time, place your other hand on the lower abdomen, just superior to the symphysis pubis. Imagine that you are pushing the uterus up from the vaginal hand to the abdominal hand. Try to move the uterus between your 2 hands. Note its size, shape, and consistency and whether manipulation causes any pain.

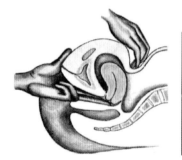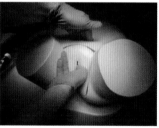

FIGURE 11-10 · **Bimanual exam of uterus.** (Left illustration: Reproduced with permission from Rishi Bhatnagar, MD. Right photo: Photo from *Practical Guide to Clinical Medicine: The Pelvic Examination.* Available from: https://meded.ucsd.edu/clinicalmed/pelvic.html.)

- A nongravid, anatomically normal uterus is typically 4 to 8 cm in length. Uterine size is often described by using the number of weeks for a correlating gravid uterus, even in a nonpregnant state. A normal uterus may be described as "6 weeks, mobile, anteverted, smooth, and regular."
- The position of the normal uterus is variable and can be:
  - Anteverted: The uterus is tipped toward the abdominal wall, and the fundus (top of uterus) will be palpated along the abdominal wall.
  - Mid-position.
  - Retroverted: The uterus is tipped toward the sacrum, and the fundus will be palpated behind the cervix in the posterior fornix.
- Palpating the adnexa can be difficult and not always possible in women with central adiposity or postmenopausal state. First, move the fingers of your internal hand to the right fornix, the space on the side of the cervix at the top of the vagina (**Figure 11-11**). Use the external hand to apply lower right quadrant pressure to sweep the right ovary toward the internal hand. Your internal fingers may palpate a walnut-sized mass, consistent with

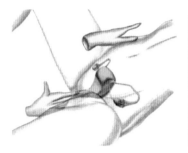 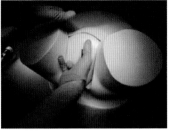

FIGURE 11-11 • **Bimanual exam of adnexa.** (Left illustration: Reproduced with permission from Rishi Bhatnagar, MD. Right photo: Photo from *Practical Guide to Clinical Medicine: The Pelvic Examination.* Available from: https://meded.ucsd.edu/clinicalmed/pelvic.html.)

normal ovary and adnexal structures. Recognize that the ovary is small and learning to identify it takes practice. Also note that palpation of the ovary can cause discomfort.

● After palpating the right side, slightly withdraw your hand and move the fingers into the left fornix. Repeat your efforts, this time trying to palpate the left ovary and adnexa.

Findings and Their Meaning

Descriptions and images of some commonly occurring physiologic and pathologic findings on the bimanual exam are provided in **Table 11-3**. For many of these pathologic conditions, workup includes a transvaginal ultrasound and β-human chorionic gonadotropin laboratory testing for diagnosis.

TABLE 11-3 • Diagnosis at a Glance: Common Pathologic Findings Identifiable on the Bimanual Exam		
Structure	**Findings**	**Pathology**
Cervix	Cervical motion tenderness	Extreme pain with upward palpation of the cervix is consistent with pelvic inflammatory disease (PID; see image of cervicitis in Table 11-2). If tubo-ovarian abscess is present, there will also be pain during exam of the adnexa and the patient typically is more ill.
	Cervix during pregnancy: The cervix changes in preparation for labor and during labor to accommodate the passage of the neonate through the birth canal	Pregnant cervix before term: Firm consistency, typically closed internal os, posterior position. Blue/purple coloration due to hypervascularity. Pregnant cervix ready for labor: Soft consistency, slightly dilated internal and external os, 1-4 cm, anterior position. Actively laboring cervix: Internal os dilated greater than 6 cm, up to 10 cm when no remaining cervical tissue can be palpated. Multipara Primigravida A B C (Reproduced with permission from Cunningham FG, Leveno KJ, Dashe JS, et al, eds. *Williams Obstetrics.* 26th ed. New York: McGraw Hill; 2022.)

(Continued)

TABLE 11-3 • Diagnosis at a Glance: Common Pathologic Findings Identifiable on the Bimanual Exam (Continued)

Structure	Findings	Pathology
Uterus	Enlarged uterus, irregular	Uterine fibroids are benign masses of the uterus. They can range in size and location, sometimes causing pain and/or abnormal uterine bleeding patterns. **Uterine fibroids** (Reproduced with permission from Brunicardi FC, Andersen DK, Billiar TR, et al, eds. *Schwartz's Principles of Surgery*. 11th ed. New York: McGraw Hill; 2019.)
		When a uterine fibroid prolapses into the vagina, it can cause significant bleeding and block the view of the cervix. It requires surgical removal. **PROLAPSING FIBROID** (Reproduced with permission from Cathy Cichon, MD.)
	Uterus during pregnancy	During pregnancy, the uterus becomes palpable externally without a bimanual exam. The top emerges above the pelvic brim at approximately 12-14 weeks' gestation. A fundal height can be recorded by measuring with a tape measure from the pubic symphysis to the palpable fundus and should correlate with the gestational age within 2 cm. **Fundal height during pregnancy** (Reproduced with permission from DeCherney AH, Nathan L, Laufer N, Roman AS, eds. *CURRENT Diagnosis & Treatment: Obstetrics & Gynecology*. 12th ed. New York: McGraw Hill; 2019.)

(Continued)

TABLE 11-3 • Diagnosis at a Glance: Common Pathologic Findings Identifiable on the Bimanual Exam (Continued)		
Structure	Findings	Pathology
Adnexa	Fallopian tube mass	Ectopic pregnancy: The pregnancy implants outside of the uterine cavity. An ectopic pregnancy is a life-threatening condition, as it can rupture with growth and cause fatal bleeding. Implantations in a prior cesarean section scar or the cervix, fallopian tube, or ovary are all ectopic pregnancy sites. **Ectopic pregnancy locations** (Reproduced with permission from Hoffman BL, Schorge JO, Halvorson LM, et al, eds. *Williams Gynecology*. 4th ed. New York: McGraw Hill; 2020.) Tubo-ovarian abscess (see description under cervical motion tenderness, earlier in this chapter) Hydrosalpinx: Damage to the fallopian tubes from infection or surgery can cause blockage, which results in filling of the tubes with sterile fluid. Distention of the tubes from this fluid can result in pain or infertility. (Reproduced with permission from Cathy Cichon, MD.)
	Ovarian mass	Physiologic (functional) ovarian cysts are usually asymptomatic but may be palpable on bimanual exam or visible on imaging. They are typically less than 3 cm and can cause mild abdominal cramping. Physiologic cysts will resolve spontaneously without treatment: • Follicular: Develops prior to ovulation • Corpus luteum: Progesterone support for potential early pregnancy

(Continued)

TABLE 11-3 • Diagnosis at a Glance: Common Pathologic Findings Identifiable on the Bimanual Exam (Continued)

Structure	Findings	Pathology
		Benign ovarian mass can develop from any of the 3 ovarian cell types, which are epithelial cells, germ cells, and sex cord stromal cells. Typically, they are <10 cm in size and can cause persistent, chronic adnexal pain or may be asymptomatic. If these masses twist around the ligaments holding the ovary, this can cause ovarian torsion. Ovarian torsion can cut off blood supply to the ovary, which is exquisitely painful and requires emergency surgery to prevent loss of the ovary. The most common benign ovarian masses include the following: • Hemorrhagic: Bleeding into a physiologic cyst; rupture of a hemorrhagic cyst can cause acute pain and peritoneal signs because the blood is irritating to the abdominal cavity • Dermoid (benign ovarian germ cell tumor, mature teratoma) • Endometrioma • Cystadenoma • Theca lutein cyst A cancerous ovarian mass may be metastatic cancer or ovarian primary cancer. Masses concerning for cancer are usually large (>10 cm), may be irregular with solid and cystic components, may be bilateral, and can be associated with pelvic ascites: Metastatic: Most commonly of breast, colon, endometrium, or gastric origin Ovarian primary from any of the 3 ovarian cell types. Various tumor markers (eg, CA-125, carcinoembryonic antigen) can help differentiate the type of tumor: epithelial carcinoma, epithelial borderline neoplasm, malignant ovarian germ cell tumor, or malignant sex cord stromal tumor. 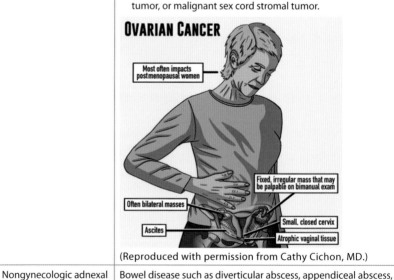 (Reproduced with permission from Cathy Cichon, MD.)
	Nongynecologic adnexal mass	Bowel disease such as diverticular abscess, appendiceal abscess, or carcinoma Pelvic kidney Bladder or ureteral diverticulum Peritoneal inclusion cyst

RECTOVAGINAL EXAM

When to Consider a Rectovaginal Exam

Especially in gynecologic cancer patients, a rectovaginal exam gives specific information regarding cancer spread between the vagina and the rectum.

How to Perform a Rectovaginal Exam

The lubricated and gloved index and middle fingers of the dominant hand are placed in the vagina and rectum (**Figure 11-12**), while the other hand simultaneously palpates the lower abdomen. Feel that the septum is smooth and mobile, or note masses or fixed areas as concerning findings. For the rectal exam alone, only the lubricated index finger is used.

Rectal and rectovaginal exams are not always indicated during a basic gynecologic exam, so it is important to consider how they might help inform your evaluation prior to conducting them.

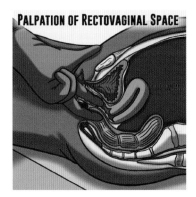

FIGURE 11-12 · **Rectovaginal exam.** (Reproduced with permission from Cathy Cichon, MD.)

Findings and Their Meaning

Commonly occurring pathologic findings on the rectal and rectovaginal exam are described in **Table 11-4**.

TABLE 11-4 • Diagnosis at a Glance: Common Pathologic Findings Identifiable on the Rectal and Rectovaginal Exam		
Exam	Findings	Pathology
Rectal exam	Blood	Benign: Internal or external hemorrhoid Malignant: Cancer of the colon (See Figure 9-15, Stool color; Chapter 9, Male Genital and Rectal Exam)
	Palpable mass	Rectal polyp, cancer (rectal, or intra-abdominal) *In a patient with peritoneal metastasis, a firm nodular rectal "shelf" may be palpated in the rectouterine pouch.
	Rectal sphincter tone	Important to evaluate in patient with flatal or fecal incontinence or with history of third- or fourth-degree perineal laceration during childbirth (see Table 11-1)
Rectovaginal exam	Septum with masses, nodularity, or immobility	Concerning for cancer spread from gynecologic organs or bowel

PREGNANT PATIENTS

The physical exam for a pregnant patient is slightly different depending on the current trimester of pregnancy (**Table 11-5**). Normal findings on exam are shown in **Figure 11-13**.

TABLE 11-5 • Gynecologic Exam for Pregnant Patients Based on Trimester	
First trimester (0-13 weeks' gestational age)	Routine pelvic exam as described earlier in chapter. Note the normal changes to the cervix during pregnancy (see Table 11-3).
Second trimester (14-27 weeks' gestational age)	Routine pelvic exam as described earlier. Uterine fundal heights described earlier. Fetal heart tones will be audible by Doppler auscultation and should be checked during each patient encounter. Place ultrasound gel at the end of the Doppler, and gently apply to the patient's abdomen to identify heart tones. Normal fetal heart rate is between 110 and 160 bpm. Differentiate from maternal heart rate by checking maternal pulse if needed. **Doppler auscultation** (Photo by Julia Cormano, MD.)
Third trimester (28-40 weeks' gestational age)	Nonlabor: Similar to second trimester. Labor: In a laboring patient, 2 fingers are inserted into the vagina for a sterile vaginal exam to check the cervix for dilation. Insert your lubricated, gloved index and middle fingers together and find the cervix. Then gently widen the gap between your 2 fingers until you feel the rim of the cervix. Approximate the distance between your 2 fingers to estimate the cervical dilation. Speculum exams are not typically done in a laboring patient due to extreme discomfort.

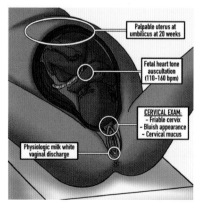

FIGURE 11-13 • **Normal exam findings during pregnancy.** (Reproduced with permission from Cathy Cichon, MD.)

Cervical swabs and pap smears can be safely collected at any time during pregnancy unless there is concern for placenta or vasa previa. Placenta previa is when the placenta implants between the fetus and the cervix, increasing risk of hemorrhage. In this situation, internal exams should be avoided unless critical to the patient's immediate care.

TRANSGENDER AND GENDER DIVERSE PATIENTS

To guide preventative medical care, any anatomic structure present that warrants screening should be screened regardless of gender identity. Create an inclusive and welcoming environment by asking patients what pronouns they use and their preferred name. See Chapter 18, LGBTQ+ Healthcare, for additional information.

Be aware of normal findings for transmasculine individuals undergoing masculinizing therapy, including the following:

- Development of facial hair
- Deepening of the voice
- Increasing body hair and muscle mass
- Redistribution of subcutaneous fat
- Male-pattern baldness
- Possible increased libido
- Possible cessation of menses (but should not be relied upon for contraception)
- Vaginal atrophy
- Increased clitoral size

CONCLUDING THE EXAM

At the end of the exam, provide the patient with privacy and tissues for wiping excess lubricant and a fresh sanitary pad if needed. After she is dressed, return to the room to answer questions, review findings, and discuss next steps in care.

TELEHEALTH TIPS

- Due to the sensitive nature of this exam, telehealth evaluation of this region is typically limited to history and counseling.
- Physical exam of sensitive organs may be completed following oral consent of the patient and agreement of the provider that use of the telehealth modality is clinically appropriate. Additionally, a chaperone is recommended for both patient and provider during the exam.
- Check with the patient to ensure they have privacy before continuing with sensitive history taking.

SUMMARY OF SKILLS CHECKLIST

- ❏ Explain rationale for exam and set up equipment, speculum, and swabs
- ❏ Give privacy while patient changes into gown
- ❏ Have a chaperone present
- ❏ Clean your hands
- ❏ Guide patient verbally to position on table with stirrups
- ❏ External exam of vulvar area

❏ Speculum exam; obtain specimens if indicated
❏ Bimanual exam
❏ Rectovaginal exam or rectal exam if indicated
❏ Clean your hands
❏ Provide patient wipes and give privacy and time to dress
❏ Return to discuss findings and plan

BIBLIOGRAPHY

American College of Obstetricians and Gynecologists. Caring for patients who have experienced trauma. Committee Opinion Number 825, April 2021. Accessed August 23, 2022. https://www.acog.org/clinical/clinical-guidance/committee-opinion/articles/2021/04/caring-for-patients-who-have-experienced-trauma.

American College of Obstetricians and Gynecologists. Diagnosis and management of vulvar skin disorders. Practice Bulletin 224. July 2020. Accessed August 23, 2022. https://www.acog.org/clinical/clinical-guidance/practice-bulletin/articles/2020/07/diagnosis-and-management-of-vulvar-skin-disorders.

American College of Obstetricians and Gynecologists. Health care for transgender and gender diverse individuals. Committee Opinion Number 823, March 2021. Accessed August 23, 2022. https://www.acog.org/clinical/clinical-guidance/committee-opinion/articles/2021/03/health-care-for-transgender-and-gender-diverse-individuals.

American College of Obstetricians and Gynecologists. Pelvic organ prolapse. Practice Bulletin Number 214. November 2019. Accessed August 23, 2022. https://www.acog.org/clinical/clinical-guidance/practice-bulletin/articles/2019/11/pelvic-organ-prolapse.

American College of Obstetricians and Gynecologists. The utility of and indications for routine pelvic examination. Committee Opinion Number 754. October 2018. Accessed August 23, 2022. https://www.acog.org/clinical/clinical-guidance/committee-opinion/articles/2018/10/the-utility-of-and-indications-for-routine-pelvic-examination.

American Medical Association. Code of Medical Ethics. Opinion 1.2.4. Use of Chaperones. 2016. Accessed August 23, 2022. https://www.ama-assn.org/delivering-care/ethics/use-chaperones.

Barnhart K. Ectopic pregnancy. *N Engl J Med.* 2009;361:379–387.

Bialy A, Wray AA. Gynecologic examination. StatPearls, May 2022. Accessed August 23, 2022. https://www.ncbi.nlm.nih.gov/books/NBK534223.

Goldberg C. Digital DDx: obstetric, gynecologic and breast symptoms or conditions. Accessed March 22, 2023. http://digitalddx.com/symptoms_list/9/.

Goldberg C. Practical guide to clinical medicine: the pelvic exam. Accessed March 23, 2023. https://meded.ucsd.edu/clinicalmed/pelvic.html.

Hoffman BL, Heinzman AB. Chapter 9. Pelvic mass. In: Hoffman BL, Schorge JO, Schaffer JI, et al, eds. *Williams Gynecology.* 2nd ed. New York: McGraw-Hill; 2012.

Hoffman BL, Sharma M. Chapter 8. Abnormal uterine bleeding. In: Hoffman BL, Schorge JO, Schaffer JI, et al, eds. *Williams Gynecology.* 2nd ed. New York: McGraw-Hill; 2012.

Lee W, Wittler M. Bartholin gland cyst. StatPearls, February 2022. Accessed August 23, 2022. https://www.ncbi.nlm.nih.gov/books/NBK532271.

Rock JA, Jone HW III. *Te Linde's Operative Gynecology.* Philadelphia: Lippincott Williams & Wilkins; 2008.

12

Neurological Exam

Sean Evans, MD

INTRODUCTION

Location, location, location. This is true in real estate and even more so in clinical neurology. Differential building and neurologic decision-making are heavily influenced by the "localization of the lesion." The lesion is the structure or system that is not functioning correctly.

Fundamentally, there are 2 primary types of localizations, focal and diffuse (**Figure 12-1**).

- In a focal lesion, there is a physical change in a specific location (eg, the left corona radiata or the right elbow). If a meningioma grows adjacent to the visual cortex, it will

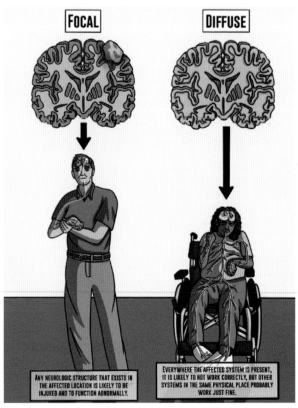

FIGURE 12-1 · **Localizing lesions.** (Reproduced with permission from by Cathy Cichon, MD.)

produce visual signs and symptoms. If the same exact tumor grew adjacent to the motor cortex, it would instead produce motor symptoms.

- In a diffuse lesion, there is a functional change of a specific system (eg, "the upper motor neurons" or "the peripheral nerves"). Everywhere that system is present, it is likely to not work correctly, but other systems in the same physical place will probably work just fine. If a neurodegenerative disorder targets cerebellar systems, then the patient will show abnormalities everywhere the cerebellar systems are active, including eye movements, speech articulation, swallowing, limb movements, gait, torso balancing, and so on, but will not show any deficits in areas where the cerebellum is not involved.

> **PEARL:** Wait a second! What about multifocal? True, most neurology texts include multifocal in addition to focal and diffuse. Conceptually, multifocal just means that a patient has more than 1 focal lesion. In each lesion, the location of the lesion, not its nature, is what determines the deficits, rather than the other way around.

Goals of the Neurologic History

- Obtain the patient's description of their symptoms, as well as pertinent absent symptoms.
- Determine which systems and structures appear to work normally and abnormally.

Goals of the Neurologic Examination

- Determine the signs of normal and abnormal neurologic function.
- Determine which systems and structures appear to work normally and abnormally.

Combine the information gathered in the history and examination to decide if the patient's problems all originate from a particular place (focal) or from a particular system (diffuse).

When Should I Engage in a Neurologic Examination?

- When patients present with symptoms suggestive of a neurologic problem
- When screening for the presence of abnormalities in patients at risk for the development of neurologic disorders
- When screening and documenting baseline function of those who are otherwise healthy

> **PEARL:** This is appropriate for individuals who have no subjective symptoms suggestive of a neurologic problem yet have systemic illnesses that might put them at risk for neurologic dysfunction (eg, patients with diabetes or thyroid disease).

What Do I Need to Do?

The major areas of the exam include the following:
- Mental status testing (covered in Chapter 13)
- Cranial nerves
- Muscle bulk, tone, and strength
- Reflexes
- Sensory function
- Coordination
- Gait

Uh, That Sounds Like a Lot … Maybe I Should Skip to the Next Chapter

This exam is perceived as being time and labor intensive. Here are some things you have probably heard and some responses:

- "The neuro exam takes too long!"
  - *It is a reasonable goal for a medical student to develop a quality basic neurologic examination that takes fewer than 5 minutes to complete.*
- "There's no way to be sure of your exam unless you do this all the time."
  - *Don't let "perfect" be the enemy of "good." Just because you're not the ultimate expert, you should still gather the information and then weigh its value appropriately.*
- "This all seems kind of subjective."
  - *True, but that's the case for many aspects of the physical exam. Ask yourself: Is the exam what I was expecting or was it a surprise? Does it seem obviously normal or obviously abnormal?*
- "There's a whole lot of neuroanatomy to know."
  - *Yes, but you don't have to be expert in everything. A basic sense of the visual system, upper and lower motor neurons, 2 sensory pathways, and how people move, gets you a very long way (all of which will be covered in this chapter!).*
- "Why not just obtain imaging?"
  - *Imaging provides data, but it doesn't tell you if those data matter. You can see the patient has a disk bulge in their spine, but without a history and examination, you don't know if it is a common incidental finding or the cause of the patient's signs and symptoms. Similarly, some patients' symptoms and signs tell that there is an abnormal structure. A subsequently normal magnetic resonance imaging (MRI) scan doesn't tell you that there is "no problem," but rather that you need to be thinking about a differential of lesions that wouldn't be identified in that particular study.*

CRANIAL NERVE TESTING

There are 12 paired cranial "nerves" (CNs). Why the quotes? CNs I and II are extensions of the central nervous system (CNS) and are not part of the peripheral nervous system (PNS) at all. Why do you care? Diseases that impact the CNS affect CNs I and II, but not CNs III-XII.

The "category" of a neurologic structure has big implications for the types of disease that should be considered. A CNS-specific disorder, multiple sclerosis commonly creates lesions in CN II (as well as in lots of other CNS structures in the brain and spinal cord) but never causes a lesion in CNs III-XII (note, that is not the same as not impacting their functions by affecting a related CNS system). Similarly, a PNS-specific disorder like Guillain-Barré syndrome will routinely cause lesions in CNs III-XII (as well as in lots of other PNS structures) but will never cause a CN II lesion because it is a CNS structure and therefore off limits.

Throughout this chapter, "Test Yourself" boxes provide opportunities for self-assessments. Answers are provided at the end of the chapter.

> **Test Yourself #1:** Which problem with vision would you predict for multiple sclerosis affecting a CN? Which problem with vision would you predict for Guillain-Barré syndrome affecting a CN?

Clinical Patterns of Cranial Nerve Dysfunction

Each CN functions as an independent structure, so you need to examine both the left and right CNs, as they can each dysfunction separately. If both the left and right CN of a pair are dysfunctional, consideration of a diffuse disorder is appropriate, and if more than one CN on one side of the body is abnormal, you would consider a focal lesion affecting that side of the brainstem.

Cranial Nerve I (Olfactory)

Assessment of ability to detect odors. This is rarely tested in clinical practice.

- Check to make sure that the patient is able to inhale and exhale through each nostril.
- Present a small test tube filled with something that has a distinct, common odor (eg, ground coffee) to the open nostril (**Figure 12-2**).
- The patient should be able to correctly identify the odor at approximately 10 cm. Each side should be checked separately.

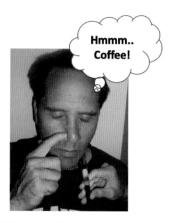

FIGURE 12-2 · **Assessing cranial nerve I.** (Photo from *Practical Guide to Clinical Medicine: The Neurological Examination.* Available from: https://meded.ucsd.edu/clinicalmed/neuro2.html.)

Findings and Their Meaning: Failure to Detect an Odor

- This can indicate a physical blockage in the nasal passages (think a tumor growing in the concha or just a whole lot of snot).
- Or this can indicate a lesion of CN I connecting the odor-sensing neurons to the brain. Due to CN I's location between the undersurface of the frontal lobe and rough orbital roof, it is often injured in traumatic brain injuries.

Cranial Nerve II (Optic)

This extension of the CNS carries visual impulses from the eye to the optical cortex of the brain. Between the eye and the optic chiasm, the pathway is called the optic nerve; from the optic chiasm to the thalamus, the path is called the optic tract. Testing involves 3 phases (also covered in Chapter 5, Eye Exam).

Acuity

- Remember, acuity is only best for the small area of vision that falls on the macula. Normal acuity is quite poor for something that you are not looking at directly.
  - Each eye is tested separately.
  - Let the patient wear their distance glasses.
  - A Snellen chart is the standard, wall-mounted device used for this assessment at a distance of 20 ft (**Figure 12-3**).
  - "Please read the smallest line you can." (Little kids identify shapes if they do not yet read.)
  - "Try the one below that."

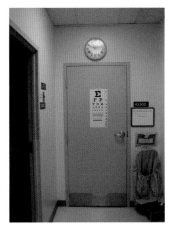

FIGURE 12-3 · **Snellen chart for measuring visual acuity.** (Photo from *Practical Guide to Clinical Medicine: The Neurological Examination.* Available from: https://meded.ucsd.edu/clinicalmed/neuro2.html.)

- Identify the last line that can be read with 100% accuracy.
- 20/20 indicates normal vision. 20/400 means that the patient's vision 20 ft from an object is equivalent to that of a normal person viewing the same object from 400 ft. In other words, the larger the denominator, the worse is the vision.
- There are handheld cards that look like Snellen charts but are positioned 14 inches from the patient (**Figure 12-4**). These are used simply for convenience. Testing and interpretation are as described for the Snellen chart.

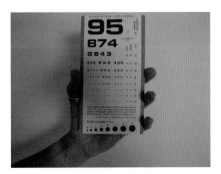

FIGURE 12-4 · **Handheld visual acuity card.** (Photo from *Practical Guide to Clinical Medicine: The Neurological Examination.* Available from: https://meded.ucsd.edu/clinicalmed/neuro2.html.)

If neither chart is available and the patient has visual complaints, some attempt should be made to objectively measure visual acuity. Can the patient read your ID badge at arm's length or at 1 ft? Can they distinguish fingers or hand movement in front of their face? Can they detect light? Failure at each level correlates with a more severe problem.

Visual Field Testing Specific areas of the retina receive input from precise areas of the visual field. This information is carried to the brain along a well-defined path (**Figure 12-5**).
- Areas of absent vision (referred to as visual field cuts) are caused by a disruption along any point in the path from the eyeball to the visual cortex of the brain.

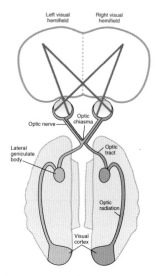

FIGURE 12-5 · **Visual pathways.** (Reproduced with permission from Kibble JD. *The Big Picture Physiology: Medical Course & Step 1 Review*. 2nd ed. New York: McGraw Hill; 2020.)

- Assessing visual fields by confrontation (**Figure 12-6**):
  - Stand in front of the patient at about arm's length.
  - Check each eye separately.
  - Cover one eye (make sure the eye is fully covered, no peeking).
  - Place your hand as far out into one quadrant (eg, upper outer, lower inner) and then provide an obvious and discrete visual stimulus, either a wiggling finger or 1, 2, or 5 fingers.
  - "Can you see my finger moving?" or "How many fingers do you see?"
  - Repeat in all 4 quadrants of each eye.

> **PEARL:** Remember, away from the very center of vision, acuity is supposed to be poor, hence the *obvious and discrete* stimuli being important.

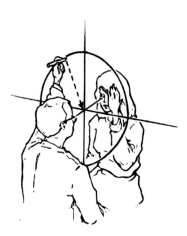

FIGURE 12-6 · **Visual field testing.** (Reproduced with permission from Manish Suneja, Joseph F. Szot, Richard F. LeBlond. Donald D. Brown: *DeGowin's Diagnostic Examination, 11e*. New York: McGraw Hill.)

Findings and Their Meaning: Visual Field Loss In most settings, diminished acuity without a loss of visual field is due to an eyeball or optic nerve lesion. A loss of visual field suggests a lesion in the visual pathway.

- If the difficulty only occurs when stimuli are provided to a single eye, the lesion is in the eyeball itself or in the optic nerve anterior to the chiasm (Figure 12-5).
- If the difficulty only occurs in the temporal field of both eyes, the lesion is at the optic chiasm.
- If the difficulty only affects the same region of vision (eg, the left upper quadrant or the right hemi-visual field), then the lesion is in the optic pathway posterior to the chiasm on the contralateral side of the brain (ie, if the visual failure is for the left fields, then the lesion is on the right side of the brain).
- A meningioma growing on the left CN II is a focal lesion and will produce a change in all the visual fields in the left eye only. Vitamin A intoxication is a diffuse disorder affecting "all the optic nerves you've got" and will produce a change in acuity of equal severity in both eyes and in all fields of vision.

Pupils The pupil has afferent (sensory) nerves that travel with CN II. These nerves carry the impulse generated by the light back toward the brain. They function in concert with efferent (autonomic motor) nerves that travel with CN III and cause pupillary constriction. See under CN III for specifics of testing.

Cranial Nerves III, IV, and VI: Assessment of Extraocular Movements

- The eyes normally move in a coordinated fashion (ie, when the left eye moves left, the right eye moves in the same direction to a similar degree).
- If both eyes are pointed at the same target, the brain forms a single 3-dimensional image. If not, the brain either suppresses one image or forms two 2-dimensional images.
- This coordinated movement depends on 6 extraocular muscles (EOMs) that insert around the eyeballs and allow them to move in all directions.
- Each muscle is innervated by one of 3 CNs: CN III, IV, or VI. Movements are described as follows (**Figure 12-7**):
  - Elevation (pupil directed upward)
  - Depression (pupil directed downward)

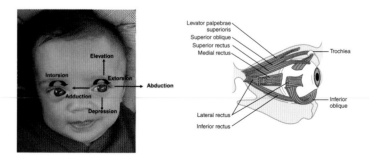

FIGURE 12-7 · **Eye movement terminology and insertion of each extraocular muscle.** (Left photo: From *Practical Guide to Clinical Medicine: The Neurological Examination*. Available from: https://meded. ucsd.edu/clinicalmed/neuro2.html. Right illustration: Reproduced with permission from Tintinalli JE, Ma OJ, Yealy DM, et al, eds. *Tintinalli's Emergency Medicine: A Comprehensive Study Guide*. 9th ed. New York: McGraw Hill; 2020.)

- Abduction (pupil directed laterally)
- Adduction (pupil directed medially)
- Extorsion (top of eye rotating away from the nose)
- Intorsion (top of eye rotating toward the nose)

The 3 CNs responsible for eye movement and the muscles that they control are as follows:
- CN IV (trochlear): Controls the superior oblique muscle.
- CN VI (abducens): Controls the lateral rectus muscle.
- CN III (oculomotor): Controls the remaining 4 muscles (inferior oblique, inferior rectus, superior rectus, and medial rectus). CN III also raises the eyelid and constricts the pupil (discussed below).

The mnemonic "SO 4, LR 6, All The Rest 3" may help remind you which CN does what (superior oblique CN IV, lateral rectus CN VI, all the rest of the muscles innervated by CN III).

EOMs and Their Function   The functions of the medial and lateral rectus muscles are simple:
- Lateral rectus: Abduction (moves the eye laterally along the horizontal plane)
- Medial rectus: Adduction (moves the eye medially along the horizontal plane)

The remaining muscles each move the eye in more than one direction (eg, some combination of elevation/depression, abduction/adduction, intorsion/extorsion). This is because they insert on the eyeball at various angles and, in the case of the superior oblique, in a different direction than expected. Review of the origin and insertion of each muscle sheds light on its actions.

Specific actions of the remaining EOMs are described below. The action that the muscle primarily performs is listed first, followed by secondary and then tertiary actions.
- Inferior rectus: Depression, extorsion, and adduction
- Superior rectus: Elevation, intorsion, and adduction
- Superior oblique: Intorsion, depression, and abduction
- Inferior oblique: Extorsion, elevation, and abduction

Although multiple EOMs move the eye in multiple directions, certain positions of the eye maximize the impact of a single muscle:
- Both the superior rectus and the inferior oblique can elevate the eye.
- Bringing the eye into full abduction disables the inferior oblique, at which point only the superior rectus elevates the eye.
- Systematically place each eye into a series of positions that are only achieved through a single muscle's function.

*Testing EOM Function (**Figure 12-8**)*
- Stand in front of the patient.
- Hold your finger up at arm's length from the patient.
- "Please follow my finger with your eyes. Try to keep your head still."
- Look at the patient's right eye only.
- Move your finger all the way to the right and watch to see if the patient's eye tracks all the way to the right.

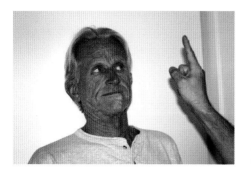

FIGURE 12-8 · **Testing extraocular movements.** (Photo from *Practical Guide to Clinical Medicine: The Neurological Examination*. Available from: https://meded.ucsd.edu/clinicalmed/neuro2.html.)

- Now move your finger up until the patient's eye is maximally elevated. Now move down until the patient's eye is maximally depressed.
- Come back to midline and move your finger all the way to the left until the patient's eye is fully adducted.
- Move all the way up and then all the way down.
- Repeat, but this time, watch the patient's left eye make the same movements.
- Make note of any movement that one or both eyes do not make completely.
- At the end, bring your finger directly in toward the patient's nose. This will cause the patient to look cross-eyed and the pupils should constrict, a response referred to as accommodation.

> **PEARL:** Many of your patients (pretty much anyone over 40) will have lost some of their ability to accommodate and focus on near objects. Placing your finger closer to the patient than arm's length will often result in a fuzzy image for them and a lot of blinking. If you're having trouble, try again with your target a bit farther from the patient!

Findings and Their Meaning: Deficits in EOM

- In general, inability to fully move an eye in a direction means that the nerve, the neuromuscular junction, or the muscle controlling that motion is abnormal or that there is a mechanical obstruction (eg, a tumor, hematoma, broken bone) to that movement.
- If all the motions that fail are related to a single nerve, then the nerve is likely the cause.

See detailed discussions in Chapter 5, Eye Exam, for more information about EOMs.

Assessing Pupils The response of pupils to light is controlled by afferent (sensory) nerves that travel with CN II and efferent (autonomic motor) nerves that travel with CN III. These innervate the ciliary muscle, which controls the size of the pupil. Testing is performed as follows:

- Shine a light into one eye. This will cause that pupil to constrict, referred to as the direct response.
- Remove the light and then shine it in the same eye, this time observing the other pupil. It should also constrict, referred to as the consensual response. This occurs because afferent impulses from one eye generate an efferent signal to constrict that is sent to both pupils.
- If the patient's pupils are small at baseline or you are otherwise having difficulty seeing the changes, turn the lights down in the room for a few minutes while you perform the rest of the exam and then recheck.

Findings and Their Meaning: Abnormal Pupillary Responses

- In general, when light is shined into a pupil, both that pupil and the opposite pupil should constrict. A lesion of the eyeball or the optic nerve on the side that the light is shined into will result in both pupils failing to constrict.
- If the afferent pathway is intact and the light signal makes it to the brainstem, then the efferent pathway uses both the left and right sides to set both pupils to the correct size.
- If only one of those pupils sets to the correct size, then the lesion is on the opposite side.
- If the abnormal pupil is too big for light conditions, the lesion is in CN III on that side.
- If the abnormal pupil is too small for light conditions, the lesion is in the sympathetic fibers on that side.

See detailed discussions in Chapter 5, Eye Exam, for more information about pupils.

> **Test Yourself #2:** Imagine a patient with a lesion of the left CN II due to microvascular stroke. What would happen to the patient's pupils when you shine a light into the right eye? What would happen when you move it to the left eye?

Cranial Nerve IV (Trochlear)

See under CN III and evaluation of EOMs.

Cranial Nerve V (Trigeminal)

This nerve has both motor and sensory components.

Assessment of Cranial Nerve V Sensory Function   The sensory limb has 3 major branches, each covering roughly one-third of the face. These are the ophthalmic, maxillary, and mandibular (**Figure 12-9**). Assessment is performed as follows:

- Brush your finger across the forehead on both sides to assess the ophthalmic branch.
- "Does this feel normal and the same on both sides?"
- Repeat on both cheeks, assessing the maxillary branch.
- Repeat on both sides of the jaw area, assessing the mandibular branch.
- If you would like to specifically assess pain fibers, you can perform the same technique with a sterile pin.
- If you would like to assess temperature sensation, you can use a metal tuning fork and ask, "Does this feel cool like metal and the same on both sides?"

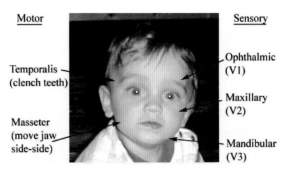

FIGURE 12-9 · **Cranial nerve V function.** (Photo from *Practical Guide to Clinical Medicine: The Neurological Examination.* Available from: https://meded.ucsd.edu/clinicalmed/neuro2.html.)

The ophthalmic branch of CN V also receives sensory input from the surface of the eye. To assess this component (**Figure 12-10**):

- Pull out a wisp of cotton.
- While the patient is looking straight ahead (this is most commonly performed on patients with decreased consciousness, so often you will be holding their eyelid up with your other hand), gently brush the wisp against the lateral aspect of the sclera (outer white area of the eye), providing the afferent limb of a reflex arc.
- This should cause the brain to trigger an efferent blink with both eyes. Blinking requires that CN VII function normally, as it controls eyelid closure.

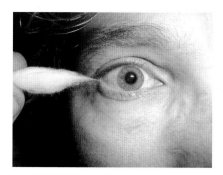

FIGURE 12-10 · **Assessing ophthalmic branch of cranial nerve V.** (Photo from *Practical Guide to Clinical Medicine: The Neurological Examination.* Available from: https://meded.ucsd.edu/clinicalmed/neuro2.html.)

Assessment of Cranial Nerve V Motor Function The motor limb of CN V innervates the temporalis and masseter muscles, both important for closing the jaw (Figure 12-9). Assessment is performed as follows:

- Place your hand on both temporalis muscles, located on the lateral aspects of the forehead.
- Ask the patient to tightly close their jaw, causing the muscles beneath your fingers to become taught.
- Then move your hands to the masseter muscles, located just in front of the temporomandibular joints (point where lower jaw articulates with skull).
- Ask the patient to tightly close their jaw, which should again cause the muscles beneath your fingers to become taught. Then ask them to move their jaw from side to side, another function of the masseter.

Cranial Nerve VI (Abducens)

See under CN III and assessment of EOMs.

Cranial Nerve VII (Facial)

This nerve innervates many of the muscles of facial expression. Assessment is performed as follows:

- First look at the patient's face. It should appear symmetric.
- There should be the same number of wrinkles on either side of the forehead.
- The nasolabial folds (lines coming down from either side of the nose toward the corners of the mouth) should be equal.

- The corners of the mouth should be at the same height.
- If there is any question as to whether an apparent asymmetry is new or old, ask the patient for a picture (eg, from a driver's license) for comparison.
- Ask the patient to wrinkle their eyebrows and then close their eyes tightly. CN VII controls the muscles that close the eye lids (CN III controls the muscles that open the lids). You will notice that when a patient closes their eyelids tightly, the roots of their eyelashes disappear, and you should not be able to open the patient's eyelids with the application of gentle upward pressure.
- Ask the patient to smile. The corners of the mouth should rise to the same height, and equal amounts of teeth should be visible on either side.
- Ask the patient to puff out their cheeks. Both sides should puff out equally, and air should not leak from the mouth.

CN VII has a precise pattern of innervation, which has important clinical implications (**Figure 12-11**).

- The lower motor neurons (LMNs) that form CN VII each control one-half of the face (right CN VII controls all of the right face).
- Upper motor neurons (UMNs) coming from either side of the cerebral cortex innervate both the right and left LMNs that allow the forehead to move up and down (left or right UMNs control right forehead movement).
- However, the UMNs that control the muscles of the lower face only innervate the LMNs traveling to the opposite side of the face (only the left UMN controls right lower face).

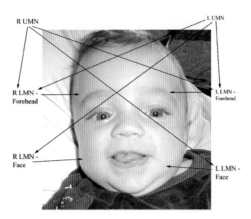

FIGURE 12-11 • Facial nerve (cranial nerve VII) pattern of innervation. (Photo from *Practical Guide to Clinical Medicine: The Neurological Examination*. Available from: https://meded.ucsd.edu/clinicalmed/neuro2.html.)

Findings and Their Meaning: Cranial Nerve VII Dysfunction in the Setting of Unilateral Facial Weakness The pattern of weakness or paralysis observed will differ depending on whether the UMN or LMN is affected. Specifically:

- UMN dysfunction: This occurs with a CNS event, such as a stroke affecting the UMNs.
- In the setting of left facial weakness caused by right UMN stroke, the patient will be able to wrinkle their forehead on both sides of their face, as the LMNs controlling the forehead on the left are innervated by UMNs from both the left and right side of the cortex.

- However, the patient would be unable to effectively close their left eye or raise the left corner of their mouth as the left CN VII LMNs for the lower face are only innervated by UMNs from the right.

- LMN dysfunction (**Figure 12-12**): This occurs most commonly in the setting of a Bell-type palsy, an idiopathic, acute CN VII peripheral nerve palsy, but can occur with any LMN injury.

- In the setting of left CN VII peripheral (ie, LMN) dysfunction, the patient will not be able to wrinkle their forehead, close their eye, or raise the corner of their mouth on the left side. Right-sided function would be normal.

- This clinical distinction is very important because central versus peripheral dysfunction carries different prognostic and treatment implications.

- A new UMN lesion would always trigger urgent imaging and evaluation of the CNS pathways in the brain.

- Although a new LMN lesion could be due to a dangerous problem, by far the most common cause is Bell palsy, a presumably autoimmune reaction to latent herpes virus infection, which has a high rate of improvement with time and a short course of anti-inflammatory steroids and antiviral medications.

> **Test Yourself #3:** A patient has weakness of the left face involving the forehead as well as the middle and lower face. Is the lesion in the UMN or the LMN? Could a CNS-specific disease such as multiple sclerosis cause this lesion? Why or why not?

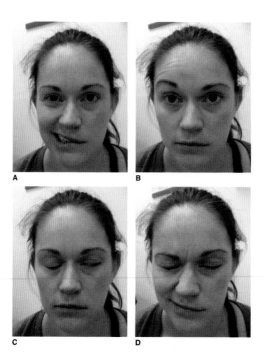

A   B

C   D

FIGURE 12-12 · **Left peripheral cranial nerve VII dysfunction.** Note loss of forehead wrinkle, inability to close eye, inability to raise corner of mouth, and decreased nasolabial fold prominence—all on left side of face. (Reproduced with permission from Berkowitz AL. *Clinical Neurology and Neuroanatomy: A Localization-Based Approach.* 2nd ed. New York: McGraw Hill; 2022, Figure 13.5.)

CN VII is also responsible for carrying taste sensations from the anterior two-thirds of the tongue, as well as signals to salivary and lacrimal glands. However, as these are rarely tested, further discussion is not included.

Cranial Nerve VIII (Acoustic)

CN VIII carries sound impulses from the cochlea to the brain. Prior to reaching the cochlea, the sound must first traverse the external canal and middle ear. A screening assessment of auditory acuity can be assessed as follows:

- Stand in front of the patient.
- Ask them to close their eyes.
- Extend your arms to full length and rub your fingers together as hard as you can without snapping.
- If the patient can hear in each ear, repeat, but this time rubbing your fingers as softly as you can hear yourself. If the patient can hear this in both ears, their hearing is likely normal.
- If the patient is unable to hear the soft rustle, bend your arms 90 degrees at the elbow and repeat.
- If they still cannot hear, repeat at one hand breadth from their ear. If they still cannot hear, repeat as close to their ear as you can without touching it.
- Report based on the distance at which the patient can hear the soft or loud rustle.

Findings and Their Meaning: Unilateral Hearing Loss
- This is a powerfully localizing finding.
- It always localizes to the side where hearing is worse and can only be localized from the cochlear nucleus in the medulla out to the ear itself, as all the more proximal CNS pathways are bilateral and redundant.

Special Testing: Tests for hearing loss (Weber and Rinne) are described in Chapter 4, Head and Neck Exam

Cranial Nerve IX (Glossopharyngeal) and Cranial Nerve X (Vagus)

CN IX predominantly provides for sensation from the inside of the soft palate of the mouth and triggers the gag reflex, a protective mechanism that prevents food or liquid from traveling into the lungs. It also contributes a small amount to the elevation of the soft palate, but most of that movement is caused by CN X. Both nerves also affect the quality of speech, with dysfunction causing a breathy or nasal sound.

Testing Elevation of the Soft Palate
- Ask the patient to open their mouth and say, "Ahhhh," causing the soft palate to rise upward. Both sides of the palate should move simultaneously and symmetrically (**Figure 12-13**).

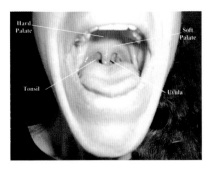

FIGURE 12-13 · **Normal position of uvula and palate.** (Photo from *Practical Guide to Clinical Medicine: The Neurological Examination*. Available from: https://meded. ucsd.edu/clinicalmed/neuro2.html.)

- Look at the uvula, a midline structure hanging down from the palate. If the tongue obscures your view, take a tongue depressor and gently push it out of the way.
- The uvula should rise up straight in the midline, but sometimes the uvula is sticky or crooked. When in doubt, trust the palate not the uvula!

Findings and Their Meaning: CN IX or X Dysfunction

- If CN IX or X on the left is not functioning (eg, in the setting of a stroke), the left side of the palate will not elevate and the uvula will be pulled to the right (**Figure 12-14**).
- The opposite occurs in the setting of left CN IX or X dysfunction.
- When patients do not have normal function of CN IX or X (or CN XII, or other motor control systems affecting the lower brainstem), they risk aspiration of food contents into the passageways of the lungs.
- Similarly, patients suffering from sudden decreased level of consciousness might no longer be able to reflexively protect their airway from aspiration by triggering their gag reflex.

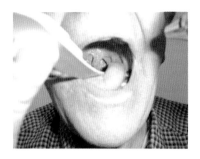

FIGURE 12-14 · Patient status post stroke affecting left cranial nerve IX. Note that the left side of the palate is lower than the right, and the uvula therefore is pulled over toward the right. (Photo from *Practical Guide to Clinical Medicine: The Neurological Examination*. Available from: https://meded.ucsd.edu/clinicalmed/neuro2.html.)

Special Testing: Assessing the Gag Reflex

- Ask the patient to widely open their mouth. If you are unable to see the posterior pharynx (ie, the back of their throat), gently push down with a tongue depressor.
- Take a cotton-tipped applicator and gently brush it against the posterior pharynx or uvula. This should generate a gag in most patients. Stimulating either side of the pharynx should provoke both sides of the palate to elevate (left CN IX in, bilateral CN X out, and vice versa).
- A small but measurable percentage of the normal population has either a minimal or nonexistent gag reflex.
- Gag testing is rather noxious. Some people are particularly sensitive to even minimal stimulation. As such, only perform this test when there is reasonable suspicion that pathology exists, such as in the setting of concerns about swallowing, speech articulation, or pharyngeal pain. If the patient has decreased mobility or decreased consciousness, be prepared to reposition and start suctioning their oropharynx if testing induces vomiting.

PEARL: Due to CN IX and CN X running so close together over their entire course, it is rare to see an isolated lesion of CN IX. Therefore, in a cooperative patient, the only time it is necessary to test CN IX by initiating the gag reflex is if the specific complaint is about sensation in the oropharynx or trouble swallowing correctly.

Cranial Nerve XI (Spinal Accessory)

CN XI innervates the muscles that permit elevation of the shoulders (trapezius) and turning the head laterally (sternocleidomastoid).

Testing
- Place your hands on top of either shoulder (**Figure 12-15**).
- "Please push up."
- Dysfunction will cause weakness/absence of movement on the affected side.

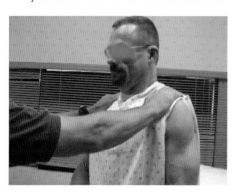

FIGURE 12-15 · **Assessing shoulder shrug (cranial nerve XI).** (Photo from *Practical Guide to Clinical Medicine: The Neurological Examination.* Available from: https://meded.ucsd.edu/clinicalmed/neuro2.html.)

Place your open left hand against the patient's right cheek (**Figure 12-16**).
- "Please turn your head against my hand."
- Repeat on the other side.
- The right sternocleidomastoid muscle (and thus right CN XI) causes the head to turn to the left, and vice versa.

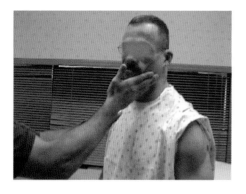

FIGURE 12-16 · **Assessing sternocleidomastoid function (cranial nerve XI).** (Photo from *Practical Guide to Clinical Medicine: The Neurological Examination.* Available from: https://meded.ucsd.edu/clinicalmed/neuro2.html.)

Cranial Nerve XII (Hypoglossal)

CN XII is responsible for tongue movement. Each CN XII innervates one-half of the tongue.

Testing
- "Please stick your tongue straight out."
- If there is any suggestion of deviation to one side or weakness, direct the patient to push the tip of their tongue into either cheek while you provide counterpressure from the outside.

Findings and Their Meaning: CN XII Dysfunction
- If the right CN XII is dysfunctional, the tongue will deviate to the right. This is because the normally functioning left half will pull the left side farther forward, bending the tip to the right.
- Similarly, the tongue would have limited or absent ability to resist against pressure applied from outside the left cheek.

MOTOR EXAMINATION

Let's quickly remind ourselves of the upper and lower motor neuron system.

- Motor control uses a 2-neuron system.
- The upper motor neuron (UMN) cell body is in the motor cortex, and its axon travels through the brain and into the spinal cord along the corticospinal (or pyramidal) tract. A UMN projects to a particular lower motor neuron (LMN) in the brainstem or spinal cord. UMNs starting on the left side of the brain typically control movements of the right side of the body, and vice versa.
- The LMN has its cell body in a brainstem nucleus if it is associated with a cranial nerve and in the anterior horn of the spinal cord if it is associated with a spinal nerve. The LMN projects out of the CNS and into the PNS, ending at a particular muscle. LMNs on the left side of the brainstem or spinal cord always control muscles on the left side of the body and vice versa.
- LMNs exit the CNS in cranial nerves or spinal nerves. If they exit as spinal nerves destined for the arms (C5-T1) or legs (L1-S2), they interconnect in the brachial and lumbosacral plexuses and then reorganize as "named" peripheral nerves, such as the radial nerve or femoral nerve (see Table 12-2).

Clinical Patterns of Motor Neuron Injury (Figures 12-17 and 12-18): Upper Versus Lower Motor Neurons

- UMNs are organized in the brain by left versus right and by body region (face vs arm vs leg).
- In the spinal cord, UMNs are organized as either above or below a particular level (ie, every UMN below T4).

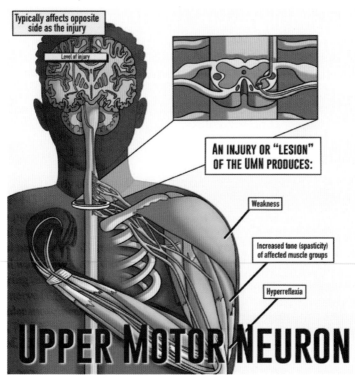

FIGURE 12-17 · **Upper motor neuron pattern of dysfunction.** (Reproduced with permission from Cathy Cichon, MD.)

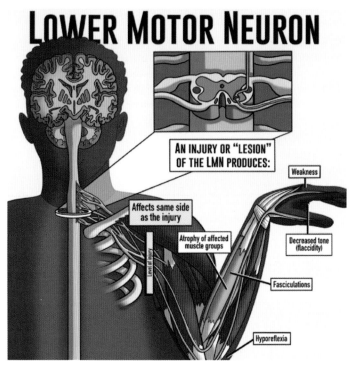

FIGURE 12-18 · **Lower motor neuron pattern of dysfunction.** (Reproduced with permission from Cathy Cichon, MD.)

- LMNs are organized by spinal level, by named peripheral nerve, or by selective vulnerability.
- If the LMN is injured at the level of the spinal nerve (ie, C7), all muscles that include C7 innervation will be abnormal.
- If the LMN is injured at the level of the named peripheral nerve (ie, radial nerve), all muscles supplied by the radial nerve, distal to the point of injury, will be affected.
- If the LMNs are injured by a selective vulnerability (ie, a toxin that damages long nerves more than short nerves), all the muscles most distant from the body will be equally affected.

> **Test Yourself #4:** Is a lesion that affects all the muscles most distant from the body a focal or diffuse lesion? Is a lesion that affects all radially supplied muscles distal to the elbow a focal or diffusion lesion?

Motor Testing

The muscle is the unit of action that causes movement. Normal strength depends on intact UMNs and LMNs, as well as a functioning neuromuscular junction and muscle. Complex movements also require input from multiple other neurologic systems. Disorders of movement can be caused by problems at any point within this interconnected system.

Muscle Bulk and Appearance

- Bulk is how large the muscle is and what it feels like when it is when it is palpated.

> **PEARL:** Worry less about the overall size of the muscle compared to other patients and more about internal comparisons to other muscles on the same patient. Is the left biceps the same as the right? Is the wrist flexor compartment the same as the extensor? Are the proximal muscles like the distal muscles?

Testing Bulk

- Using your eyes and hands, carefully examine the major muscle groups of the upper and lower extremities (**Figure 12-19**).
- With experience, you will get a sense of the normal range for given age groups, factoring in their activity levels, and overall states of health.

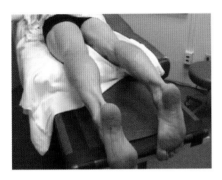

FIGURE 12-19 · **While both legs have well-developed musculature, the left has greater bulk.** (Photo from *Practical Guide to Clinical Medicine: The Neurological Examination*. Available from: https://meded.ucsd.edu/clinicalmed/neuro2.html.)

> PEARL: Healthy muscle, regardless of the age and fitness of the patient, has a firm texture, like uncooked steak, whereas dystrophic or atrophic muscle often has a soft, stringy texture, like cooked pot roast or carnitas.

Tone

- When a muscle group is relaxed, the examiner should be able to easily manipulate the joint through its normal range of motion. This movement should feel fluid, but not floppy.
- For the screening examination, both arms and legs should be tested.

Testing Tone

- "Please let your arm (or leg) go as loose as you can. I'll move it gently."
- Carefully move the limb through its normal range of motion. Do not maneuver it in any way that is uncomfortable or generates pain.

Findings and Their Meaning: Abnormalities of Tone

- If the examiner moves the joint (patient relaxed) and there is increased resistance, this is referred to as increased tone, which can be further characterized as rigid or spastic based on the presence of other signs.
- Spasticity is used to describe increased tone in the setting of UMN signs such as hyper-reflexia and weakness.
- Rigidity is used to describe increased tone in the setting of basal ganglia signs such as resting tremor and bradykinesia.
- Flaccidness is the complete absence of tone. This occurs when the LMN is cut off from the muscles that it normally innervates. A flaccid limb is often easily identified simply by looking at it move under the effect of gravity, as it will have an overtly abnormal "floppiness."

> PEARL: Rating tone is highly subjective and requires lots of manipulation of normal limbs prior to feeling confident about abnormalities. If you are a neuro-novice, practice, but don't stress over it!

Strength

- Strength is the absolute power that the patient can generate when contracting a muscle group.
- As with muscle bulk (described earlier), worry less about the overall strength of the muscle compared to other patients and more about internal comparisons to other muscles on the same patient. Is the left biceps the same as the right? Is the wrist flexor compartment the same as the extensor? Are the proximal muscles similar to the distal muscles?
- Interpretation must also consider the expected strength of the muscle group being tested. The quadriceps group, for example, should be much more powerful than the biceps.

The 0 to 5 rating scale for muscle strength is described in **Table 12-1**.

TABLE 12-1 • Scale for Rating Strength	
0/5	No movement.
1/5	Barest flicker of movement of the muscle, although not enough to move the structure to which it is attached.
2/5	Voluntary movement that is not sufficient to overcome the force of gravity. For example, the patient would be able to slide their hand across a table but not lift it from the surface.
3/5	Voluntary movement capable of overcoming gravity, but not any applied resistance. For example, the patient could raise their hand off a table, but not if any additional resistance were applied.
4/5	Voluntary movement capable of overcoming "some" resistance.
5/5	Normal strength.

- + and – can be added to allow for more nuanced scoring of 4/5 strength (eg, 4+ or 4–).
- A patient who can overcome "moderate but not full resistance" might be graded 4+. This is subjective, with a fair amount of variability among clinicians.
- Ultimately, it is most important that you develop your own sense of what these gradations mean, allowing for internal consistency and interpretability of serial measurements.

Testing Strength

- In the screening examination, it is reasonable to check only the major muscles and muscle groups.
- For each muscle group being tested, stabilize the limb above and below the joint in motion and ask the patient to make a single discrete movement (ie, "Push up" or "Push down," "Push me away," or "Pull me toward you").
- More detailed testing can be performed in the setting of discrete or unexplained weakness.
- The names of the major muscles and muscle groups along with the spinal roots and peripheral nerves that provide their innervation are provided in this section (also see Table 12-2).
- While the muscles can be tested in any order and in many different positions, the following are easily reproduced patterns for seated and supine patients.

Intrinsic Muscles of the Hand (C8, T1)

- "Please spread your fingers apart" (**Figure 12-20**).

> PEARL: The muscles that control adduction and abduction of the fingers are called the interossei, all of which are innervated by the ulnar nerve. As such, you do not see patients with isolated trouble adducting or abducting and do not need to test both.

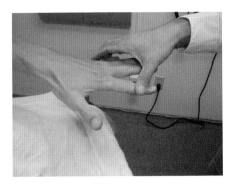

FIGURE 12-20 · **Assessing strength of the interossei.** (Photo from *Practical Guide to Clinical Medicine: The Neurological Examination*. Available from: https://meded.ucsd.edu/clinicalmed/neuro2.html.)

Flexors of the Fingers (C7, C8, T1)

- Finger flexion is a compound movement with different muscles active at each joint. The lumbricals flex at the metacarpal-phalangeal, the flexor digitorum superficialis flexes at the proximal interphalangeal, and the flexor digitorum profundus flexes at the distal interphalangeal.
- While each of these can be tested by holding above and below each joint and asking the patient to flex the distal portion of the finger, most screening exams use the following simple movement.
- "Please push down with your fingers."
- Test each hand separately.
- The muscle groups that control flexion are innervated by the median and ulnar nerves.

PEARL: If the patient's complaint is about trouble gripping or if they have penetrating trauma to the hand or forearm, the more detailed testing of each muscle at each joint becomes important. Look it up or ask for expert help!

Wrist Flexion (C7, C8, T1)

- "Please push down" (**Figure 12-21**).
- Test each hand separately.
- The muscle groups that control flexion are innervated by the median and ulnar nerves.

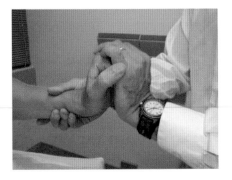

FIGURE 12-21 · **Assessing wrist flexion strength.** (Photo from *Practical Guide to Clinical Medicine: The Neurological Examination*. Available from: https://meded.ucsd.edu/clinicalmed/neuro2.html.)

Wrist Extension (C6, C7, C8)

- "Please push up" (**Figure 12-22**).
- Test each hand separately.
- The extensor radialis muscles control extension and are innervated by the radial nerve.

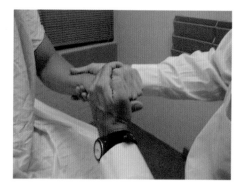

FIGURE 12-22 • Assessing wrist extension strength. (Photo from *Practical Guide to Clinical Medicine: The Neurological Examination*. Available from: https://meded.ucsd.edu/clinicalmed/neuro2. html.)

Elbow Flexion (C5, C6)

- The main flexor (and supinator) of the forearm is the brachialis muscle (along with the biceps muscle).
- "Please pull back" (**Figure 12-23**).
- Test each arm separately.
- These muscles are innervated by the musculocutaneous nerve.

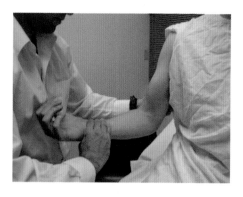

FIGURE 12-23 • Assessing elbow flexion strength. (Photo from *Practical Guide to Clinical Medicine: The Neurological Examination*. Available from: https://meded.ucsd.edu/clinicalmed/neuro2. html.)

Elbow Extension (C7, C8)

- The main extensor of the forearm is the triceps muscle.
- "Please push out" (**Figure 12-24**).

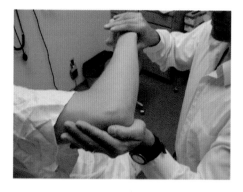

FIGURE 12-24 • Assessing elbow extension strength. (Photo from *Practical Guide to Clinical Medicine: The Neurological Examination*. Available from: https://meded.ucsd.edu/clinicalmed/neuro2. html.)

- Test each arm separately.
- The triceps is innervated by the radial nerve.

> **PEARL:** All extensors of the elbow, wrist, and fingers are supplied by the radial nerve. Damage to the radial nerve (with a resultant "wrist [and finger] drop") often results from compression of the radial nerve against the humerus for a prolonged period. This can occur when a person loses consciousness (eg, from intoxication) with the inside aspect of the upper arm resting against a solid object (known as a "Saturday night palsy" – see Table 12-2)

Shoulder Abduction (C5, C6)

- The deltoid muscle is the main muscle of abduction.
- Have the patient flex at the elbow while the arm is held out from the body at 45 degrees.
- "Please push out" (**Figure 12-25**).
- Test each shoulder separately.
- The deltoid is innervated by the axillary nerve.

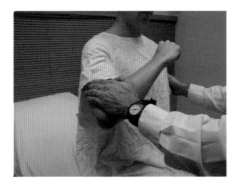

FIGURE 12-25 · **Assessing shoulder abduction strength.** (Photo from *Practical Guide to Clinical Medicine: The Neurological Examination.* Available from: https://meded.ucsd.edu/clinicalmed/neuro2.html.)

Hip Flexion (L2, L3)

- With the patient seated, place your hand on top of one thigh.
- "Please push up" (**Figure 12-26**).
- The main hip flexor is the iliopsoas muscle, innervated by the femoral nerve.

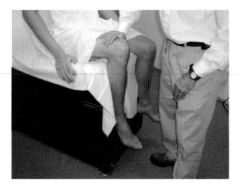

FIGURE 12-26 · **Assessing hip flexion strength.** (Photo from *Practical Guide to Clinical Medicine: The Neurological Examination.* Available from: https://meded.ucsd.edu/clinicalmed/neuro2.html.)

Hip Extension (L5, S1)

- Place your hand under the back of the knee.
- "Please push down."
- Test each leg separately.
- The main hip extensor is the gluteus maximus, innervated by inferior gluteal nerve.

Hip Abduction (L4, L5, S1)

- Place your hands on the outside of both knees.
- "Please push your knees apart" (**Figure 12-27**).
- This movement is mediated by multiple muscles.

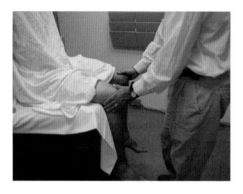

FIGURE 12-27 · **Assessing hip abduction strength.** (Photo from *Practical Guide to Clinical Medicine: The Neurological Examination*. Available from: https://meded.ucsd.edu/clinicalmed/neuro2. html.)

Hip Adduction (L2, L3, L4)

- Place your hands on the inner aspects of the thighs.
- "Please push your knees together" (**Figure 12-28**).
- A number of muscles are responsible for adduction.
- They are innervated by the obturator nerve.

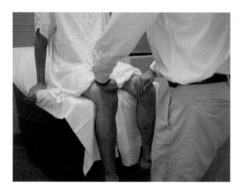

FIGURE 12-28 · **Assessing hip adduction strength.** (Photo from *Practical Guide to Clinical Medicine: The Neurological Examination*. Available from: https://meded.ucsd.edu/clinicalmed/neuro2. html.)

Knee Extension (L2, L3, L4)

- Have the seated patient steadily press their lower extremity into your hand against resistance. If supine, place one hand under their knee, lifting it 1 ft off the bed. Ask the patient to push their ankle up against resistance.

- "Push out against me" (**Figure 12-29**).
- Test each leg separately. Extension is mediated by the quadriceps muscle group, which is innervated by the femoral nerve.

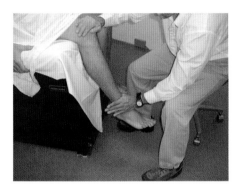

FIGURE 12-29 · **Assessing knee extension strength.** (Photo from *Practical Guide to Clinical Medicine: The Neurological Examination.* Available from: https://meded.ucsd.edu/clinicalmed/neuro2. html.)

Knee Flexion (L5, S1, S2)

- Hold the top of the patient's thigh and the back of their ankle, and ask them to pull their ankle back toward the examination table. If supine, lift the patient's knee 1 ft off the bed, and tell the patient to keep their heel on the bed against the resistance of your other hand.
- "Pull back against my hand."
- Each leg is tested separately.
- Flexion is mediated by the hamstring muscle group, via branches of the sciatic nerve.

Ankle Dorsiflexion (L4, L5)

- "Please bend your ankle up" (**Figure 12-30**).
- Each foot is tested separately.
- The muscles that mediate dorsiflexion are innervated by the deep peroneal nerve.

> PEARL: The peroneal nerve is susceptible to injury at the point where it crosses the head of the fibula (laterally, below the knee). If injured, the patient develops "foot drop," an inability to dorsi-flex the ankle (see Table 12-2).

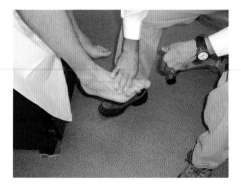

FIGURE 12-30 · **Assessing ankle dorsiflexion strength.** (Photo from *Practical Guide to Clinical Medicine: The Neurological Examination.* Available from: https://meded.ucsd.edu/clinicalmed/neuro2. html.)

Ankle Plantar Flexion (S1, S2)

- "Please bend your ankle down" (**Figure 12-31**).
- Test each foot separately.
- The gastrocnemius and soleus, the muscles that mediate this movement, are innervated by a branch of the sciatic nerve.
- Plantar flexion and dorsiflexion can also be assessed by asking the patient to walk on their toes (plantar flexion) and heels (dorsiflexion).

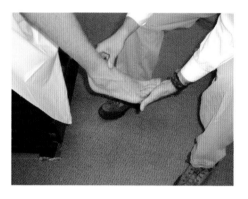

FIGURE 12-31 · **Assessing ankle plantar flexion strength.** (Photo from *Practical Guide to Clinical Medicine: The Neurological Examination.* Available from: https://meded.ucsd.edu/clinicalmed/neuro2. html.)

Findings and Their Meaning: Patterns of Weakness

Weakness means that there is a lesion in the UMN, LMN, neuromuscular junction, or muscle being tested. While that sounds like a big differential, it is important to recall that for any muscle in the body, it is easy to look up the exact location of the specific UMN, LMN, and neuromuscular junction involved, so it is highly localizing. Determining the likely localization is based on the pattern of weakness, as well as other testing (eg, tone, reflexes).

If there is weakness, try to identify a pattern, which might provide a clue as to the etiology of the observed decrease in strength. In particular, note differences between the following (**Figure 12-32**):

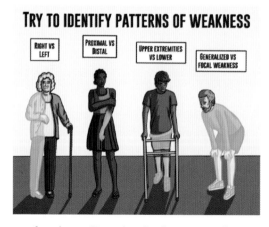

FIGURE 12-32 · **Patterns of weakness.** (Reproduced with permission from Cathy Cichon, MD.)

- Right versus left. The brain is organized right versus left. If all the involved muscles are on the right side, especially if they span more than one body region (face, arm, and/or leg), then the brain (UMN) is the likely localization.
- Proximal muscles versus distal. Diffuse injuries of LMNs tend to impact distal muscles much more than proximal muscles. Diffuse injuries of muscle tend to impact large proximal muscles more than small distal muscles.
- Upper extremities versus lower extremities. The spinal cord is organized as vertical segments. If all of the involved muscles are below a certain level, especially if on both the left and right, the lesion is likely in the spinal cord (UMNs).
- Is the weakness generalized, or is it a focal group with a commonality? Generalized weakness will be bilateral and often involve multiple body regions, suggesting a diffuse lesion of muscle, neuromuscular junctions, LMNs, or UMNs. Focal weakness will often be on only one side and in only one body region, involving "all the muscles supplied by X nerve," or "only muscles supplied by X spinal nerve."
- Sudden neurologic lesions due to lack of blood supply, or strokes, happen in lots of different locations but produce very different patterns of deficits. If a stroke happens in the left motor cortex, then we would predict right body weakness, with increased tone and largely normal bulk. If a stroke happens across the spinal cord at T6, we would expect weakness and increased tone of both legs and largely normal bulk. If a stroke happens in the right sciatic nerve as it exits the pelvis (yes, strokes happen in peripheral nerves!), then we would expect weakness of all the muscles supplied by the right sciatic nerve (knee flexors, ankle extensors and flexors, toe extensors and flexors, to name a few), but we would expect abnormally low tone, atrophy, and fasciculations.

Fasciculations

- There should be no muscle movement when the limb is at rest. Quick, spontaneous twitches of the muscle or segments of the muscle are called fasciculations. While all patients have occasional benign fasciculations and some patients have many benign fasciculations, they are more common in the setting of LMN injuries.

> **PEARL:** If a muscle has fasciculations (even a lot of them) but has normal tone, bulk, and strength when tested, it is highly likely to be a benign condition. A muscle that has fasciculations and is weak, flaccid, and/or atrophic is highly likely to represent a significant LMN injury.

> **Test Yourself #5:** A patient suffers a CNS motor system injury due to severe global hypoperfusion. Can you predict their motor examination findings?

SENSORY EXAM

Reminder of How the Sensory System Works

- Sensory information uses 2 different major input pathways, each of which uses 3 neurons, referred to as first-, second-, and third-order neurons.
- The first-order neuron's cell body is in the PNS, on the same side of the body as the sensations it detects. Its most distal projection is to the skin or viscera where it detects a particular sensory modality. Its most proximal projection is into the spinal cord or brainstem.
- The second-order neuron's cell body is in the spinal cord or brainstem on the same side as the sensations it carries, and its axon projects across the midline before traveling to the thalamus on the other side of the body from the place the sensation was detected (from left to right or vice versa).

- The third-order neuron's cell body is in the thalamus on the opposite side of the body from the original sensation and projects to the sensory cortex. Thus, the right thalamus sends sensory information from the left side of the body to the right cortex.
- The first input pathway is called the dorsal column system and carries information regarding discriminative touch and proprioception (body position). Its first-order neuron enters the spinal cord and immediately travels up to the level of the medulla before synapsing onto the second-order neuron, which crosses to the other side of the medulla before ascending to the thalamus on the opposite side of the body. There is an equivalent system for information from the face called the trigeminothalamic system.
- The second input pathway is called the spinothalamic system and carries information regarding pain and temperature perception. Its first-order neuron enters the spinal cord and immediately synapses on the second-order neuron, which crosses to the other side of the spinal cord and then ascends through the rest of the spinal cord and brainstem prior to reaching the thalamus on the opposite side of the body. There is an equivalent system for information from the face called the descending spinal tract of the trigeminal nerve (that's a mouthful!).

Clinical Patterns of Injury

- Because of the complexity of having 2 different primary sensory systems, each conveying different modalities, as well as an equivalent but separate set of systems conveying information from the face, there are multiple sensory patterns of abnormality, some of which are represented in **Figure 12-33**.
- Because of the variety of possible clinical patterns, efficient sensory testing often depends on the examiner having a hypothesis about a potential injury comparing the patient's responses to the predicted pattern.

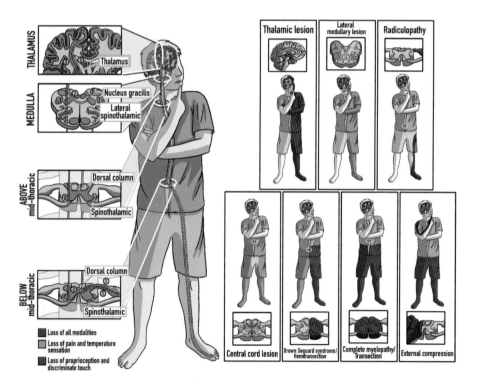

FIGURE 12-33 • **Patterns of sensory deficits.** (Reproduced with permission from Cathy Cichon, MD.)

Sensory Testing

Sensory testing of the face is discussed in the section on cranial nerves. Testing of the extremities focuses on the 2 main afferent pathways: spinothalamic and dorsal columns.

Spinothalamic Testing

- The patient's ability to perceive the touch of a sharp object is used to assess the spinothalamic pain pathway.
- To do this, use a disposable sterile pin with a blunt surface on the other side (or use a blunt object, like a cotton applicator).
- Start in an area of the body that feels normal to the patient.
- Orient the patient by informing them that you are going to first touch them with the sharp end and then with the dull end.
- Verify that the patient can distinguish between the 2 sensations of sharp and dull (**Figure 12-34**).

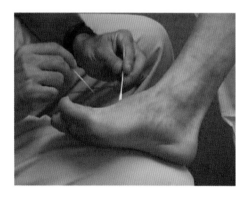

FIGURE 12-34 · **Assessing spinothalamic function.** (Photo from *Practical Guide to Clinical Medicine: The Neurological Examination.* Available from: https://meded.ucsd.edu/clinicalmed/neuro2.html.)

- Now, if you have a sensory hypothesis (you predict a pattern of sensory change based on the history or other examination elements), explore the affected areas of the body by choosing locations and asking the patient if they can identify the difference between the sharp and dull stimuli.
- For example, if your hypothesis is that they sustained a stroke, leading to the left hemibody having a sensory deficit, you would compare sensation on the left to the right in multiple body regions and expect to see a consistent deficit on the left.
- If you are performing a full neurologic screening exam without expectation of a sensory deficit, performing quick hypotheses testing is most efficient.
- "Is this the same on your left side and your right side?"
- "Is this the same on your fingers and your arm?"
- "Does this stay the same as I move up your leg?"

PEARL: Remember, you learn the most by applying the sharp stimuli, where the correct answer is "That's sharp." If you imagine testing skin that is numb to sharp stimuli, applying the dull stimulus and having the patient say, "That's dull," would not teach you the same thing as applying the sharp stimulus and the patient saying, "That's dull."

- Spinothalamic tract function can also be assessed by checking the patient's ability to detect differences in temperature.
- Hold a tuning fork against the affected limb.
- "Does it feel cool, like metal?"
- "Is it the same on the left and the right?"
- "Does it change as I move it up your leg?"

> **PEARL:** Verify that the tuning fork feels cool by touching it against your inner wrist. Beware of the warm tuning fork that has been in your pocket!

Dorsal Columns

Proprioception

This refers to the body's ability to know where it is in space. As such, it contributes to balance. Normal proprioception is very sensitive and is very well preserved with age.

Testing

- "Please close your eyes. I'm going to gently move your toe up and down."
- With one hand, grasp either side of the great toe at the interphalangeal joint. Place your other hand on the lateral and medial aspects of the great toe distal to the interphalangeal joint (**Figure 12-35**).

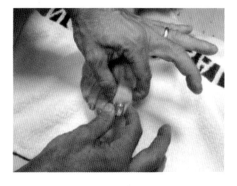

FIGURE 12-35 · **Testing proprioception.** (Photo from *Practical Guide to Clinical Medicine: The Neurological Examination.* Available from: https://meded.ucsd.edu/clinicalmed/neuro2.html.)

- Orient patient to up and down as follows:
  - Dorsiflex the toe (pull it upward). "This is up."
  - Plantarflex the toe (pull it downward). "This is down."
  - Make very small but discrete movements.
- Deflect the toe up or down without telling the patient in which direction you are moving it. They should be able to correctly identify the movement and direction. "Which way did I move it?"
- Both great toes should be checked in the same fashion. If normal, no further testing needs to be done.
- If the patient is unable to correctly identify the movement/direction, move more proximally (eg, to the ankle joint) and repeat (eg, test whether they can determine whether the foot is moved up or down at the ankle).
- Similar testing can be done on the fingers. This is usually reserved for those settings when patients have distal findings and/or symptoms in the upper extremities.

Vibratory Sensation

Vibratory sensation also travels to the brain via the dorsal columns. Thus, the findings generated from testing this system should corroborate those of proprioception. Vibratory perception is also very sensitive but much less well preserved with age compared with proprioception.

Testing

- Start at the toes, with the patient seated. You will need a 128-Hz tuning fork.
- Grasp the tuning fork by the stem and strike the forked ends against your hand, causing them to softly vibrate.
- Place the stem on top of the interphalangeal joint of the great toe. Put a few fingers of your other hand on the bottom side of this joint (**Figure 12-36**).

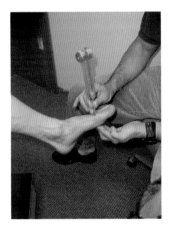

FIGURE 12-36 · **Testing vibratory sensation with 128-Hz tuning fork.** (Photo from *Practical Guide to Clinical Medicine: The Neurological Examination.* Available from: https://meded.ucsd.edu/clinicalmed/neuro2.html.)

- "Can you feel this vibrating?" You should be able to feel the same sensation with your fingers on the bottom side of the joint.
- The patient should be able to determine when the vibration stops, which will correlate with when you are no longer able to feel it transmitted through the joint.
- Repeat testing on the other foot.

Special Testing: Assessing the Perineum and Perianal Region

- Testing of the sacral nerve roots, serving the anus, is important if the patient complains of incontinence or inability to defecate/urinate, or there is otherwise reason to suspect that these roots may be compromised. In the setting of cauda equina syndrome, for example, multiple sacral and lumbar roots become compressed bilaterally (eg, by posteriorly herniated disk material or a tumor).
- Test for normal or abnormal anal sphincter tone, which can be appreciated on rectal exam (see section on rectal exam; Chapter 9, Male Genital and Rectal Exam).
- Test for spinothalamic pain sensitivity by asking the patient to detect pin pricks in the perineal and perianal areas.

Findings and Their Meaning: Patterns of Sensory Impairment—First-, Second-, or Third-Order Nerve Dysfunction (Figure 12-37)

- Decide if the pattern of abnormality seems focal or diffuse.
- A focal lesion in the first-order neurons (PNS) will affect all of the skin that sends its sensory input through that structure (ie, all of the skin supplied by the right radial nerve or all of the skin supplied by the left L5 spinal nerve) and will generally affect all sensory modalities evenly.
- A focal lesion in the third-order neurons (traveling from the thalamus to the sensory cortex) will affect all of the body regions on the opposite side (ie, all of the right body, or the right leg and arm more than face) and will generally affect all sensory modalities evenly.
- A focal lesion in the second-order neurons (in the spinal cord or lower brainstem) might cause dysfunction of all the body regions below the lesion if it is complete, but also has the ability to affect different modalities differently, as the spinothalamic pain and temperature fibers will be traveling on a different path than the dorsal column proprioception

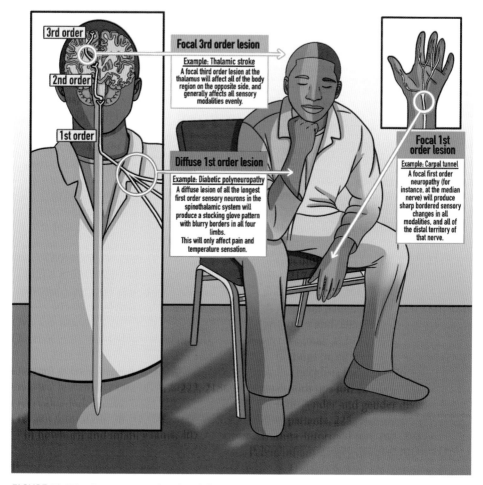

FIGURE 12-37 · Patterns associated with first-, second-, and third-order nerve impairment. (Reproduced with permission from Cathy Cichon, MD.)

and vibration fibers, leading to "crossed" patterns with different dysfunction on the left and right sides of the body or involvement of some modalities but not others.

• A diffuse lesion affecting predominantly long fibers will cause sensory changes in distal body parts.

• A diffuse lesion selectively targeting pain fibers will only affect pain perception but will do so on both sides of the body and in multiple body regions.

• A diffuse lesion selectively targeting pain fibers and long fibers will only cause pain abnormalities in the feet and fingertips. This is often called a "stocking glove" pattern and is typical for common causes of polyneuropathy, such as diabetes.

• A focal first-order neuropathy, such as right carpal tunnel syndrome compressing the right median nerve, will produce sharp bordered sensory changes in all modalities and all the distal territory of the right median nerve (**Table 12-2**). A focal lesion of all the third-order neurons on the right, such as a stroke in the right thalamus, will produce sensory changes in all modalities on the left side of the body. A diffuse lesion of all the longest first-order sensory neurons in the spinothalamic system will produce a stocking glove pattern with blurry borders in all 4 limbs, but only for pain and temperature sensation, not for discriminative touch or proprioception.

Table 12-2 provides additional information about common sensory and motor findings associated with specific peripheral nerve dysfunction.

TABLE 12-2 • Common Peripheral Nerves, Territories of Innervation, and Findings Associated With Their Dysfunction				
Peripheral Nerve	Sensory Innervation	Motor Innervation	Contributing Spinal Nerve Roots	Clinical
Radial nerve	Back of thumb, index, middle, and 1/2 ring finger; back of forearm	Wrist extension and abduction of thumb in palmer plane	C6, 7, 8	At risk for compression at humerus, known as "Saturday night palsy"
Ulnar nerve	Palmar and dorsal aspects of pinky and 1/2 of ring finger	Abduction of fingers (intrinsic muscles of hand)	C7, 8, and T1	At risk for injury with elbow fracture. Can get transient symptoms when inside of elbow is struck ("funny bone" distribution)
Median nerve	Palmar aspect of the thumb, index, middle, and 1/2 ring finger; palm below these fingers	Abduction of thumb perpendicular to palm (thenar muscles)	C8, T1	Compression at carpal tunnel causes carpal tunnel syndrome
Lateral cutaneous nerve of thigh	Lateral aspect thigh		L1, 2	Can become compressed in obese patients, causing numbness over its distribution
Peroneal nerve	Lateral leg, top of foot	Dorsiflexion of foot (tibialis anterior muscle)	L4, 5, and S1	Can be injured with proximal fibula fracture, leading to foot drop (inability to dorsiflex foot)

PEARL: If you are struggling with focal sensory patterns, refer to Figure 12-37 to test your under-standing. Keep in mind that most clinicians have not memorized the distributions of all peripheral nerves or spinal nerve roots. In most clinical settings, you can consult a reference to see if the mapped territory matches a specific nerve distribution.

PEARL: Occasionally, the history or screening examination will suggest a discrete anatomic region that has sensory impairment. When this occurs, it is important to map out the territory involved, using careful pin testing to define the medial/lateral and proximal/distal boundaries of the affected region. You may even make pen marks on the skin to clearly identify where the changes occur, especially if symptoms are occurring in an inpatient setting where serial team members will be evaluating the patient.

Special Testing: Assessing for Early Diabetic Neuropathy

- A careful foot examination should be performed on all patients with symptoms suggestive of sensory neuropathy or at particular risk for this disorder (eg, anyone with diabetes).
- Loss of sensation in this area can be particularly problematic as the feet are a difficult area for the patient to evaluate on their own.
- Small wounds can become large, deep, and infected, unknown to the insensate patient.
- Sensory testing, as described earlier, can detect this type of problem.
- Disposable monofilaments (known as the Semmes-Weinstein aesthesiometer) are spe-cially designed for a screening evaluation. These small nylon fibers are designed such that the normal patient should be able to feel the ends when they are gently pressed against the soles of their feet.
- Have the patient close their eyes so that they do not receive any visual cues.
- Touch the monofilament to 5 to 7 areas on the bottom of the patient's foot. Pick locations so that all of the major areas of the sole are assessed. Avoid calluses, which are relatively insensate.
- The patient should be able to detect the filament when the tip is lightly applied to the skin.
- Patients with normal sensation should be able to detect the monofilament when it is lightly applied (**Figure 12-38**, left). If the force required to provoke a sensory response is strong enough to bend the monofilament (Figure 12-38, right), then sensation is impaired.
- Patients with impaired sensation should pay particular attention to foot care (eg, not walking around shoeless) and directed to check their feet on a daily basis. This can both prevent problems from occurring and allow early identification and treatment of small wounds, before they become more complicated issues.

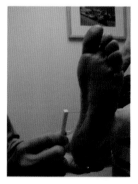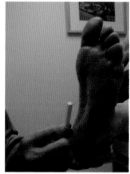

FIGURE 12-38 · **Assessing findings of monofilament testing.** (Photos from *Practical Guide to Clinical Medicine: The Neurological Examination.* Available from: https://meded.ucsd.edu/clinicalmed/neuro2.html.)

REFLEX TESTING

Reflex testing lets you interrogate a circuit including both sensory and motor pathways. It is simple, yet informative, and can give important insights into the integrity of the nervous system at many different levels.

Physiology and Anatomy of Reflexes (Figure 12-39)

- Deep tendon stretch reflexes are hardwired in the brainstem or spinal cord and are intended to keep muscle length constant. When a tendon is rapidly stretched by being struck, sensory afferent fibers carry the information to the spinal cord, and an automated signal is sent back through efferent LMNs, triggering contraction of the muscle (and sometimes other muscles as well).
- Pathologic processes affecting afferent (sensory) or efferent (LMN) fibers will cause the reflex to be diminished or absent.
- UMNs generally inhibit the function of the hardwired reflexes. An injury to a UMN will allow the LMN it normally projects onto to become disinhibited and hyperreflexive.
- A normal response generates an easily observed shortening of the muscle. This, in turn, causes the attached structure to move.

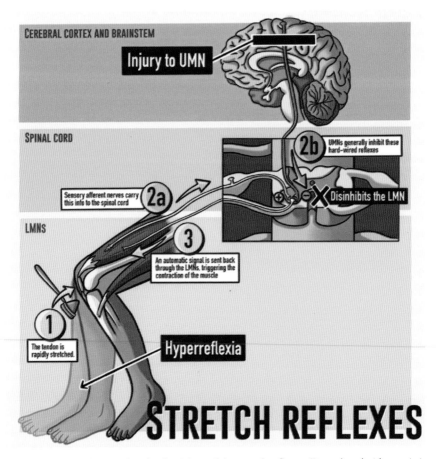

FIGURE 12-39 · **Physiology and pathophysiology of the stretch reflexes.** (Reproduced with permission from Cathy Cichon, MD.)

The vigor of contraction is graded using the scale in **Table 12-3**.

TABLE 12-3 • Rating Scale for Assessing Reflexes	
0	No evidence of contraction
1	Decreased, but still present (hyporeflexive)
2	Normal
3	Super-normal (hyperreflexive)
4	Clonus: Repetitive shortening of the muscle after a single stimulation

The Reflex Hammer

- You will need to use a reflex hammer when performing this aspect of the exam.
- Generally, hammers with heavy heads and/or long flexible handles are easiest to work with.
- For any style of hammer, a quick, firm strike, in which the head of the hammer bounces off the tendon, is superior to a small, slow, "tapping" motion.

Testing

- The muscle group to be tested must be in a neutral position (ie, neither stretched nor contracted).
- The tendon attached to the muscle that is to be tested must be clearly identified. The extremity should be positioned such that the tendon can be easily struck with the reflex hammer. The goal is to transmit energy to the tendon and rapidly stretch it.
- In most cases, it is easiest to palpate the tendon, compressing any overlying soft tissue, and then strike the backs of your fingers, allowing energy to be transferred to the tendon and not absorbed in the subcutaneous tissue.
  - If you have difficulty identifying a tendon, ask the patient to flex the appropriate muscle. The tendon should become taut and thus readily apparent.
- Strike the tendon with a single brisk stroke. Ideally, the hammer will strike and bounce away from your fingers in one movement. While this is done firmly, it should not elicit pain.
- Occasionally, due to other medical problems (eg, severe arthritis), you will not be able to position the patient's limb in such a way that you are able to strike the tendon. If this occurs, do not cause the patient discomfort. Simply move on to another aspect of the exam.
- The reflex grading system described in Table 12-3 is somewhat subjective. Additional levels of response can be included by adding a + or a − to any of the numbers. As you gain more experience, you will have a greater sense of how to grade responses.

Specifics of Reflex Testing

The peripheral nerves and contributing spinal nerve roots that form each reflex arc are provided below.

Brachioradialis (C5, C6; Radial Nerve)

- This is most easily done with the patient seated. The lower arm should be resting loosely on the patient's lap (**Figure 12-40**).
- The tendon crosses the radius (thumb side of the lower arm) approximately 10 cm proximal to the wrist on the dorsal surface of the arm.
- Roll your fingers over the radius and feel for the tendon snapping over the edge of the bone.
- Strike your fingers with your reflex hammer.

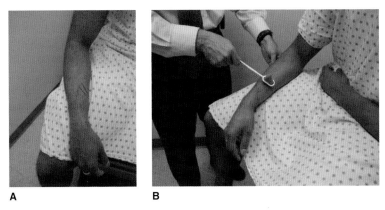

A   **B**

FIGURE 12-40 · **Assessing brachioradialis reflex. (A)** Brachioradialis tendon outlined. **(B)** Eliciting brachioradialis reflex. (Photos from *Practical Guide to Clinical Medicine: The Neurological Examination.* Available from: https://meded.ucsd.edu/clinicalmed/neuro2.html.)

- Observe the lower arm and body of the brachioradialis for a response.
- A normal reflex will cause the lower arm to flex at the elbow and the hand to supinate (turn palm upward) while extending slightly at the wrist.

Biceps (C5, C6; Musculocutaneous Nerve)

- This is most easily done with the patient seated (**Figure 12-41**).
- Identify the location of the biceps tendon. To do this, have the patient flex at the elbow while you observe and palpate the antecubital fossa. The tendon will look and feel like a thick cord.
- Allow the arm to rest in the patient's lap, forming an angle of slightly more than 90 degrees at the elbow.
- A normal response will cause the biceps to contract, drawing the forearm upward.

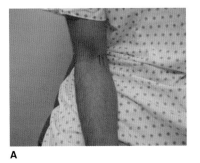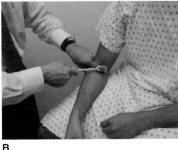

A   **B**

FIGURE 12-41 · **Assessing biceps reflex. (A)** Biceps tendon outlined. **(B)** Biceps reflex testing. (Photos from *Practical Guide to Clinical Medicine: The Neurological Examination.* Available from: https://meded.ucsd.edu/clinicalmed/neuro2.html.)

Triceps (C7, C8; Radial Nerve)

- This is most easily done with the patient seated (**Figure 12-42**).
- Have the patient place their hands on their hips and let the weight of their arms fall on their hands ("as if you're frustrated that this is taking so long"). Place your fingers on the medial epicondyle of the humerus and roll your fingers superiorly and medially into

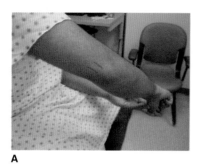
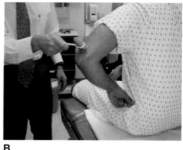

A   B

FIGURE 12-42 · **Assessing triceps reflex. (A)** Triceps tendon outlined. **(B)** Triceps reflex, arm unsupported. (Photos from *Practical Guide to Clinical Medicine: The Neurological Examination*. Available from: https://meded.ucsd.edu/clinicalmed/neuro2.html.)

the fossa just above, compressing the soft tissue and identifying the triceps tendon, a discrete, broad structure that can be palpated (and often seen) as it extends across the elbow to the body of the muscle, located on the back of the upper arm.

- Strike your fingers with your reflex hammer.
- If the patient's hands are on their hips, the normal reflex will make the muscle visibly shorten and the arm will slightly adduct backward toward the midline of the body.

Patellar (L3, L4; Femoral Nerve)

- This is most easily done with the patient seated and feet dangling over the edge of the exam table. If they cannot maintain this position, have them lie supine (**Figure 12-43**).

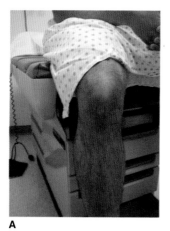
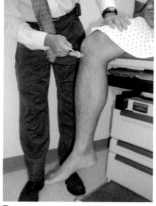

A   B

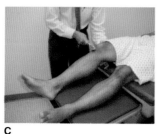

C

FIGURE 12-43 · **Assessing patellar reflex. (A)** Patellar tendon outlined. **(B)** Patellar reflex testing (seated). **(C)** Patellar reflex (supine). (Photos from *Practical Guide to Clinical Medicine: The Neurological Examination*. Available from: https://meded.ucsd.edu/clinicalmed/neuro2.html.)

- Identify the patellar tendon, a thick, broad band of tissue extending down from the lower aspect of the patella (kneecap), by placing your thumb and finger on either side of the patient's patella and running them inferiorly until they meet on top of the tendon, compressing any subcutaneous tissue.
- If you are not certain where it is located, ask the patient to extend their knee. This causes the quadriceps (thigh muscles) to contract and makes the attached tendon more apparent.
- Strike your fingers, which will then transmit the impulse.
- For the supine patient, support the back of their thigh with your hands such that the knee is bent and the quadriceps muscles relaxed, ideally with your thumb on the tendon. Then strike the back of your thumb as described above.
- In the normal reflex, the lower leg will extend at the knee.

Achilles (S1, S2; Sciatic Nerve)

- This is most easily done with the patient seated and feet dangling over the edge of the exam table (**Figure 12-44**).

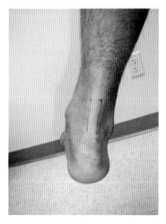

FIGURE 12-44 · **Achilles tendon outlined, patient seated.** (Photo from *Practical Guide to Clinical Medicine: The Neurological Examination*. Available from: https://meded.ucsd.edu/clinicalmed/neuro2.html.)

- If they cannot maintain this position, have them lie supine, crossing one leg over the other in a figure 4. Or, failing that, arrange the legs in a frog-type position (**Figure 12-45**).
- Identify the Achilles tendon, a taut, discrete, cord-like structure running from the heel to the muscles of the calf.
- If you are unsure, ask the patient to plantar flex, which will cause the calf to contract and the Achilles to become taut.
- Position the foot so that it forms a right angle with the rest of the lower leg. You will need to support the bottom of the foot with your hand.
- Strike the tendon directly with your reflex hammer (this is the one commonly tested tendon reflex in which the examiner does not strike their own fingers).
- A normal reflex will cause the foot to plantar flex (ie, move into your supporting hand).

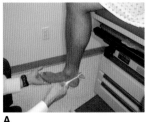
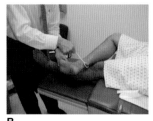

A   **B**

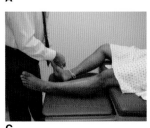

FIGURE 12-45 · (A-C) Various positions for checking Achilles reflex. (Photos from *Practical Guide to Clinical Medicine: The Neurological Examination.* Available from: https://meded. ucsd.edu/clinicalmed/neuro2. html.)

C

Reflex Troubleshooting

If you are unable to elicit a reflex, stop and consider the following:

- Are you striking in the correct place? Confirm the location of the tendon by observing and palpating the appropriate region while asking the patient to perform an activity that causes the muscle to shorten, making the attached tendon more apparent.
- Make sure your patient is relaxed. Remind them to let the limb be loose in a calm and reassuring manner (ie, don't say, "Relax, relax, relax"; rather, calmly say, "Try to let your arm go as loose as you can").

> **PEARL:** When in doubt about your ability to elicit the patient's reflex, check the other reflexes. If you can easily elicit all but the left triceps, it suggests that the left triceps is abnormal, not that you are incompetent. If the left reflexes are difficult to elicit and the right reflexes are very easy to elicit, and the patient is reporting trouble moving the right side of their body, then likely the right reflexes are pathologically overactive, rather than that you are not performing the correct technique. Conversely, if the right reflexes are easier to elicit than the left, and the patient is reporting weakness in the left arm, then the left arm reflexes are likely pathologically decreased.

Findings and Their Meaning: Abnormal Reflexes

Normal reflexes require that every aspect of the system function normally. Disease can cause specific patterns of dysfunction. These can be interpreted as follows:

- Disorders in the sensory limb will prevent or delay the transmission of the impulse to the spinal cord. This causes the resulting reflex to be diminished or completely absent.
- Abnormal LMN function will result in decreased or absent reflexes.
- If the UMN is completely disrupted, the arc receiving input from this nerve becomes disinhibited, resulting in hyperactive reflexes.
- Primary disease of the neuromuscular junction or the muscle itself will result in a proportional diminishment of the reflexes, as disease at the target organ (ie, the muscle) precludes movement.

- A patient has diffusely difficult to elicit reflexes and is also mildly weak in all 4 limbs, with decreased muscle tone, but has normal sensory function. This strongly suggests a diffuse disorder of LMNs, such as spinal muscular atrophy. Another patient has the same diffusely difficult to elicit reflexes but has normal strength and tone and has difficulty determining the position of their toes and trouble distinguishing a pin from a cotton swab. This strongly suggests a diffuse disorder of sensory neurons, such as might be seen in a sensory axonal polyneuropathy due to alcohol use disorder.

> **PEARL:** Of note, immediately following a UMN injury, the reflexes are transiently diminished, with hyperreflexia developing hours or days later.

> **Test Yourself #6:** A patient is unable to extend their right elbow, wrist, and fingers on history and examination. The rest of their arm muscles are normal. Predict their reflex pattern for the right triceps, biceps brachii, and brachioradialis.

Babinski Response

The Babinski response is a test used to assess for UMN dysfunction (although it is not a tendon stretch reflex, but rather the reemergence of a primitive behavior, which is normally suppressed by healthy UMNs) and is performed as follows:

- Use the handle end of your reflex hammer, which is solid and comes to a point.
- The patient may either sit or lie supine.
- Start at the lateral aspect of the foot, near the heel. Apply gentle, steady pressure with the end of the hammer as you move up toward the ball (area of the metatarsal heads) of the foot.
- When you reach the ball of the foot, move medially, stroking across this area.
- Then test the other foot.
- Some patients find this test to be particularly uncomfortable. Tell them what you are going to do and why. If they are still averse, you may have to omit it.
- If the great toe flexes and the other toes flair, the Babinski response is said to be "present." If not (ie, normal), it is recorded as "absent."
- Referring to the Babinski response as "up-going" or "down-going" is slang but is consistently understood, whereas reporting the response as + or – is problematic because it is unclear if + means "the abnormal sign is present" or if it means "all is well."
- Withdrawal of the entire foot (due to unpleasant stimulation) is not a positive response.

Findings and Their Meaning: Babinski Responses

- In the normal patient, the first movement of the great toe should be downward (ie, plantar flexion).
- If there is an upper motor neuron injury (eg, spinal cord or brain injury), then the great toe will dorsiflex and the remainder of the other toes will fan out (**Figure 12-46**).

> **PEARL:** Because UMNs in the corticospinal tract are incompletely myelinated at birth, newborns normally have a Babinski sign present (and are notably not good at walking.) As myelination proceeds, the Babinski sign becomes absent at around 6 months, and parents need to get ready to start chasing the kid around.

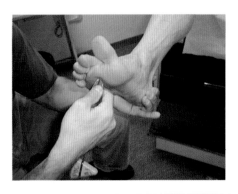

FIGURE 12-46 · Babinski response present. (Photo from *Practical Guide to Clinical Medicine: The Neurological Examination.* Available from: https://meded.ucsd.edu/clinicalmed/neuro2.html.)

COORDINATION

- Coordination testing looks for difficulty with accurately guiding a body part to a target, either perceived (seen, heard, felt, or smelled) or otherwise conceived (thought of). This function is predominantly performed with the help of the cerebellar circuitry.
- Coordination testing also looks for the smoothness, speed, and rhythmicity of movements. This function is predominantly performed with the help of the basal ganglia circuitry.
- Coordination testing looks for spontaneous rhythmic movements, referred to as tremors. The dominant distinction in tremors is whether the tremor occurs while the limb is in use (an action tremor) or while the limb is at rest (a resting tremor).

> **PEARL:** Holding your head up while seated or standing or holding your hands out in front of you is an "action," while letting your arms swing at your side while walking is "rest."

- Cerebellar circuitry includes inputs from the PNS, projecting through the spinal cord up to the cerebellum, as well as pathways from the cerebral cortex down to the cerebellum and back up from the cerebellum to thalamus and back on to the cerebral cortex, so multiple localizations can cause dysfunction.
- The left cerebellar hemisphere controls the left side arm and leg, and vice versa, whereas the cerebellar vermis controls body posture and gait.
- Basal ganglia circuitry is largely confined to subcortical regions of the cerebral hemispheres and upper brainstem. The left side of the basal ganglia affects the right side of the body and vice versa.

Testing

- The patient is asked to perform repetitive "targeted" and "rapid alternating" movements, and the examiner watches for the accuracy, smoothness, speed, and rhythmicity of the movements.
- Tremor is simply observed during periods of rest and action.
- A suspected action tremor can be provoked by asking the patient to "hold their hands out like they are stopping traffic."

Targeted Movements

Finger to Nose Testing

- With the patient seated, position your index finger at around arm's length in front of the patient (**Figure 12-47**).
- Instruct the patient to move their index finger between your finger and their nose. Watch several cycles.
- Then test the other hand.

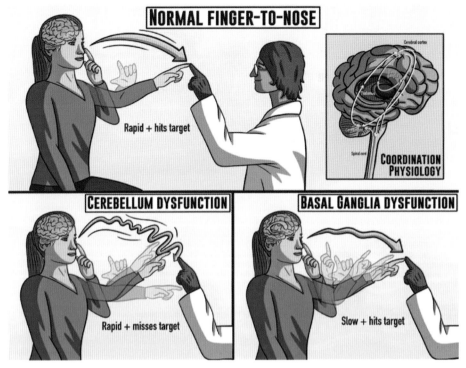

FIGURE 12-47 · **Assessment and findings associated with targeted movements.** (Reproduced with permission from Cathy Cichon, MD.)

Heel to Shin Testing

- Direct the patient to move the heel of one foot up and down along the top of the other shin, in a straight line.
- Then test the other foot.

Rapid Alternating Movements

Rapid Alternating Finger Movement Testing

- "Please touch your thumb to your fingers in turn, 1, 2, 3, 4."
- Test both hands.

Rapid Alternating Hand Movements

- "Please alternate patting your palm and the back of your hand one after the other on your thigh."
- Then test the other hand.

Rapid Foot Taps

- "Please tap your foot on the ground."
- Test both feet in turn.

Findings and Their Meaning: Targeted Movements

Regardless of the targeted movement chosen, having the body part strike in a different location than aimed for or following an unpredictable path (being "sloppy," called dysmetria) suggests ipsilateral cerebellar dysfunction (Figure 12-47).

The cerebellar circuitry is widely distributed and includes 2 primary inputs to the cerebellum and 1 output from the cerebellum.

- One input pathway involves information moving from the periphery into the cerebellum and includes peripheral nerves signaling to the spinal cord and spinocerebellar tracts projecting to the cerebellum.
- The other input pathway takes information from the premotor cortex regarding planned motor movements and projects to the cerebellum through the pons.
- The output pathway gives guidance from the cerebellum to the motor cortex and travels through the midbrain, thalamus, and subcortical cerebral hemisphere.
- A lesion anywhere in these paths produces ataxia, but the pattern of body parts involved will differ depending on the location. A few examples:
  - A patient with diabetic polyneuropathy will have a diffuse lesion of distal nerves, such that the spinal input to the cerebellum from distal feet and fingers will be impaired. The patient will have ataxia for distal foot and finger movements.
  - A patient with compression of the spinal cord at T2 due to a bulging disk will have interruption of the spinocerebellar pathways from the legs, but not from the arms, and will have trouble with ataxic gait, but not ataxic arm movements.
  - A patient with a multiple sclerosis plaque in the right cerebral hemisphere will have interrupted communication between the left cerebellum and the right motor cortex and end up with ataxia of the left arm and left leg and possibly speech dysarthria.

In each of these examples, cerebellar circuitry is interrupted and a cerebellar sign, ataxia, can be predicted, although none of these lesions are in the cerebellum.

Findings and Their Meaning: Abnormalities in Rapid Alternating Movements

Regardless of the rapid alternating movement chosen, moving too slow or too fast and varying the length of the movement (sometimes the tap is big, sometimes small, sometimes the hand fully pronates and sometimes it does not), referred to as dysdiadochokinesia, suggests contralateral basal ganglia dysfunction.

Findings and Their Meaning: Tremors

- An action tremor is typically benign and is often due to diffuse cerebellar/basal ganglia dysfunction due to intoxication, endocrinologic dysfunction (eg, hyperthyroidism), or degeneration.
- A rest tremor strongly suggests contralateral basal ganglia dysfunction and is unlikely to be benign.
- A resting tremor, occurring when the patient is not using the limb, is strongly suggestive of basal ganglia motor dysfunction. If this is also associated with some element of increased tone (rigidity), as well as dysdiadochokinesia (slowness, lack of rhythmicity of movement), it is called "parkinsonism." If it is exclusively unilateral, it could be a focal lesion (eg, a tumor) in the contralateral basal ganglia. If it is purely symmetric bilaterally, it is likely due to a toxin affecting the basal ganglia diffusely. For reasons that remain unclear, Parkinson disease, despite being a degenerative disorder that you would predict would be diffusely symmetric, is always bilateral but significantly asymmetric.

PEARL: If weakness due to a primary muscle, neuromuscular junction, UMN, or LMN disease limits the patient's ability to move a limb, they will likely not be able to show smooth accuracy on these tests. Imagine yourself performing the test while holding 20 pounds (or 50 pounds, assuming you are super strong!). As such, coordination testing should be performed after strength testing and should look for dysmetria or dysdiadochokinesia out of proportion to observed weakness.

Test Yourself #7: Both a patient with cerebellar dysfunction and a patient with basal ganglia dysfunction will have "abnormal coordination testing." Compare and contrast the expected findings on both targeted and rapid alternating movements.

Bonus Test Yourself #7a: Compare and contrast targeted movements and rapid alternating movement testing for a patient with a UMN lesion and a patient with a sensory lesion affecting the same body region.

PEARL: If a patient has a sensory deficit (eg, vision loss), then substitute a different modality. Try it yourself. Touch an object in space in front of you, close your eyes, and then touch your nose and reach back out to the prior target. Surprised yourself, didn't you? Turns out your cerebellum can accurately target your finger back to the "conceived" (in this case, a recalled location) target nearly as well as it can target your finger to a visually "perceived" target. Want to really scramble your noodle? Close your eyes. Stick your left hand out somewhere randomly. Hold it still. Keep your eyes closed and use your right hand to touch your left fingertip. The brain is pretty cool, isn't it?

GAIT TESTING

- The ability to stand and walk normally is dependent on input from several systems, including visual, vestibular, cerebellar, motor, and sensory.
- A lot of information about neurologic (and other) disorders can be gained from simply watching a patient stand and then walk.

Testing

- Ask the patient to stand. If they are very weak or unsteady, make sure that you are in position to, and able to, catch and support them if they begin to fall. Enlist the help of a colleague if you need an extra pair of hands. If you are still unsure as to whether standing/walking can be performed safely, skip this area of testing. No test result is worth a broken hip!
- Once you have decided that it is safe to ask the patient to walk unsupported, ask the patient to walk, typically in a hallway where you can see them take 5 to 10 strides in a row as they walk away from you and then back toward you. Use a mental checklist to make sure you assess each component of walking. When first practicing or observing a patient with complicated gait mechanics, you will likely need the patient to make several laps up and down the hall.

PEARL: Remember, the patient likely walked several hundred strides to get into the building to see you, so having them go a little farther so you can get the correct assessment is a good investment of time and energy!

- Observe their stance, the width that they keep their feet apart as they walk. Most patients with normal neurologic function will place each foot nearly directly in front of the other (assuming their habitus allows this placement), such that their footprints on a beach would appear one in front of the other, rather than one next to the other.

- Observe their stride length. Most people have a natural walking stride that is about 2.5 times the length of their foot.
- Observe the placement of their foot falls. Each foot should appear to touch down in a predictable location, directly in front of where it touched down previously. If the foot seems to unpredictably hit closer or farther from the patient, or more to the left or right than expected, it is abnormal.
- Observe the symmetry of the stride. The time spent standing on each foot should be the same, and the movement of the limb should be the same on each side. If not, the patient will "limp." When you see a limp, try to decide what is different about the cadence (eg, "the patient is spending more time standing on the right foot than the left, and winces each time they put weight on the left leg").
- Observe the foot strike. This is easiest if the patient is barefoot. Normal gait involves the heel striking first, followed by a smooth transition to the ball of the foot with the toes coming down in a smooth motion, followed by a lift of the heel, and then the ball of the foot off the ground.
- Observe the rest of the body's movement. Do they stand up straight or stoop? Do their arms swing symmetrically? Do they begin tremoring?
- If the patient is walking stably, it is fine to attempt provocative maneuvers such as asking them to walk on their toes or walk on their heels. These movements place increased demand on balance systems and stress certain muscle groups (ankle plantar flexors and dorsiflexors, respectively). You can also provoke their balance systems by asking them to walk one foot directly in front of the other, as if on a tightrope, called tandem gait. Walking is like riding a bike, it is easier to balance if you are going a bit quicker and looking where you are going.

> PEARL: If a patient was already keeping their stance wide-based, be suspicious that they will struggle with tandem gait.

- If the patient can walk in a tandem gait, ask them to stand with their feet together and balance with their eyes open (like balancing on a bike that is not rolling). If they are unsteady, ask them to widen their feet until they are steady. Once they are steady, ask them to close their eyes and see if they remain steady. Widening the feet as necessary controls for midline ataxia, and closing the eyes removes vision, placing the rest of the onus on vestibular function. This is called the Romberg test, and each phase of the positioning is important, as each tells you a different thing.

Findings and Their Meaning: Gait Abnormalities (Figure 12-48)

- A wider than expected base (the distance between the patient's feet as they walk) suggests midline ataxia, a failure of the sensory apparatus or the cerebellar circuitry that keeps the torso balanced.
- A shorter than expected stride length suggests too small and slow a movement, an element of parkinsonism and a function of basal ganglia motor circuitry.
- Unpredictable foot placement suggests dysmetria of the leg in motion, a failure of cerebellar targeting circuitry.
- Abnormal foot strike and asymmetric movements often suggest a particular muscle group's weakness or pain related to neurologic or nonneurologic disease states.

> Test Yourself #8: Can you predict the gait abnormality of a patient with a diffuse lesion of their cerebellum? A focal UMN lesion affecting the left arm and leg? A focal lesion of the right femoral nerve? A diffuse lesion of the distal sensory nerves in bilateral legs? A focal lesion affecting the optic chiasm?

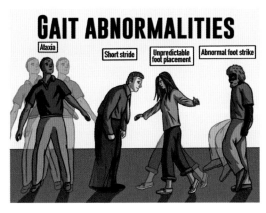

FIGURE 12-48 · **Gait abnormalities.** (Reproduced with permission from Cathy Cichon, MD.)

MAKING SENSE OF NEUROLOGIC FINDINGS

The neurologic examination has a lot of components, and it is easy to get bogged down in the data collection and recording. If at the end of the encounter, what you have is a long list of muscles that are 4+ or 5−, deep tendon reflexes that are 1s or 2s, and toes that are either up or down, you will be frustrated and confused. Keep in mind that your goal is to understand your patient's signs and symptoms in a way that lets you move forward in their management. With that in mind, here are some useful tips.

For a patient without neurologic signs and symptoms, in whom you are performing a screening examination:

- Are they pretty much the same on the left and the right?
  - Does it seem like all the abnormalities are one side and not the other?
  - This strongly suggests a brain lesion, as the brain is organized left versus right.
- Are they pretty much the same top and bottom?
  - Does it seem like all the abnormalities are below a certain point on the body?
  - This strongly suggests a spinal cord lesion, as the spinal cord is organized in segments from top to bottom.
- Are all the body regions about the same (each arm, each leg, each side of the face)?
  - Does it seem like all the abnormalities are in one body region?
  - This strongly suggests a focal lesion, likely in the PNS, as the peripheral nerves exiting into one body region never travel to another region (ie, the CNs going to the right face never travel to the right arm, and the nerves going to the right leg never travel to the right arm).
- Are all the abnormalities in a single system?
  - Are they present all over the body, wherever that system is represented?
  - This strongly suggests a diffuse dysfunction of that system.

> **PEARL:** Are you trying to decide if you really found an unexpected lesion? Does it seem like part of a logical grouping of signs, or does it seem totally out of the blue? Most neurologic structures or systems do more than one thing. If you discover an abnormal reflex in one spot, do you also find that the associated muscle is weak or the associated skin region is numb? Or do you find that only that solitary reflex is out of whack? If multiple correlated systems are abnormal at the same time, there is a lot higher likelihood that you have discovered a true lesion.

For a patient with neurologic symptoms, in whom you are performing a diagnostic examination:

- Perform a complete examination, but when you are attempting to assign a localization, focus on possibilities that would align with the patient's symptoms.
  - If they came to you with a concern about their right arm, focus on the abnormalities you found affecting the right arm, and then worry about incorporating other data afterward.
- Put your highest importance on the examination elements that are most obviously abnormal.
  - If one limb has obviously hyperactive reflexes and is markedly weak, then it is highly likely that the UMNs affecting that limb are abnormal, so focus on that first, rather than worrying a ton about whether the exactly correct sensory pattern is present.
- When findings are in conflict for multiple systems, generally put the most emphasis on the strength exam, followed by the reflex exam, followed by the CN exam, followed by the coordination and gait exam, followed by the sensory exam.
- Trust your gut. Does the exam feel correct?
  - This likely means that your formal exam coordinates with your hypotheses from your history and with your subconscious expectations from having been in the room with the patient and observing them interact with you.
  - If you are startled by the findings on examination, something is probably going wrong!

> **PEARL:** If your "gut" is not well developed yet, reverse engineer it. When you are with a patient who you know has abnormalities (eg, your attending just showed you the massive stroke affecting their left arm and leg), take a break from "examining" them, and simply observe them interact with you and their environment. You will quickly develop a sense of how a person with a neurologic deficit moves and behaves differently than a person without such a deficit.

Clinical Correlation 1: In the setting of a patient who presents and reports that for the past 2 months they have been noticing that both their legs feel strange and that they are having trouble balancing and walking, you would be suspicious that you are hearing about either:
- A diffuse problem of all the legs you've got

or

- A focal problem of a structure in the spinal cord because all the problems seem to be on the lower half of the body

---

If your exam then showed:

Cranial nerves:	Normal
Sensation:	Absence of ability to sense pin prick, vibration, or proprioception below the level of the umbilicus
Strength:	Weakness of all the major muscle groups of the lower extremities
Tone:	Increased tone of the lower extremities
Reflexes:	Hyperreflexia in both legs
Babinski:	Toes up-going bilaterally (ie, Babinski response is present)
Coordination:	Stiff-legged, wide-based, slow, and unsteady gait. Trouble with performing smooth movements of either leg. Arms normal.

You would then conclude this is likely a spinal cord lesion above the legs because you see a UMN pattern of motor dysfunction (weakness, increased tone, increased reflexes). Your first thought that "maybe this is a diffuse problem of all the legs you've got" is probably wrong because, "hey, the legs aren't really all that much different than the arms," but more concretely wrong because, "hey, there aren't any UMNs in the legs, so if the lesion was in the legs, I'd see LMN signs instead."

Clinical Correlation 2: What about a patient who presents and reports that they are having trouble using their left hand since they woke up this morning? The hand seems numb to them, as well as clumsy and weak. They are walking fine and can use their right arm without difficulty. They have not noticed any trouble moving their face, and they can speak and see without difficulty. You would say:

- "Sounds like a focal problem in the left arm, certainly not a diffuse problem of all the arms they've got."

and

- "Sounds like it's probably a peripheral problem of just the left arm because it is unlikely that a brain lesion would affect just one body region or that a spinal cord problem would affect just one side of the body."

If your exam then showed:

Cranial nerves:	Normal
Sensation:	Decreased sensation on the back of the left hand and the backs of the left fingers for pin, light touch, and temperature, but otherwise normal sensory function
Strength:	Inability to extend the left wrist, thumb, or fingers, but otherwise normal strength
Tone:	A floppy left wrist and fingers, but otherwise normal tone
Reflexes:	Absent reflex at the left brachioradialis, but otherwise normal reflexes
Babinski:	Down-going toes bilaterally
Coordination:	Normal gait; normal movements of the right arm and bilateral legs

---

You would conclude this was a lesion of the left radial nerve because all the muscles that are weak are supplied by that nerve, and all the skin that is numb is supplied by that nerve. You would localize it to distal to the innervation of the triceps because if it was proximal to the triceps, elbow extension would have also been weak, and the triceps reflex would have been abnormal and above the elbow, because if it were below, the brachioradialis reflex would have been normal. You'd feel good that you're likely correct because you saw LMN signs of low tone in the affected limb and you didn't see abnormalities anywhere else.

⚕ TELEHEALTH TIPS

Cranial Nerves

- For visual acuity, ask the patient to show you their device and note how large they have set the font. Ask them if they can read it at arm's length with either eye.
- Do not ask a patient to follow your finger with their eyes. No matter how far you move it on your side of the screen, it is not moving very far on their screen. Ask them to move their own finger and watch it themselves. You watch their eyes.

- Ask them to smile and close their eyes tightly.
- Ask them to rub their fingers by either ear. Does it sound the same on both sides?
- Ask them to speak and wag their tongue side to side.

Motor Examination
- Ask them to make symmetric movement. Ask them to lift both arms over their head, move both arms side to side, and open and close their hands. Watch for symmetry. If not symmetric, decide which side is abnormal, and how so. Too sloppy? Too droopy? Too slow?

Sensory Examination
- Ask the patient to trace the area that feels abnormal with one finger.
- Ask them to touch the same area gently on both sides of their body and tell you if it feels the same.

Reflexes
- Show the patient where to tap with their fingers and have them tap firmly. If you see a huge reflex, it is likely abnormally hyperreflexive.

Coordination and Gait
- Have the patient point at the camera lens and then touch their nose and repeat with each hand.
- Have them do the same movement with each hand or foot while you observe.
- Have them set the camera on something and walk away from the camera for as many steps as possible and then turn around and walk back toward you.

TEST YOURSELF ANSWERS

Test Yourself #1: Which problem with vision would you predict for multiple sclerosis affecting a CN? *Multiple sclerosis a CNS disorder and would cause lesions in CN II or in the brain and spinal cord. This would affect the actual transmission and processing of vision, causing deficits such as monocular blindness or a homonymous hemianopia.*

Which problem with vision would you predict for Guillain-Barré syndrome affecting a CN? *Guillain-Barré affects PNS structures, and if it attacked cranial nerves III, IV, and/or VI, it could produce abnormal eye movements, leading to dysconjugate gaze and binocular diplopia (double vision).*

Test Yourself #2: Imagine a patient with a lesion of the left CN II due to microvascular stroke. What would happen to the patient's pupils when you shine a light into the right eye? *When you shine the light into the "good" eye, CN II on that side transmits all of the light signal into the brain. Both pupils are then constricted appropriately.*

What would happen when you move it to the left eye? *When you move the light to the "bad" eye, CN II on that side does not transmit all of the light signal into the brain, and the pupils are reset to what the brain perceives is the new, lower light condition. To the observer, the pupil paradoxically dilates when the light is moved to it, but this is really just the predictable physiologic response of a defect in the afferent limb of the pupillary reflex.*

Test Yourself #3: A patient has weakness of the left face involving the forehead as well as the middle and lower face. Is the lesion in the UMN or the LMN? *This is a lesion of the LMN because it affects all of the fibers traveling to the muscles of the left side of the face. If the lesion was in the right UMNs, it would not affect the forehead, as the left UMNs are redundant for that region and could send an alternate signal.*

Could a CNS-specific disease such as multiple sclerosis cause this lesion? Why or why not? *Yes. Remember, the cell body and very beginning of the axons for LMNs are part of the CNS (in this case, CN VII's cell bodies are in the facial nucleus in the caudal pons). Therefore, a multiple sclerosis plaque in or near the facial nucleus could produce a LMN pattern of facial weakness.*

Test Yourself #4: Is a lesion that affects all the muscles most distant from the body a focal or diffuse lesion? *Diffuse. It is selectively targeting muscles that share the feature of being far removed from central vascular and nervous supplies and that fire for precision and control, rather than for power and stability.*

Is a lesion that affects all radially supplied muscles distal to the elbow a focal or diffusion lesion? *Focal. All muscles beyond a certain point are affected, regardless of their other characteristics. If you wanted to argue that there is something special and different about radially innervated muscles beyond the elbow and that it was just a coincidence that they were supplied by the radial nerve, you would at least be making a viable point!*

Test Yourself #5: A patient suffers a CNS motor system injury due to severe global hypoperfusion. Can you predict their motor examination findings? *This would be a diffuse injury of all the UMNs a patient has. You'd expect the UMN phenotype of weakness, spasticity, and hyperreflexia, affecting face, arm, and leg evenly on both the left and the right, and you'd expect better preservation of the arm flexors and leg extensors.*

Bonus question: Would you see forehead preservation in this UMN injury? *No. Because both the left and the right UMNs are equally injured, you would not see preservation of the forehead innervation.*

Test Yourself #6: A patient is unable to extend their right elbow, wrist, and fingers on history and examination. The rest of their arm muscles are normal. Predict their reflex pattern for the right triceps, biceps brachii, and brachioradialis. *All the extensor muscles of the arm are supplied by the radial nerve. The absence of any other weakness in other locations suggests this is a focal LMN lesion of the radial nerve proximal to the triceps innervation. The triceps and brachioradialis are both radial innervated muscles and will have hyporeflexia. The biceps reflex is innervated by the musculocutaneous nerve and will be normal in this setting.*

Test Yourself #7: Both a patient with cerebellar dysfunction and a patient with basal ganglia dysfunction will have "abnormal coordination testing." Compare and contrast the expected findings on both targeted and rapid alternating movements. *Cerebellar dysfunction will lead to ataxia, and you will see difficulty getting to the correct target (dysmetria) and trouble with controlling the smoothness and rhythmicity of the movements (dysdiadochokinesia). Basal ganglia dysfunction will cause too few or too many movements, lead to increased tone (rigidity), and cause trouble starting movements and keeping the appropriate speed up (akinesia and bradykinesia). Many patients with basal ganglia dysfunction will also have trouble with rhythmicity.*

Bonus Test Yourself #7a: Compare and contrast targeted movements and rapid alternating movement testing for a patient with a UMN lesion and a patient with a sensory lesion affecting the same body region. *For the patient with weakness, they will be both slower and sloppier with the movement than one would expect, and the degree of the changes will be proportional to the weakness. A severe sensory lesion will impair fine movements that require sensory feedback to execute, whereas a mild sensory lesion will leave movements unimpaired.*

Test Yourself #8: Can you predict the gait abnormality of a patient with a diffuse lesion of their cerebellum? *They would have trouble accurately placing their feet, leading to a wider, shorter, more cautious stride, known as an ataxic gait.*

A focal UMN lesion affecting the left arm and leg? *They would have weakness of the leg and would tend to keep it more extended. They would spend less time standing on that weaker leg, so they would appear to limp, and they would need to swing the weak leg in a wider arc to clear their toe from stubbing on the ground. This is a circumduction gait.*

A focal lesion of the right femoral nerve? *They would have trouble fully extending the knee against resistance. Walking on flat ground could be near normal, but trying to run or climb stairs would disclose the weakness.*

A diffuse lesion of the distal sensory nerves in bilateral legs? *If it was severe enough, the patient would lose their ability to sense where their feet were relative to their body, and their cerebellum would not be able to function normally. They would end up with an ataxic gait, as described above.*

A focal lesion affecting the optic chiasm? *They would have a bilateral temporal hemianopia and would have trouble seeing either side of their environment. They would walk normally but likely bump into lots of things that they did not see.*

✓ SUMMARY OF SKILLS CHECKLIST

- ❏ Wash your hands
- ❏ Cranial nerves:
  - CN I (olfactory): Smell
  - CN II: Visual acuity (Snellen chart or handheld card)
  - CN II: Visual fields (confrontation)
  - CN II and III: Pupillary response to light—direct and consensual
  - CN III, IV, and VI: Extraocular movements
  - CN V (trigeminal): Facial sensation; muscles mastication (clench jaw, chew); corneal reflex (with CN VII)
  - CN VII (facial): Facial expression
  - CN VIII (auditory): Hearing
    - *If hearing decreased: Weber (assessing if lateralizes w/tuning fork mid-line)
    - *If hearing decreased: Rinne (bone vs air)
  - CN IX, X (glossopharyngeal, vagus): Raise palate ("ahh")
  - CN XI (spinal accessory): Turn head against resistance, shrug shoulders
  - CN XII (hypoglossal): Tongue movement
- ❏ Motor testing:
  - Muscle bulk
  - Tone
  - Strength of major groups: shoulders, elbows, wrists, hand, hips, knees, ankles
- ❏ Sensory testing, in distal lower and upper extremities:
  - Spinothalamic (sharp vs dull)
  - Dorsal columns (proprioception, vibration with 128-Hz tuning fork)
- ❏ Reflexes:
  - Achilles
  - Patellar
  - Brachioradialis
  - Biceps
  - Triceps
  - Babinski assessment
- ❏ Coordination
  - Targeted movements (eg, finger→ nose)
  - Rapid alternating movements (eg, rapid foot taps)
- ❏ Gait
- ❏ Wash your hands

BIBLIOGRAPHY

Bhattacharyya S. Spinal cord disorders: myelopathy. *Am J Med.* 2018;131:1293-1297.

Bowley M, David W, Cho S, et al. A 57 year old woman with hypoesthesia and weakness in the legs and arms (copper deficiency). *N Engl J Med.* 2017;377(20):1977-1984.

Caputo GM, Cavanagh PR. Assessment and management of foot disease in patients with diabetes. *N Engl J Med.* 1994;331:854-860.

Charles A. Migraine. *N Engl J Med.* 2017;377:553-561.

Chiles BW, Cooper PR. Acute spinal injury. *N Engl J Med.* 1996;334:514-520.

Cornbluth D. Peripheral neuropathy. *N Engl J Med.* 1982;307:1457.

Crawford P, Zimmerman E. Differentiation and diagnosis of tremor. *Am Fam Phys.* 2011;83(6):697-702.

D'Arcy C, McGee S. The rational clinical examination: does this patient have carpal tunnel syndrome? In: Simel D, Drummond R, eds. *The Rational Clinical Exam.* New York: McGraw-Hill; 2009:111-124.

Dawson DM. Current concepts: entrapment neuropathies of the upper extremities. *N Engl J Med.* 1993;329:2013-2018.

Deyo R, Weinstein J. Low back pain. *N Engl J Med.* 2005;344:363-370.

Dyck PJ. Current concepts in neurology. The causes, classification and treatment of peripheral neuropathy. *N Engl J Med.* 1982;307:283-286.

Frohman E, Wingerchuk DM. Transverse myelitis. *N Engl J Med.* 2010;363:564-572.

Ganz D, Bao Y, Shekelle PG, et al. Will my patient fall? *JAMA.* 2007;297:77-86.

Goldberg C. Practical guide to clinical medicine: the neurological exam. https://meded.ucsd.edu/clinicalmed/neuro2.html.

Goldstein L, Simel D. Is this patient having a stroke? *JAMA.* 2005;293:2391-2402.

Gorson KC. Case 9-2001: a 64 year old woman with peripheral neurophathy, paraproteinemia and lymphadenopathy (peripheral neuropathy/mono-neuritis multiplex/amyloidosis). *N Engl J Med.* 2001;344:917-923.

Griffith D, Liff DA, Ziegler TR, et al. Acquired copper deficiency: a potentially serious and preventable complication following gastric bypass surgery. *Obesity.* 2009;17(4):827-831.

Grubb B. Neurocardiogenic syncope. *N Engl J Med.* 2005;352:1004-1010.

Harney D, Patijn J. Meralgia paresthetica: diagnosis and management strategies. *Pain Med.* 2007;8(8):669-677.

Kapoor R, Saint S, Kapoor JR, et al. D is for delay (niacin deficiency). *N Engl J Med.* 2014;371:2218-2223.

Katz JN, Simmons BP. Carpal tunnel syndrome. *N Engl J Med.* 2005;346:1807-1811.

Katz T, Lyons J. Peripheral nervous system manifestations of infectious diseases. *Neurohospitalist.* 2014;4(4):230-240.

Kiernan M, Vucic S, Cheah BC, et al. Amyotrophic lateral sclerosis. *Lancet.* 2011;377:942-955.

Koike H, Sobue G. Paraneoplastic neuropathy. *Handb Clin Neurol.* 2013:115:713-726.

Lacomis D. Neurosarcoidos. *Curr Neuropharmacol.* 2011;9(3):429-436.

Larsen P. NeuroLogic examination videos and descriptions: an anatomical approach. https://neurologicexam.med.utah.edu/adult/html/home_exam.html.

Lessell S. Optic neuropathies. *N Engl J Med*. 1978;299:533-536.

Louis ED. Essential tremor. *N Engl J Med*. 2001;345:887-891.

Nobuhiro Y, Hartung H. Guillain-Barre syndrome. *N Engl J Med*. 2012;366:2294-2304.

Noseworthy J, Lucchinetti C, Rodriguez M, Weinshenker BG. Multiple sclerosis. *N Engl J Med*. 2000;343:938-952.

Nutt J, Wooten G. Diagnosis and initial management of Parkinson's disease. *N Engl J Med*. 2005;353:1021-1102.

Poncelet A. An algorithm for the evaluation of peripheral neuropathy. *Am Fam Physician*. 1998;57(4):755-764.

Rao G, Fisch L. Srinivasa S. Does this patient have Parkinson disease? In: Simel D, Drummond R, eds. *The Rational Clinical Exam*. New York: McGraw-Hill; 2009:505-525.

Ropper A, Ropper AH. Acute spinal cord compression. *N Engl J Med*. 2017;376:1358-1369.

Ropper AH, Samuels MA. Klein JP. Chapter 5. Ataxia and disorders of cerebellar function. In: Ropper AH, et al, eds. *Adams & Victor's Principles of Neurology*. 12e. New York: McGraw-Hill; 2023.

Ropper AH, Samuels MA. Klein JP. Chapter 6. Disorders of stance and gait. In: Ropper AH, et al, eds. *Adams & Victor's Principles of Neurology*. 12e. New York: McGraw-Hill; 2023.

Ropper AH, Samuels MA. Klein JP. Chapter 35. Multiple sclerosis and other neuroimmunologic disorders. In: Ropper AH, et al, eds. *Adams & Victor's Principles of Neurology*. 12e. New York: McGraw-Hill; 2023.

Ropper AH, Samuels MA. Klein JP. Chapter 45. Diseases of muscle. In: Ropper AH, et al, eds. *Adams & Victor's Principles of Neurology*. 12e. New York: McGraw-Hill; 2023.

Scully E, Klompas M, Morgan EA, et al. Waiting for the other foot to drop (mixed motor and sensory peripheral neuropathy). *N Engl J Med*. 2013;368:2220-2225.

Stabler S. Vitamin B12 deficiency. *N Engl J Med*. 2013;368(2):149-160.

Tiemstra J, Khatkhate N. Bell's palsy: diagnosis and management. *Am Fam Physician*. 2007;76:997-1002.

Vinod E. Off balance (visual field cuts/ataxia/cerebellar dysfxn). *N Engl J Med*. 2014;370:e37.

Weaver L. Carbon monoxide poisoning. *N Engl J Med*. 2009;360:1217-1225.

Yuki N, Hartung H. Guillain-Barre Syndrome. *N Engl J Med*. 2012;366:2294-2300.

13

Mental Status Exam

Savita G. Bhakta, MD, DFAPA and Jessica Bailis, PsyD

INTRODUCTION

The mental status examination (MSE) is the quantitative and qualitative assessment of behavior, thought, emotion, and cognition at a specific point in time. It can be viewed as the psychological equivalent of the physical exam. According to the Association of Directors of Medical Student Education in Psychiatry, the MSE is categorized as a core competency for undergraduate medical education and a key component of coursework in clinical psychiatry. While neurologists and psychiatrists primarily conduct a formal MSE as part of their evaluations, statistics reveal that 1 in 5 adults in the United States experience mental illness each year. Moreover, 29% of adults with medical conditions have comorbid mental illness, and 68% of adults with mental illness have comorbid medical conditions. These staggering figures underscore the need for all physicians across specialties to possess the fundamental knowledge and skills to conduct an MSE because they are likely to encounter individuals requiring a nuanced understanding of their mental status. This chapter aims to empower the reader with critical tools for enhanced clinical reasoning and diagnosis by offering practical insights and tips for conducting an MSE.

Key Considerations in the Approach to the Mental Status Exam

- Like physical exam findings, the results of a well-performed MSE (coupled with the medical and psychiatric history) guide clinical diagnosis and treatment planning for an array of mental and medical issues.
- Several components of the MSE are based on observations that begin when the clinician first meets the patient and continues throughout the course of the interview.
- The way in which the patient relates their history of present illness will reveal much about behavior, alertness, speech, thought process, affect, and attitude. The MSE provides a language and structure for describing and discussing these features.
- To avoid misinterpretation, it can help to write down key patient responses (eg, mood, thought process) verbatim and the order in which they were expressed.
- Informal observations made during the interview about the patient's mental state are woven together with the results of specific testing. For example, the clinician will gain considerable information about memory, organization of thought, and attention span from the general interview, whereas the formal cognitive assessment measures the degree of attention or memory dysfunction.

- The sensitivity of the entire medical history is dependent on the mental state of the patient.
- Usually, the formal portion of the MSE is conducted toward the end of the evaluation, to compile specific data about the patient's cognitive functioning. However, in patients with cognitive impairment (eg, dementia or delirium), it is beneficial to conduct a cognitive assessment early in the interview to identify and characterize the level of impairment.
- In some instances, the patient's condition (eg, markedly depressed level of consciousness, intoxication) will preclude a complete, ordered evaluation of mental status. As such, flexibility is important when gathering these data, which includes knowing when to "cut your losses" and abandon a more detailed examination. This will come with experience.
- It is worth noting that findings from the MSE may identify normal responses (eg, anxiety when in an unfamiliar environment), medical conditions (eg, agitation from intoxication), primary mental health disorders (eg, hallucinations from schizophrenia), and/or some combination of explanations. It is the sum of all the findings (medical and psychiatric history, physical exam, and MSE), coupled with judicious testing, that empowers the clinician to draw conclusions and make diagnoses.
- The MSE provides a "snapshot" of the patient, a picture as they exist at one point in time. Frequently—and this applies to many aspects of the clinical exam—several interactions are necessary (often along with collateral information about the patient's usual level of functioning) before drawing meaningful conclusions about the patient's condition.

> PEARL: It is easy to confuse the MSE with the Mini-Mental State Exam (MMSE). The latter is a neuropsychological screening test for cognitive impairment and suspected dementia. It is mentioned under cognitive testing.

COMPONENTS OF THE MENTAL STATUS EXAM

The mnemonic ASEPTIC can be used to remember the components of the MSE:
- A – Appearance and behavior
- S – Speech
- E – Emotion (mood and affect)
- P – Perception (auditory/visual hallucinations)
- T – Thought content (suicidal/homicidal ideation) and process
- I – Insight and judgment
- C – Cognition

If not done already, start by introducing yourself and stating the reason for the evaluation. Do your best to make the patient comfortable.

Note that the potential explanations/diagnoses for findings provided throughout this chapter for each category of the MSE are not intended to be exhaustive or fully inclusive. Rather, they represent a few common examples so that the reader will have a better understanding of how this information might be utilized in the clinical environment.

Appearance and Behavior

Abnormalities in appearance can provide insight into a patient's life and ability to care for themselves. Such abnormalities can be the first indicator of several psychiatric conditions.

> **PEARL:** In your description, use language that is specific, constructive, and useful. Avoid stigmatizing and/or patronizing words such as "odd," "crazy," "attention seeking," or "good."

Appearance: While assessing a patient's *physical appearance*, pay attention to the following features:

- Age: Estimated age by physical appearance compared with the patient's stated age.
- Body habitus: For example, well built, average, tall, petite.
- Body mass index (BMI): For example, high BMI (>25), low BMI (<18), or average BMI (18-25).
  - Low BMI may indicate.
    - An eating disorder such as anorexia
    - Depression-related weight loss (ie, disinterest in eating)
    - Catabolic state (eg, hyperthyroidism, malignancy, chronic infection)
    - Lack of access to food or food insecurity
  - High BMI may indicate:
    - An eating disorder such as binge eating
    - Recognize that approximately 70% of adults in the United States are overweight (BMI 25 to <30) and approximately 40% are obese (BMI ≥ 30).
- Visible physical features: Can include physical abnormalities (eg, marfanoid habitus, ptosis) and other observable characteristics (eg, wounds, scars, tattoos, piercings).

> **PEARL:** Superficial cut marks or needle markings on the flexor side of the forearm could suggest self-harm behavior or substance use, respectively.

- Hygiene and grooming: For example, kempt, unkempt, disheveled, body odor and/or halitosis, meticulously shaved, or excessively scruffy.
  - Appearing unkempt, disheveled, or malodorous may indicate:
    - Economic/social challenges, such as lack of access to shower, adequate shelter, or clothing
    - Depression: Lack of energy or interest in usual self-care
- Dress: The amount and type of clothing used by the patient, taking into consideration the patient's cultural norms. A change from a patient's usual dress may indicate:
  - A manic or hypomanic episode: Patient starts wearing brightly colored, flamboyant clothing
  - A psychotic episode: Patient appears overdressed, wearing multiple layers of clothes in summer

Behavior: Abnormalities in behavior can provide insight into an individual's mental state. Such abnormalities should guide how, where, and when the interview is conducted to ensure the safety of the patient and interviewer.

> **PEARL:** If a patient is agitated, it is important to ensure the interview is conducted in an open space using a low voice. Allow the patient to calm down before proceeding. Consideration for your own safety must be a priority.

Behavior assessment is done by paying attention to the following:
- Attitude toward the interviewer: For example, friendly, cooperative, indifferent, evasive, defensive, or seductive. A patient who is hostile, defensive, uncooperative, or guarded may indicate:
  - Mania, paranoia, or substance use
  - Potentially normal behavior in response to a stressful situation (eg, someone brought by law enforcement involuntarily)
- Posture: For example, stooped, hunched, or sustained uncomfortable posturing. Slouched or stooped posture may indicate:
  - Depression, Parkinson's disease
- Facial expressions: For example, angry, sad, anxious, tearful, or pleasant.
- Eye contact: For example, staring, avoiding, or intense.
  - No eye contact or decreased eye contact may indicate:
    - Depression
    - Autism spectrum disorder
    - In certain cultures, it could be a norm to not make eye contact with authority figures.
  - Intrusive eye contact (eg, prolonged staring) may indicate:
    - Paranoid schizophrenia, mania
- Motor behavior: Gestures, mannerisms, psychomotor activity, abnormal movements.
  - Psychomotor retardation/bradykinesia (slow or little movement) may indicate:
    - Depression or Parkinson's disease
    - Medication side effects (eg, from an antipsychotic)
  - Psychomotor agitation/hyperkinesia (excessive movement) may indicate:
    - Acute stimulant intoxication (eg, cocaine use)
    - Manic behavior associated with bipolar disorder
    - Akathisia (a common side effect of antipsychotics)
  - Fidgeting may indicate:
    - Anxiety or attention deficit hyperactivity disorder (ADHD)
    - Mania, delirium, dementia (see end of chapter)
- Disinhibited behavior: Disregard of social conventions may indicate:
  - Mania, delirium, dementia (see end of chapter)
- Engagement and rapport: A strong doctor-patient therapeutic relationship is built on engagement and rapport. It also affects the course of the interview.
  - Disengaged/distant may indicate:
    - Simply lack of interest in participation
    - Paranoid thinking

- Rapport that is difficult to establish may indicate:
  - Patient is not able to trust the interviewer, which could be normal in certain societies or cultures
  - A by-product of intimate partner violence or other abuse
  - A psychiatric disorder, such as schizophrenia, mania, or personality disorder
- Level of distress: A patient may be distressed (mild, moderate, or severe) as a result of:
  - Underlying medical problems causing discomfort (eg, breathless from heart failure, pain from an injury)
  - Being brought in for evaluation against their will
  - Hallucinations or paranoia of sufficient severity that they are upsetting to the patient
- Level of arousal: A patient may be vigilant, alert, drowsy, lethargic, or in a fluctuating state of arousal.
  - Drowsiness, lethargy, or otherwise being unusually subdued may indicate substance intoxication (eg, alcohol), drug overdose (eg, opioid, benzodiazepine), or delirium.
  - Hypervigilance (ie, very alert, on edge) may indicate:
    - Posttraumatic stress disorder (PTSD), anxiety, mania
    - Intoxication (eg, with a stimulant like cocaine), agitated delirium (see end of chapter)

PEARL: Very lethargic patients may need acute medical attention, interventions, and support (eg, airway protection, fluids, antidotes to treat an overdose). Assessing vital signs and getting medical assistance may become the priority. If a patient can answer questions, at a minimum, assess their orientation (ie, do they know who they are, where they are, and date and time).

Sample Description of Appearance and Behavior in a Patient With Untreated Schizophrenia: "*The patient appeared older than his stated age of 45. He had a high BMI of 38 and was disheveled and overdressed in multiple layers of soiled winter coats that seemed inappropriate for the hot, summer weather. His hair appeared dirty and matted. Although alert and cooperative with the interviewer, he appeared distant, sat tensely in his chair, avoided eye contact, and had facial grimacing throughout the interview.*"

A summary of behavior and appearance descriptors is provided in **Figure 13-1**.

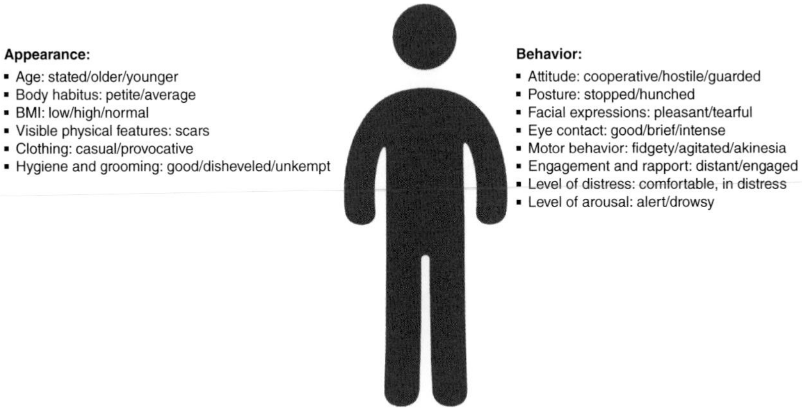

Appearance:
- Age: stated/older/younger
- Body habitus: petite/average
- BMI: low/high/normal
- Visible physical features: scars
- Clothing: casual/provocative
- Hygiene and grooming: good/disheveled/unkempt

Behavior:
- Attitude: cooperative/hostile/guarded
- Posture: stopped/hunched
- Facial expressions: pleasant/tearful
- Eye contact: good/brief/intense
- Motor behavior: fidgety/agitated/akinesia
- Engagement and rapport: distant/engaged
- Level of distress: comfortable, in distress
- Level of arousal: alert/drowsy

FIGURE 13-1 • Summary of descriptors of behavior and appearance. BMI, body mass index.

Speech

Speech is evaluated passively throughout the psychiatric interview. The qualities to be noted are the amount of verbalization, fluency, rate, rhythm, volume, tone, and latency (time to respond).

> **PEARL:** Certain speech patterns can indicate a neurocognitive or psychiatric disorder. Speech can also provide a window into the thought form and content (more on this later in the chapter) of the patient as well as demographic background.

Speech is characterized as follows:

- Quantity of speech: Talkative, spontaneous, expansive, poverty of speech (ie, very little is said)
  - Speaking too little (ie, poverty or paucity of speech) may indicate:
    - Mutism: An inability to speak seen in structural or motor dysfunction of the vocal apparatus
    - Akinetic mutism: An individual's unwillingness to speak despite having an intact vocal apparatus
    - Alogia: Reduced speech output (eg, always replying to questions with one-word answers) as seen in schizophrenia or depression
  - Speaking too much (ie, logorrhea) can be indicative of mania or anxiety.
- Rate of speech: Fast, slow, normal, pressured
  - Speaking too slow can be indicative of depression or neurocognitive disorders (eg, Parkinson's disease).
  - Pressured speech (ie, difficult to interrupt or redirect) can be indicative of mania or acute substance intoxication.
- Volume of speech: Loud, soft, whisper, inaudible
  - Speaking too low (eg, inaudible or in a whisper) may be indicative of depression or schizophrenia if patient believes someone is listening.
  - Speaking too loudly can be seen with:
    - Agitation in mania, substance intoxication, delirium, or schizophrenia
    - Neurocognitive disorders or hearing difficulties that make it difficult to control the volume of their voice
- Tone of speech: Nasal tone, monotone
  - Monotone can be seen in schizophrenia, depression, or neurocognitive disorder (eg, Parkinson's disease).
  - Child-like tone may indicate developmental delay (depending on the patient's age).
- Fluency and rhythm of speech: Slurred, clear, with appropriately placed inflections, stutter, hesitant, good articulation, aphasic
  - Nonfluent in English could indicate:
    - English may not be their first language (appropriate to use a medical interpreter service)
    - Word-finding difficulty due to neurocognitive disorder or delirium (eg, stroke, intoxication)
  - Dysarthria: The impaired articulation of words resulting from motor dysfunction of the vocal apparatus can be seen in:
    - Neurocognitive disorders (eg, stroke)
    - Alcohol intoxication (slurred speech) or primary cerebellar dysfunction

- Response latency: The length of time it takes for the patient to respond
  - This can be increased, decreased, or with no latency. Increased latency (delays) may indicate:
    - Thought blocking in psychosis (eg, schizophrenia)
    - Depression or neurocognitive disorders (eg, Parkinson's disease)

Example of Speech of a Depressed Patient: *"The patient responds in monosyllables in a low volume, monotone at a slow rate, with increased latency, and lacks spontaneous speech."*
A summary of speech descriptors is provided in **Figure 13-2.**

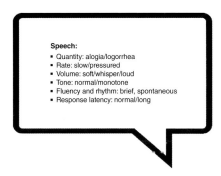

Speech:
- Quantity: alogia/logorrhea
- Rate: slow/pressured
- Volume: soft/whisper/loud
- Tone: normal/monotone
- Fluency and rhythm: brief, spontaneous
- Response latency: normal/long

FIGURE 13-2 • Summary of speech descriptors.

Emotion (Consists of Mood and Affect)

Mood: Mood refers to the patient's subjective assessment of their emotions over a period when asked how they feel. Most psychiatric conditions are associated with some degree of mood alteration.

> PEARL: Mood should be described using the patient's own words (eg, numb, happy, ecstatic, sad, guilty, angry, exhausted, frustrated, frightened) and placed within quotation marks.

- Mood described as "marvelous," "ecstatic," or "great" may indicate mania, hypomania, or substance intoxication.
- Mood described as "I feel sad," "I feel nothing at all," or "I feel numb" may indicate depression.
- Mood described as "frightened," "embarrassed," or "stressed" may indicate anxiety disorder (eg, PTSD, generalized anxiety disorder).

Affect: Affect refers to the clinician's objective assessment of a patient's emotions conveyed both verbally and nonverbally during an interview. Affect is based on the facial expressions observed throughout the interview in the context of the topics discussed. The clinician does not ask any questions when assessing affect because it is purely observational. It is important to assess a patient's affect during the MSE because changes in affect are characteristic of many psychiatric conditions.

Affect can be described as follows:
- Quality: Dysphoric, neutral, euthymic, detached, anxious, irritable, hostile, sad, angry, or euphoric
  - Ecstatic or euphoric affect may be seen in individuals experiencing mania or acute substance intoxication.
  - Fixed and/or constricted affect may be seen in individuals with severe depression.

- Congruency: Congruent or incongruent with stated mood. Note if there is congruency between mood and affect. An incongruent affect is when patient describes their mood as sad but is laughing, or patient appears sad but describes their mood as happy.
- Range: Flat, blunted, full, or exaggerated
  - Blunted or flat affect may be seen in individuals with schizophrenia or Parkinson's disease.
- Mobility: Fixed, constricted, labile, or mobile
  - Labile mood, described as fluctuations in mood from sudden crying to laughing, may indicate:
    - Mania
    - Neurocognitive disorders (eg, frontal lobe syndrome, frontal dementia)
- Appropriateness to situation: Appropriate versus inappropriate emotions
  - Inappropriate to the content that is being discussed (eg, smiling while talking about a traumatic experience). May be seen in mania or individuals with cluster B personality traits/disorders.

Sample Description of Emotion: "*LM describes their mood as 'I feel on top of the world!' While their affect is observed to be euphoric, congruent to the mood, it is labile and inappropriate to the situation at times during the interview.*"

Perception

Perception is defined as the process of becoming aware of external stimuli through the senses. Disturbance in the process of becoming aware results in perceptual abnormalities.

Perceptual abnormalities can be illusions, hallucinations, or dissociative phenomena such as depersonalization or derealization.

- Illusions are misperceptions of actual stimuli and are either a misinterpretation or clear error in perception (eg, a person believes that they have seen a snake when it is actually a rope, heard whispers when it is really the wind blowing, or observes figures moving in the dark at night when really leaves on a tree are blowing).
  - Illusions are nonpathologic: Most individuals can point to a time when they had a misperception or fleeting perception (eg, thinking there is someone standing in the dark at night when it is a coat hanging on a rack).
- Hallucinations are perceptions in the absence of sensory stimuli in any of the 5 senses (auditory, visual, gustatory, olfactory, and tactile) (**Table 13-1**).

TABLE 13-1 • Hallucinations Affecting the 5 Senses					
Perception	👃	👁👁	👂	👄	✋
Type of hallucination	Olfactory	Visual	Auditory	Gustatory	Tactile
Description	Smell in absence of any smell	See things in absence of visual stimuli	Hear things in absence of auditory stimuli	Taste things in the absence of stimuli	Feel things on body in the absence of stimuli

(Continued)

TABLE 13-1 • Hallucinations Affecting the 5 Senses (Continued)					
How to assess?	If smell things others can't smell	If see things or have visions others can't see	If hear things that others can't hear	If taste things others can't taste	If they feel any bodily sensations such as touch or movement without known cause
Examples of medical or psychiatric disorders	Temporal lobe epilepsy, delusional disorder	Migraines, auras from seizures, Lewy body dementia, delirium due to alcohol withdrawal	Schizophrenia, postpartum psychosis, mania, depression	Schizophrenia, delusional disorder, Parkinson disease, kidney failure	Cocaine intoxication, schizophrenia, delusional disorder

Patients often conceal these experiences. To identify them, ask leading questions, such as, "Have you ever seen or heard things that other people could not see or hear?" or "Have you ever seen or heard things that later turned out not to be there?"

Likewise, it is necessary to interpret affirmative responses conservatively, as mistakenly hearing one's name being called or experiencing hypnagogic hallucinations (occur while falling asleep) is within the realm of normal experience. If the patient responds in affirmation that they are hearing voices, follow-up questions should be asked, such as: "Do you hear one or several voices?" "Are the voices male or female?" "Are the voices of people you know, or are they unfamiliar?" "Are these voices simple statements or complex sentences?" "Do the voices engage in a conversation with you or comment on your thoughts?" Other types of hallucinations include the following:

- Command auditory hallucinations (ie, voices instructing the patient to do things). This can be a psychiatric emergency if the voices are telling the patient to harm self or others, especially if the patient often follows these commands. This may be seen in patients with schizophrenia, postpartum psychosis, manic episode, or depression.
- Lilliputian hallucinations: This is a type of visual hallucination in which items, people, or animals seem visually smaller or larger than they would be in reality, as might be seen with delirium secondary to hepatic encephalopathy or alcohol withdrawal.
- Reflex hallucinations: Stimuli in one sensory modality cause a hallucination in a different sensory modality (eg, music causing visual hallucinations). These may be seen with hallucinogen use.
- Derealization: Perception that one's surrounding and events are experienced as if the person is detached from them or that they are distorted, changed, or unreal. Often described by the patient as "things around me are unreal" or "I am seeing the surroundings through a tunnel."
- Depersonalization: Perception that one is standing outside oneself as a detached observer to surroundings, experiences, and events that occur. Ask the patient, "Do you ever feel you are not in your own body or you are looking from the outside in?" Derealization or depersonalization may be seen among individuals with:
  - PTSD, anxiety, or acute stress reaction
  - Complex partial seizures

Sample Description of Perception: *"Mr. Y reports hearing voices daily for several years. There are usually several people conversing, both men and women, who are unfamiliar to him, and he is usually able to ignore them. However, for the past several days, he has been hearing a male voice that he believes is his neighbor's which has been commenting on his every move and telling him what to do. Mr. Y reports that this voice has been difficult to ignore. Yesterday, the voice told him to buy a gun, and he started researching where to purchase one."*

Thought

Thought is assessed by paying attention to the responses to the questions asked. A clinician should consider how a patient shares their thoughts (also known as thought form/process) and what kind of thoughts they are sharing (also known as thought content).

Thought Form/Process: Thought form/process is assessed using the following descriptors:
- Logic, coherence, and relevance: Are the ideas strung together in a relatively linear fashion? Do they follow conventional grammar and syntax? Is the response relevant to the questions asked? If yes, then the thought form is considered linear and goal directed.
- Organization and thought stream/flow: What are the quantity and speed of thoughts?

Table 13-2 summarizes thought distortions seen in various neuropsychiatric disorders along with examples.

Thought Content: While assessing thought content, consider the totality of your conversation with the patient, including what is being said as well as what is *not* said! While obtaining the history, look for signs of depression (eg, increased speech latency, apathy, stooped posture), psychosis (eg, loosening of association, internally preoccupied, guarded, constantly checking surroundings), or mania (eg, pressured speech, racing thoughts). Use the sample questions that follow to elicit specific thought content.

Delusions: Defined as fixed, false beliefs. These are unshakable beliefs that are held despite evidence against them, with no logical support, and not in keeping with the person's societal, cultural, and educational background.
- Delusions may have themes such as erotomanic, grandiose, jealous, persecutory, and/ or somatic. They can also be bizarre.
- Also consider if there's an extensive delusional belief system that supports the delusion (eg, patient may have a very intricate and detailed explanation of why they believe they are being targeted).
- It is important to corroborate these beliefs with people who know the patient in order to determine if they are factual. For instance, if the patient states that their life is in danger and that they are being targeted by a group of people, clinicians should corroborate this information before considering it as a persecutory delusion.

Persecutory delusion: Fixed belief that someone is trying to harm them (eg, "The next-door neighbor is an FBI agent trying to kill me"). To assess, ask, "Do you feel like someone is out there to hurt you or spy on or plot against you?" Can be seen in patients with psychosis, substance intoxication, or dementia and in survivors of domestic violence.

TABLE 13-2 • Summary of Thought Form Distortions

Thought Form Distortion	Description	Psychiatric Disorder	Example
Circumstantial	Overinclusive response eventually getting to the original point	Attention deficit disorder, anxiety disorder	"I was in the shop today to buy strawberries because I like strawberries, more of the sweet kind, which you can get if you buy the xx brand, and then a kind lady gave her box of strawberries to me for free, so my mood has been good."
Tangential	Response veers off from the target of the question and is irrelevant	Schizophrenia, dementia, delirium	When asked, "How is your mood today?" the person might respond, "I hate strawberries. I think they make me sick."
Loosening of association (ie, derailment)	Overall breakdown of logical connection between ideas/words	Schizophrenia, delirium	"I sang for my sister. For this I went to hell. How long is the road?"
Clang associations (type of loosening of association)	Words that sound alike are lumped together	Schizophrenia, delirium	"Where are the knees keys please to sneeze?"
Neologism	A new word is created that does not have any meaning to others	Schizophrenia, delirium, dementia, aphasia from stroke or head injury, considered normal in children	"Cranium sock" to mean hat
Word salad	A mixture of seemingly random words and phrases that make the thoughts unintelligible and confusing	Schizophrenia, delirium, dementia, receptive aphasia	"Winter camera hay catching gold house."
Flight of ideas	A rapid jumping ("flight") from topic to topic without completing each train of thought	Mania	"It is sunny, sun is hot, you look hot, red juice."
Thought block	A sudden interruption in the flow of thought seen as loss of the goal of a communication and not being able to return to the topic	Schizophrenia	"I know the FBI is spying because…"; break in thinking as if mind goes blank, also described as "I don't have any thoughts."
Perseveration	Persistent inappropriate repetition of same thoughts	Delirium, dementia	"I have 2 daughters. I have 2 daughters. I have 2 daughters."
Echolalia	An involuntary repetition of words, phrases, or noises one hears	Schizophrenia, delirium, autism	When asked, "What's your name?" instead of saying their name, the person might repeat, "Your name"
Palilalia	An involuntary repetition of words or phrases with increasing rapidity	Tourette syndrome, dementia, autism	Repeating "chicken wings" rapidly

291

Grandiose delusion: Fixed belief of having talents or abilities that no one else has (eg, "I am HIM, here to heal you" and then touches a random patient/person on their head, gesturing to heal them). Ask, "Do you feel like you have abilities that no one else has?" Can be seen in patients with mania, psychosis, or substance intoxication, especially methamphetamine and phencyclidine.

Delusion of reference: The belief that everything one perceives in the world relates to one's own destiny (eg, thinking that the newspaper or TV is sending messages or hints to them). Ask, "Do you feel like people, particularly strangers, are talking about you or looking at you?" Can be seen in patients with mania or psychosis.

Thought control/withdrawal/insertion: Fixed belief that thoughts are being controlled by external force often described as someone trying to insert unwanted thoughts or extract thoughts. To assess, ask, "Do you think someone is controlling your thoughts or taking them away or inserting them in your brain against your will?" Can be seen in patients with schizophrenia.

Nihilistic delusion: Fixed belief that the mind, body, or the world at large or parts thereof does not exist (eg, the person might say their organs have stopped functioning). Can be seen among patients with severe depression with psychotic features.

Overvalued ideas: An unreasonable and sustained belief that is maintained with less than delusional intensity (ie, the person can acknowledge the *possibility* that the belief is false). For example, the person might say, "Whenever I go out, I see a white car. I think people in white cars are following me." However, when probed further and asked if it could be a coincidence, the person might briefly consider it as a coincidence. These ideas are usually in keeping with the person's societal, cultural, and educational background.

Obsession: Repetitive, persistent, intrusive, and unpleasant thoughts or images that cause severe distress and anxiety. These are frequently accompanied by compulsive rituals (eg, a person might have intrusive thoughts about their hands being dirty and have the compulsion to wash them multiple times). To assess for obsessive thinking, ask, "Do you have repetitive thoughts or images that are intrusive in nature? Do you engage in any specific behavior to get rid of these persistent thoughts?" Can be seen among patients with obsessive compulsive disorder.

Phobia: A persistent (≥6 months) and intense fear of one or more specific situations or objects (phobic stimuli) (eg, a person might avoid traveling by plane due to fear of something bad happening while in midair and not being able to escape [aviophobia]). To assess for phobias, ask, "Are you scared of anything specific? For example, are you afraid of enclosed places (claustrophobia), spiders (arachnophobia), or blood (hematophobia)? If so, for how long has this fear affected you?"

Preoccupied: A state of being self-absorbed and "lost in thought," which ranges from transient absent-mindedness to a symptom characterized by withdrawal from external reality and turning inward upon self. This is assessed mainly by observing the patient's behavior during the interview. Can be seen among patients with Attention-Deficit/Hyperactivity Disorder (ADHD) (transient absent-mindedness) or psychosis (withdrawn from external reality).

Ruminations: Sustained and passive thinking about something bad, harmful, or unhopeful that dominates the patient's attention (eg, a person might constantly think that "No one is ever going to be attracted to me. I am so fat. I will end up alone."). To assess for ruminative thinking, you might ask, "What is generally on your mind? How do you feel about yourself, life, and the future?" Can be seen among patients with depression.

Suicidal thinking: Thoughts an individual has about ending their own life. Suicidal thinking can be passive (meaning wishing something would kill them) or active (meaning actively planning to kill themselves). Universal screening for suicide risk is important. That is, all patients age 12 and older who are medically and developmentally able to answer questions should be screened for suicide risk. This practice promotes equity and addresses bias by ensuring screening across all demographics, communities, and care settings.

- Studies have shown that people who have died of suicide visited a healthcare provider in the weeks or months before their death, representing a potential opportunity for intervention.
- Asking about suicide can be a way to identify someone at risk and get them help.
- To assess for suicidal thinking, ask the following:
  - Passive suicidal ideations: "Do you ever think what is the point in living or that you would be better off dead?" (If yes to passive, then ask for active.)
  - Active suicidal ideations: "Do you have any thoughts of hurting or harming yourself?"
  - If yes to suicidal ideations, then ask about intent, plan, and means:
    - "How strongly do you feel that you want to hurt or harm yourself?" (intent)
    - "Have you thought of a plan about how you will hurt yourself?" (plan)
    - "Do you have the resources to carry out your plan?" (means)
- Suicide risk can be assessed using the Columbia Suicide Severity Rating Scale (CSSRS). It is administered at different points in time to determine risk reduction and treatment response. CSSRS is available for free online.
- If a patient voices suicidal ideation but has no intent or plan, the focus should be on crisis management, providing a suicide hotline number (eg, 988), and coming up with a safety contract. In such cases, it is important to collaborate with the patient's social support (eg, relatives or friends) to help ensure the safety of the patient.
- If suicidal ideations are accompanied by intent, plan, and means, then it is important to admit the patient to a psychiatric hospital or an intensive outpatient program for appropriate interventions and to ensure their safety.
- If a patient with active suicidal ideations with intention and plan refuses psychiatric care, then involuntary psychiatric hospitalization should be considered to ensure their safety.

Homicidal thinking: Having thoughts about ending someone else's life. Again, assess for intent, plan, means, and whom the patient plans on hurting.

- Ask "Do you have any thoughts of hurting others?" If yes: "Tell me more. How and why you plan on hurting others?" "Do you have the means to carry out your plan?" "Whom do you plan on hurting?" "When and where would you carry out your plan?"

> **PEARL:** If a patient voices homicidal ideations with intent and plan, then it is important to obtain information about the person or people toward whom the violence will be directed. If the thoughts are directed toward a specific individual, then according to the Tarasoff law, the clinician must notify both the police and the person against whom the threat of violence is directed.

- Both active suicidal and homicidal ideations with intent and plan are psychiatric emergencies and are reasons for involuntary psychiatric hospitalizations if the patient refuses voluntary psychiatric care.
- It is important to ask about suicidal and homicidal ideations during the assessment, as patients are often hesitant to share these thoughts voluntarily.

Sample Description of Thought Process and Content: "*Patient ZY had circumstantial thought process with occasional linear and goal-directed thoughts. They were preoccupied with internal stimuli, reporting paranoid and persecutory delusions that the CIA was following them and that their life was in danger. They were also thinking of ending their life before the CIA could get to them by overdosing on their medications.*"

Insight and Judgment

Insight: Insight is the awareness of one's clinical situation. Insight can be assessed by asking the following questions:
- "What is your understanding of your diagnosis?"
- "Do you agree with this diagnosis?"
- "Do you think treatment (medications or therapy) is important?"

Depending on the patient's response to the above questions, insight could be described as:
- Good insight
  - Overall, the patient has a good intellectual and emotional understanding of their symptoms or difficulties. The patient is acutely aware of their symptoms or illness and also of their own limitations and strengths. Their symptoms are likely to be in remission, and they know when to reach out for help and when to rely on themselves.
- Partial insight
  - The patient may understand their symptoms or diagnosis intellectually "on paper" but fails to understand it emotionally or fully grasp the impact of it on their life.
- Poor insight
  - The patient may be in complete denial of their symptoms or diagnosis, or there may be only slight awareness.
  - Anosognosia is the clinical term for the lack of ability to perceive the realities of one's own diagnosis. This can be seen among patients with schizophrenia, dementia, or stroke.

> PEARL: Assessment of insight is critical because it will determine the level of treatment engagement and compliance.

Judgment: Judgment is described as the general ability to problem solve.
- It can be assessed by asking about the following common scenario: "What would you do if you found a sealed, addressed, stamped envelope on the ground?" The response to this scenario can give you an idea of how the individual would solve the problem.
- Judgment is also assessed throughout the interview and based on the patient's recent actions, such as if they have done anything to put themselves or other people in harm's way.

- Based on the assessment, an individual's judgment could be described as either:
  - Grossly intact
  - Grossly impaired

Sample Description of Insight and Judgment: *"Mr. YM has partial insight. He states that his doctors have diagnosed him with schizophrenia, but he doesn't know what that means and does not believe he has it. However, he takes his prescribed medications regularly as this helps him stay calm. His judgment is grossly intact. He states he usually doesn't pick up things from the street meant for others, such as sealed envelopes."*

Cognition

- A complete MSE includes the cognitive exam as described in this section.
- The cognitive assessment follows a hierarchic ordering of cortical function, starting with basic functions such as orientation, attention, general fund of knowledge, and memory (assessed as part of every MSE). It is followed by assessment of higher-order abilities of language, constructional ability, and abstract thinking.
- This can be overwhelming and even threatening for some patients. For this reason, it is conducted at the end of the MSE, after rapport has been established.
- Ensure that the room is quiet.
- Inform the patient that this portion of the exam will require them to do simple math or counting, spell words, recall, and draw.
- Let them know that they should just try their best and that it is okay if they are not able to complete all of the tasks.
- Ask the patient about their education level to get a sense of what their baseline cognition and intellectual function might be.

> **PEARL:** For certain patients (eg, suspected dementia), cognitive assessment should be conducted using structured screening tools, such as the following:
> - Montreal Cognitive Assessment (MoCA): Open access and can easily be found online
> - Saint Louis University Mental Status Examination (SLUMS): Also open access and easily found online
> - Mini-Cog: Proprietary but can be reprinted with author permission for clinical use
> - Mini-Mental Status Exam (MMSE): Proprietary

Orientation: Provides a very rough sense of the person's overall cognition but is only a start. Assess a person's orientation to time, place, person, and situation—often documented as alert and oriented (AO) × 4 in the electronic health record. The following questions can be used to assess orientation:

- "Can you tell me today's day, date, and year?"
- "Can you tell me where you are currently and what are you doing here?"
- "Do you know who I (the interviewer) am?"

Attention and Concentration: The ability of an individual to focus and sustain their thoughts on a specific task or topic. This can be assessed by asking the patient:

- To spell a word (eg, "world") backward (ie, "d-l-r-o-w")
- To subtract 7 from 100, and keep subtracting 7 from the result for 5 times (ie, 93, 86, 79, 72, 65)
- If they have noticed any problems balancing their checkbooks or calculating correct change when making purchases using money

Memory: The process of recalling information. It is classified according to the length of time a particular piece of information can be recalled.

- Immediate memory: The shortest type of information storage.
  - This can be assessed by asking the patient to repeat a set of unrelated words and/or numbers in the original order. For example, ask the patient to repeat the following: "Red," "25," and "pretzel."
- Short-term memory: Information that is stored for a few minutes to be processed and used while performing a task.
  - This can be assessed by listing 3 unrelated objects for immediate memory and then asking the patient to remember the 3 objects and repeat them to you after 5 minutes in no specific order.
- Long-term memory: Information is stored for days to years.
  - This can be assessed by asking about an objectively verifiable personal or historical fact (eg, the patient's place of birth, where they were raised)
- Amnesia: Loss of memory
- Retrograde amnesia: Inability to recall memories and/or information acquired prior to an incident. Can be seen in patients with:
  - Head Injury, stroke
  - Dissociative fugue, where an individual cannot recall any information about their past or their own identity, usually preceded by an emotional trauma
- Anterograde amnesia: Inability to recall memories and/or information acquired after the incident. Can be seen in patients with:
  - Head Injury, stroke, dementia
  - Alcohol-induced Wernicke-Korsakoff syndrome
- Transient global amnesia: Sudden inability to recall memories and/or information acquired prior to and after the incident, usually lasting 24 hours. Can be seen after:
  - Head injury, stroke
- Confabulation: Filling in lapses of memory with fabricated events, without the intention of deceiving the interviewer. Can be seen in patients with:
  - Alcohol-induced Wernicke-Korsakoff syndrome

Fund of Knowledge: An individual's awareness/knowledge of current events. This can be assessed by asking the individual to name the current and past president or governor of the state they reside in. Or simple geography questions, such as naming bordering states. Fund of knowledge can increase with education and decrease in patients with dementia.

Abstract Thinking: The ability to analyze information, detect patterns and connections between different pieces of data, and then apply that knowledge to practice. This can be assessed by asking the patient:

- The meaning of the phrase, "People in glass houses should not throw stones"
- To list similarities and differences between an orange and a ball
- To list similarities and differences between a painting and a poem
- A concrete response (eg, "Don't throw stones because it will break the glass") may be seen in patients with schizophrenia, dementia, autism spectrum disorder, stroke, or intellectual disabilities.

Cultural Considerations

- A patient's cultural background can affect many aspects of the MSE.
- Clinicians must be cognizant that their own culture and life experiences can affect their observation and interpretation of a patient's behavior. This awareness is necessary when differentiating between cultural norms and psychopathology.
  - For example, seeing visions and communicating with deceased loved ones may be common experiences in one culture yet considered symptoms of a psychotic disorder in another.
- Furthermore, patients from different cultures may communicate and/or manifest symptoms in a variety of ways. For example, patients from Asian cultures may be more likely to endorse somatic symptoms rather than emotional symptoms.
- In addition, a patient's behavioral presentation, including eye contact, emotional expression, and willingness to provide personal or family information, may vary and requires culturally sensitive interpretation.
- It is important to account for other factors such as the patient's education history when assessing general fund of knowledge. Renn and John (2019) note that nonwhite and ethnic minorities often perform comparably to their white counterparts on performance-based assessments but may experience a disadvantage on assessment measures that have been developed using white-only samples.
- English language abilities should also be considered if the MSE is conducted in English, as language fluency may confound the verbal aspects of the MSE. Questions and items used to assess abstract thinking may be unfamiliar or have different significance to patients from different cultures or those with limited English fluency. For example, a patient's inability to interpret a proverb may indicate a different upbringing rather than impaired intellectual function.

The Role of Bias in the Mental Health Assessment

- Similar to managing biases that affect other aspects of care, the first step is recognizing that biases exist and that we have to consider what role they might be playing when gathering and interpreting data.
- The reasons behind abnormalities in mental status are many and often require careful consideration of contributing factors before identifying their root cause.
- As with any aspect of clinical care, it is important for a clinician to take their own history, review primary data, and obtain collateral information (eg, from family members, friends), as is relevant and permitted by the patient. Diagnoses mentioned in a patient's record are not always fully supported, and it is easy to accept or be influenced by what others have written. Mental health issues are particularly susceptible to these forces, as diagnoses are based on history and behaviors and rarely depend on imaging, labs, and objective data that are a prominent feature of other aspects of healthcare.
- As with any area of wellness and disease, patients may have their own biases toward mental health. This can affect their willingness to engage in an assessment and/or accept that they may have problems in this domain.

Pitfalls to Consider When Assessing Mental Status

- It is common for diseases in other organ systems to have psychiatric manifestations. Mental status changes can be the initial presentation of, or occur secondarily to, disorders that are based elsewhere in the body.

- Organ system-based illnesses (eg, vascular disease, cancer) can contribute to mental health disorders (eg, depression or anxiety). And symptoms related to mental health conditions (eg, anxiety) can have organ system-based manifestations (eg, shortness of breath, chest pain).
- Time course and evolution are particularly important to note. An acute change in behavior and thinking might indicate an organic cause compared to the gradual changes in thinking and behavior more commonly seen in psychiatric disorders.
- Appropriate engagement in an MSE requires that the patient is able to understand the questions and report back their responses.
  - Interpreters should be utilized if there are language issues. If patients have impaired speech (eg, from a prior stroke), then other means may need to be employed in order to gauge their responses (eg, writing out answers to questions).
  - Patients need to be able to hear the questions being asked, which can be challenging if they have auditory deficits.
  - Multiple simultaneous challenges (eg, to speech, hearing, and/or understanding a foreign language) can create the appearance of impaired mental status when in fact the problems lie elsewhere.
  - It may take longer than anticipated to complete the MSE, requiring patience to gather accurate information.

DIAGNOSES AND INSIGHTS BASED ON THE MENTAL STATUS EXAM

Diagnoses are made and insights drawn based on the pattern of responses to the MSE. Responses suggestive of delirium, dementia, depression, mania, and schizophrenia are provided on the following pages, as these are common clinical conditions where the MSE is key in establishing the diagnosis. Note that the order in which the MSE is presented differs from how the specific elements were described earlier for several of the case examples. The sequence provided in the examples for delirium and dementia follows a common approach used in clinical practice—to check for orientation early in the MSE in order to determine the accuracy of patient report.

DIAGNOSIS OF DELIRIUM

Delirium is characterized by an abrupt change in prior behaviors resulting in a broad range of mental impairments. This results in confused thinking and a range of other deficits, often in a fluctuating pattern. It is caused by one or more insults (eg, infection, metabolic disorder, intoxication) that manifest as impairments in mental function. Identifying and treating the underlying process is the best way of addressing the patient's acute mental impairment.

Clinical Scenario

A 55-year-old man with a history of alcohol use disorder and depression is admitted to the medicine service for hematemesis. He is refusing treatment and wants to leave against medical advice. The psychiatric team is consulted to evaluate the patient's decision-making capacity, as the medical team needs to perform multiple interventions. Upon evaluation, the key MSE findings (below), along with this patient's psychiatric history, suggest that he lacks decision-making capacity at the time of the evaluation.

Key MSE Findings

- Appearance: Unkempt, unshaven, wearing hospital gown, dozing off while talking
- Attitude: Withdrawn, partly cooperative
- Eye contact: Poor
- Motor behavior: Picking at clothes, unsteady gait, flapping of outstretched hand at the wrist (ie, asterixis)
- Orientation: Disoriented to time and situation but oriented to place and person
- Speech: Incoherent, fluctuating volume between loud and whisper
- Mood: "I want to leave"
- Affect: Angry, congruent with mood
- Perception: "Those tiny people in the corner will kill me" (lilliputian visual hallucinations)
- Thought process: Tangential, perseveration
- Thought content: Persecutory delusions
- Insight: Poor
- Judgment: Grossly impaired based on not being able to understand the severity of symptoms, the risks and benefits of recommended treatment, and what would happen if he did not undergo the recommended treatments
- Attention: Distracted, unable to perform serial subtraction or spell the word "world" backward
- Memory: Unable to recall 3 objects immediately in the same order and after 5 minutes; confabulating answers to questions related to long-term memory
- Fund of knowledge: Unable to answer the current President of United States.
- Abstract thinking: Unable to describe the similarity between apple and orange; when asked to explain what the saying "An acorn never falls far from the tree" means, he replies, "I hate falling."

DIAGNOSIS OF DEMENTIA

Dementia is a disorder characterized by an impaired ability to remember, think, or make decisions that interferes with doing everyday activities. It typically develops slowly over time and is progressive.

Clinical Scenario

A 75-year-old woman with history of Alzheimer dementia for the past 7 years was brought in by her daughter for an urgent follow-up psychiatric outpatient appointment as she has been refusing to eat food cooked by home aide.

Key MSE Findings

- Appearance: Frail looking, appears older than stated age, casually dressed, fairly groomed
- Attitude: Partly engaged, defensive
- Eye contact: Brief, looking around the room
- Motor behavior: Hand tremors, fidgety
- Orientation: Alert, oriented to person and place but not to time or situation
- Speech: Speaks softly, almost whispering, answers in 1 or 2 words
- Mood: "Don't know"
- Affect: Flat, congruent to mood

- Perception: Denies hallucinations but appears responding to internal stimuli
- Thought process: Tangential, occasionally linear, goal-directed
- Thought content: "Food is tampered" paranoid delusion
- Insight: Poor, doesn't think she has an illness or any other problem
- Judgment: Grossly impaired; responds "What envelope?" "What envelope?"; gets agitated
- Attention: Inattentive, able to do one serial subtraction by 3 starting at 20 but not after 17
- Memory: Impaired immediate and short-term memory but able to recall 9/11 events
- Fund of knowledge: When asked to name the current President replies George H.W. Bush and same answer for past President, unable to answer California's neighboring states.
- Abstract thinking: Able to say similarity between apple and orange but not difference; responds to the expression "The grass always looks greener on the other side" as "The grass is dying. I don't know."

DIAGNOSIS OF DEPRESSION

Depression is a disorder characterized by feeling sad, hopeless, or empty and having related symptoms on a daily basis, with a lack of interest in life. It lasts for 2 weeks or longer.

Clinical Scenario

A 35-year-old with a past psychiatric history of major depressive disorder currently not on psychiatric medications presents to their primary care provider for worsening depression.

Key MSE Findings

- Appearance: High BMI, wearing weather- and age-appropriate clothing, unbrushed hair, stooped posture
- Attitude: Cooperative, withdrawn
- Eye contact: Brief eye contact mostly looking downward
- Motor behavior: Psychomotor retardation
- Speech: Slow rate, low volume, pauses, sighs, decreased production, monotonous
- Mood: "Bit fed up"; "Everything seems black"
- Affect: Dysphoric, tearful, congruent to mood
- Perception: Denies any hallucinations
- Thought process: Linear, goal-oriented
- Thought content: No evidence of delusional thought content; exhibits ruminative themes related to guilt, loss, and death; passive suicidal ideations ("What's the point really?") but denies active suicidal ideations, intent, and plan
- Insight: Good
- Judgment: Grossly intact
- Orientation: Oriented to person, place, time, and situation
- Attention: Mild impairment; able to subtract 7 from 100 until 86, then long pause and required prompting to continue
- Memory: Intact remote memory, able to repeat 3 objects but unable to recall after 5 minutes, mild impairment in recent memory.
- Fund of knowledge: Consistent with post-secondary education
- Abstract thinking: Grossly intact

DIAGNOSIS OF BIPOLAR DISORDER

Bipolar disorder is characterized by mood swings between manic episodes and depressive episodes. The MSE below is a description of an individual experiencing mania.

Clinical Scenario

A 27-year-old with past psychiatric history of bipolar I disorder who was lost to follow-up for 8 months presents to the walk-in clinic wanting to "heal everyone."

Key MSE Findings

- Appearance: Wearing brightly colored, provocative outfit; mildly unkempt; appears stated age; well nourished
- Attitude: Excited initially but becomes irritable and hostile toward the end
- Eye contact: Intense
- Motor behavior: Psychomotor agitation: pacing, fidgeting
- Speech: Rapid rate, loud at times, uninterruptible, pressured, increased production
- Mood: "Wonderful!"
- Affect: Euphoric, labile, irritable at times, congruent to mood
- Perception: Auditory hallucination, "The Lord is talking to me"
- Thought process: Flight of ideas, jumping from one topic to another, "hungry, food, fish"; clang associations; using rhyming words, "names, games," "dingly dang"; circumstantial
- Thought content: Grandiose delusions; "I am here to heal everyone"; delusions of reference, preoccupation
- Insight: Poor
- Judgment: Grossly impaired
- Orientation: Oriented to person, place, time, and situation
- Attention: Impaired, easily distractible, and requires redirection
- Memory: Able to recall 2 of 3 objects but gets distracted and adds various objects; remote memory is intact
- Fund of knowledge: Consistent with post-secondary education.
- Abstract thinking: Able to provide similarity and difference between apple and orange; responds to the expression "Rome was not built in a day" as "I can build Rome in few days. I have the power to build anything."

DIAGNOSIS OF SCHIZOPHRENIA

Schizophrenia is a chronic disorder characterized by delusions, hallucinations, disorganized thinking/behavior, and cognitive impairment.

Clinical Scenario

A 40-year-old man was brought in by the police for psychiatric evaluation to the emergency department after they received a 911 call that he was wandering the streets, yelling at passersby, and gesturing aggressively.

Key MSE Findings

- Appearance: Patient with high BMI, malodorous, appearing older than stated age, wearing multiple coats on a warm day
- Attitude: Guarded, hypervigilant, hostile

- Eye contact: Staring
- Motor behavior: Restless, hand tremor
- Speech: Loud, incoherent
- Mood: "Happys**t"
- Affect: Angry, mood incongruent
- Perception: Hearing command auditory hallucinations
- Thought process: Word salad, neologisms; "cranium sock" to refer to hat; tangential
- Thought content: Persecutory delusions, thought insertion, "The aliens are inserting messages through the hole in this cranium sock"; homicidal ideations, "I have been asked to eliminate the Indians"; when asked further, has intent and plan to shoot but no access to means
- Insight: Poor
- Judgment: Impaired
- Orientation: Oriented to person, place, time, and situation
- Attention: Grossly impaired, unable to perform serial subtractions, preoccupied with internal stimuli
- Memory: Too agitated and preoccupied to complete word repeat and recall
- Fund of knowledge: Gets angry when asked to name the current US President and refuses to answer two states bordering Arizona.
- Abstract thinking: Grossly impaired; when asked what "People who live in glass houses should not throw stones" means, he responds, "I will throw a stone at you if you try to hurt me."

🖥️ TELEHEALTH TIPS

An exponential rise in video telehealth for mental health and other clinical specialties was observed in many healthcare systems at the outset of the COVID-19 pandemic. Since then, more than half of the mental health visits are now delivered via telehealth. While evidence indicates that videoconference-based mental healthcare produces outcomes and benefits similar to those of traditional in-person care, it is important to consider several factors while conducting an MSE via telehealth:

- In general, providers should follow the policies and procedures of their healthcare system regarding consent requirements prior to a telehealth visit. At minimum, consider obtaining verbal consent prior to the first telehealth visit to review privacy, emergency procedures, and possible limitations of the modality. Prior to beginning each visit, discuss a backup modality (eg, telephone) in case of technology failure or poor connectivity.
- Make sure you obtain the location, address, and phone number at the start of (or prior to) the visit. Should a patient safety or emergency medical/psychiatric situation arise during the course of the telehealth visit, providers should be aware that calling 911 will necessitate specifying the location of the patient; otherwise, 911 call recognition software may direct services toward the caller's location.
- Make sure the patient has privacy, a secure place, and feels comfortable proceeding with the MSE. People experiencing domestic violence, for example, may be overheard by their abuser if engaging in teletherapy at home or other places to which the abuser has access.
- Individuals experiencing mania, ADHD and/or those who are hypervigilant may get distracted by various aspects of the video platform. It may be helpful to build strategies to manage distraction during the MSE.

- Individuals with dementia, young children, and patients with physical disabilities may need assistance using technology, and it is important to obtain consent from the caregiver prior to the exam.
- Building rapport via telemedicine can be challenging. Providers may need to put in extra effort to form bonds and devise ways of connecting with their patients, such as by maintaining eye contact by looking at the web camera (rather than at the patient on the screen), speaking more slowly, and allowing for longer pauses during conversation. You can ask a patient about a picture in their background or compliment them on room décor in order to help create an environment that indicates interest and promotes dialogue.
- Individuals who do not have legal status, engage in behavior that is criminalized (eg, sex work, illicit drug use), and/or are refugees from oppressive governments or gang activity may fear being recorded and have questions about media storage.
- The appearance and behavior component of the MSE can be limited depending on how much of the patient is visible on camera. Several observational elements of the MSE might need follow-up questions to obtain a complete evaluation. For example, you might ask the patient to stretch their hands straight in front of the camera and spread their fingers to assess for tremors.
- If the patient experiences emotional distress or a panic attack during the MSE, clinicians can help by identifying grounding strategies to bring them back to the here and now. If another person is in the home, clinicians can ask that person for assistance if the situation is becoming unsafe for the patient. Having a dog or cat in the room may help pet owners regulate when in distress.
- Individuals who experience significant dysregulation, such as being severely oppositional or aggressive or manifesting behaviors that other people experience as aggressive, may not be able to safely engage in an MSE via telehealth. Clinicians will have to remind the patient about acceptable behavior and terminate the session and alert emergency services if needed.

✅ SUMMARY OF SKILLS CHECKLIST

- ❏ Appearance: Hygiene? Dress? Grooming?
- ❏ Behavior
  - Attitude: Engaged? Disengaged? Distant?
  - Eye contact: Good? Poor? Staring?
  - Cooperative? Hostile? Defensive? Uncooperative? Guarded?
  - Motor behavior: Seated quietly? Fidgety? Psychomotor agitation?
- ❏ Speech quality: Clear with normal tone and volume? Brief? Mute? Increased production?
- ❏ Mood: "I feel…"
- ❏ Affect: Congruent with mood and ranges appropriately? Incongruent? Labile?
- ❏ Perception: Evidence of hallucinations? Illusions? Derealization? Depersonalization?
- ❏ Thought process: Linear, organized, and goal directed? Disorganized? Circumstantial? Tangential? Flight of ideas?
- ❏ Thought content: Evidence of psychotic process? Delusions? Obsessions?
  - Suicidal ideation?
  - Homicidal ideation?
- ❏ Insight: Awareness of clinical situation? Good, partial or poor
- ❏ Judgment: Grossly intact or impaired? "What would you do if you found a stamped, sealed, and addressed envelope on the ground?"
- ❏ Orientation: To person, place, time, and situation?
- ❏ Attention/concentration: Perform serial 7 subtractions
- ❏ Memory: Intact for immediate, recent (eg, repeat 3 objects at 5 minutes) and remote
- ❏ Fund of knowledge: Name current and past US Presidents; name 2 bordering states
- ❏ Abstract thinking: Describe difference between ball and orange, painting and a poem, meaning of an expression/proverb

BIBLIOGRAPHY

American Psychiatric Association. *Diagnostic and Statistical Manual of Mental Disorders (DSM) 5.* Washington, DC: American Psychiatric Association; 2014.

Busch AB, Sugarman DE, Horvitz LE, et al. Telemedicine for treating mental health and substance use disorders: reflections since the pandemic. *Neuropsychopharmacology.* 2021;46:1068-1070.

Caplan JP, Stern TA. Mnemonics in a nutshell: 32 aids to psychiatric diagnosis. *Curr Psychiatry.* 2008;7(10): 27-33. https://www.mdedge.com/psychiatry/article/63313/mnemonics-mnutshell-32-aids-psychiatric-diagnosis.

Center for Behavioral Health Statistics and Quality, Substance Abuse and Mental Health Services Administration. Data collections. https://www.samhsa.gov/data/.

Daniel M, Carothers T. Mental status examination. In: Hersen M, Thomas J. *Handbook of Clinical Interviewing with Adults.* New York: SAGE Publications; 2007:49-75.

DeMartini J, Patel G, Fancher TL. Generalized anxiety disorder. *Ann Intern Med.* 2019;170(7):ITC50 63.

Froehlich TE, Robison JT, Inouye SK. Screening for dementia in the outpatient setting: the time and change test. *J Am Geriatr Soc.* 1998;46:1506-1511.

Goldberg C. Digital DDx: mental health symptoms or conditions. Accessed February 11, 2023. http://digitalddx.com/symptoms_list/14/.

Goldberg C. Practical guide to clinical medicine: mental status exam. Accessed February 11, 2023. https://meded.ucsd.edu/clinicalmed/mental.html.

Hirschfeld RMA, Russell JM. Assessment and treatment of suicidal patients. *N Engl J Med.* 1997;337:910-915.

Hirschfeld RM, Williams JB, Spitzer RL. Development and validation of a screening instrument for bipolar spectrum disorder: the Mood Disorder Questionnaire. *Am J Psychiatry.* 2000;157(11): 1873-1875.

Inouye S. Delirium in older persons. *N Engl J Med.* 2006;354:1157-1165.

Lipowski ZJ. Delirium (acute confusional states). *JAMA.* 1987;258:1789-1792.

Lipowski ZJ. Delirium in the elderly patient. *N Engl J Med.* 1989;320:578-582.

Maurer D. Screening for depression. *Am Fam Physician.* 2012;85(2):139-144.

Mayeux R. Early Alzheimer's disease. *N Engl J Med.* 2010;362:2194-2201.

McCarron RM, Vanderlip ER, Rado J. Depression. *Ann Intern Med.* 2016;165(7):ITC49-ITC64.

Mitchell S, Teno JM, Kiely DK, et al. The clinical course of advanced dementia. *N Engl J Med.* 2009;361:1529-1538.

Patel G, Fancher T. Generalized anxiety disorder. *Ann Intern Med.* 2013;159(11):ITC6-1.

Petersen R. Mild cognitive impairment. *N Engl J Med.* 2011;364:2227-2234.

Rabins P, Blass DM. Dementia. *Ann Intern Med.* 2014;161(3):ITC1.

Renn BN, John SE. Mental status examination. In: Segal DL. *Diagnostic Interviewing.* 5th ed. New York: Springer International Publishing; 2019:77-102.

Robinson E. Mental health. In: Jackson Y. *Encyclopedia of Multicultural Psychology.* New York: SAGE Publications; 2006:295-305.

Saitz R. Unhealthy alcohol use. *N Engl J Med.* 2005;352:596-560.

Sapira JD. *The Art and Science of Bedside Diagnosis.* Baltimore: Williams and Wilkins; 1990:516-522.

Schuckit M. Recognition and management of withdrawal delirium (delirium tremens). *N Engl J Med.* 2014;371:2109-2113.

Snyderman D. Mental status examination in primary care: a review. *Am Fam Phys.* 2009;80(8):809-814.

Substance Abuse and Mental Health Services Administration. Key substance use and mental health indicators in the United States: results from the 2020 National Survey on Drug Use and Health (HHS Publication No. PEP21-07-01-003, NSDUH Series H-56). Rockville, MD: Substance Abuse and Mental Health Services Administration; 2021.

Taylon D. Depression in the elderly. *N Engl J Med.* 2014;371:1228-1236.

Venna N, Gonzalez RG, Camelo-Piragua SI. A 69-year-old woman with lethargy, confusion, and abnormalities on brain imaging (PML). *N Engl J Med.* 2010;362:1431-1437.

Wilson J. Alcohol use. *Ann Intern Med.* 2009;150(5): ITC3-1.

14

Knee Exam

Michal Kalli Hose, MD

INTRODUCTION: CORE PRINCIPLES OF THE JOINT EXAM

Detailed examination of the joints is usually not included in the routine medical examination. However, joint-related complaints are very common, and understanding anatomy and physiology of both normal function and pathologic conditions is critically important when evaluating the symptomatic patient. By gaining an appreciation for the basic structures and function of the joint, the exam becomes more intuitive, and even if you cannot remember the eponym attached to each specific test, you will be able to perform the maneuvers based on your knowledge of the structures that are being tested. A well-performed and well-interpreted joint exam helps to make the correct diagnosis and avoid unnecessary lab and imaging tests.

Historical Clues When Evaluating Any Joint-Related Complaint

- Did the joint pain start acutely, or was it slowly progressive?
- If traumatic, what was the mechanism of injury?
- What is the functional limitation of the joint?
- Are there symptoms within a single joint, or do they affect multiple joints?
- Were there prior problems with the affected area?
- Are there associated systemic symptoms?

Common Approach to the Examination of All Joints

- Make sure the area is well exposed, with no shirt, pants, or other coverings on either side. Use a gown as necessary.
- Understand the normal functional anatomy. What does this joint normally do?
- Carefully inspect the joint(s) in question. Are there signs of inflammation or injury (swelling or redness)? Is there deformity? Because many joints are symmetric, compare with the opposite side.
- Observe the joint while the patient attempts to perform normal activity. What can they do and not do? What specifically limits them?
- Palpate the joint in question. Is there warmth or point tenderness? If so, over what anatomic structure(s)?
- Assess the range of motion (ROM). Check active ROM (patient moves the joint). Then check passive ROM (you move it) if active ROM is limited or causes pain.

- Perform a strength and neurovascular assessment. See chapters on the cardiovascular (Chapter 6) and neurologic (Chapter 12) exams for details.
- Proceed with joint-specific provocative maneuvers related to pathology occurring in the affected joint (see descriptions in this chapter as well as Chapter 15, the shoulder exam).
- In the setting of acute injury and pain, it is often very difficult to assess a joint because the patient "protects" the affected area, limiting movement and thus your examination. It helps to examine the unaffected side first, as this gains the patient's confidence and allows you to develop a sense of their normal.

> PEARL: Exposure of the area to be examined is vital.

NORMAL ANATOMY AND FUNCTION OF THE KNEE

The knee is a hinge-type joint, with most of the movement related to flexion and extension via the use of powerful muscles in the upper leg. There is also some degree of rotational movement (**Figures 14-1** and **14-2**).

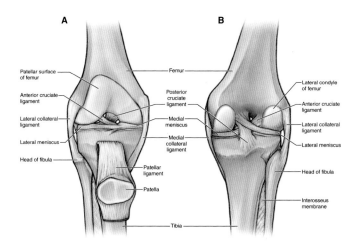

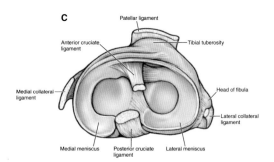

FIGURE 14-1 · **Knee anatomy.** (Reproduced with permission from Morton DA, Foreman KB, Albertine KH. *The Big Picture: Gross Anatomy, Medical Course & Step 1 Review.* 2nd ed. New York: McGraw Hill; 2019.)

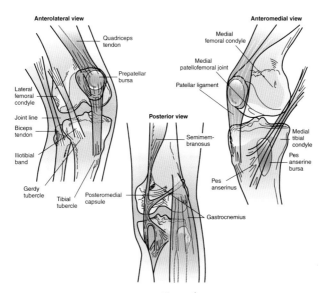

FIGURE 14-2 · Functional Anatomy of the knee. (Reproduced with permission from Gross A, Ma C. Approach to the patient with knee pain. In: Imboden JB, Hellmann DB, Stone JH, eds. *Current Diagnosis & Treatment: Rheumatology*. 3rd ed. New York: McGraw-Hill; 2013.)

Key Anatomic Structures

- Patella
- Patellar tendon/ligament
- Quadriceps, hamstring, and calf muscles
- Femur and tibia
- Medial and lateral joint lines
- Tibial tuberosity
- Anterior cruciate ligament (ACL), posterior cruciate ligament (PCL), lateral collateral ligament (LCL), and medical collateral ligament (MCL)
- Medial and lateral meniscus
- Bursae: suprapatellar, prepatellar, infrapatellar, and pes anserine (**Figure 14-3**)

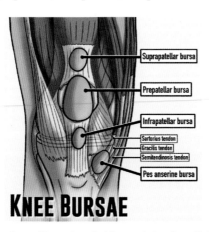

FIGURE 14-3 · **Bursae of the knee.** (Reproduced with permission from Cathy Cichon, MD.)

Knee Exam Flow for Main Components

- Inspection/observation
- Palpation with knee extended
- ROM and strength
- Palpation with the knee flexed at 90 degrees
- Ligament exam
- Meniscal exam

INSPECTION/OBSERVATION

- You may gain important insights by watching the patient walk.
  - Do they limp or appear to be in pain?
  - When standing, is there evidence of any deformity?
- There is a predilection for degenerative joint disease to affect the medical aspect of the knee, a common cause of bowing.
- Observe for knee alignment and document if there is bowing (varus) or knock-kneed (valgus) deformity (**Figure 14-4**).

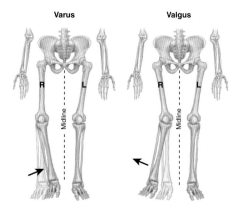

FIGURE 14-4 · Knee alignment. (Reproduced with permission from Parks E. *Practical Office Orthopedics.* New York: McGraw Hill; 2017.)

- Chronic/progressive damage, as in degenerative joint disease, may lead to abnormal contours and appearance. Observe for scars, asymmetry, focal swelling, and erythema (suggesting inflammation). Is there obvious generalized swelling as would occur with an effusion?
- Observe for bony abnormalities (osteophytes) or quadriceps muscle atrophy.
- Observe for swelling or inflammation of the knee bursae (Figure 14-3).
  - Suprapatellar
  - Prepatellar: located directly over the patella
  - Infrapatellar: located over tibial tuberosity
  - Pes anserine

Findings and Their Meaning: Pain and Inflammation of the Bursa

- Bursae are small pouches of fluid that lie between bony prominences and the tendons that surround joints. Their presence allows the tendons to move without generating a lot of friction.

- The bursae do not communicate with the joint space itself. In the normal setting, the bursae are not visible on exam.
- Inflammation of a bursa, most commonly due to overuse of the tendon or direct trauma, can cause pain and swelling. Examination of the affected area reveals focal pain, often with swelling, warmth, and redness.
- Prepatellar and infrapatellar bursitis (often related to infection) most frequently results from repeated direct trauma and abrasions, as may occur with people who spend a lot of time on their knees (eg, carpet layers, carpenters).

PALPATION WITH KNEE EXTENDED

- If the knee is injured, start by examining the unaffected side. This allows for comparison and relaxes the patient, as you are not performing maneuvers that cause discomfort from the outset.
- Evaluate for an effusion, a collection of fluid within the joint space.
  - With a large effusion, you can visualize the fluid in the distended suprapatellar pouch (**Figure 14-5**; photo on left, left knee). You may also be able to ballot the patella. Place one hand on the suprapatellar pouch and use the other to gently push the patella down. With a sizable effusion, the patella will float or bounce back up.
  - To palpate for a smaller or more subtle effusion, milk the fluid superiorly up into the suprapatellar pouch and toward the lateral aspect of the joint. Then gently push on the superolateral aspect of the joint. The fluid will move down into the medial aspect of the knee, and you will see a bulge or fluid wave (Figure 14-5; photo on right).
  - The effusion itself makes the knee feel somewhat unstable or floating and may limit ROM.

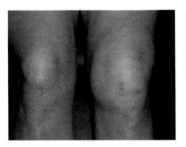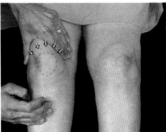

FIGURE 14-5 · **Observation and palpation for a knee effusion.** (Left photo: From Usatine RP, Smith MA, Mayeaux EJ Jr, Chumley HS. *The Color Atlas and Synopsis of Family Medicine.* 3rd ed. New York: McGraw Hill; 2019, Figure 97-4. Reproduced with permission from Richard P. Usatine, MD. Right photo: Reproduced with permission from Lawry GV. *Systematic Musculoskeletal Examinations.* New York: McGraw Hill; 2012, Figure 5-30.)

Findings and Their Meaning: Effusions

- Intense inflammation within the joint space, such as from infection, gout, or rheumatoid arthritis, can cause an effusion.
- The joint and overlying skin are usually warm and red. In addition, there is significant pain with any active or passive movement.

- The more intense the inflammation, the more severe is the pain and the more limited the ROM.
- Identifying the precise cause of inflammatory arthritis is critical as it directs the clinician toward the best treatment, limiting permanent damage to the joint. This usually requires aspiration and examination of the joint fluid.
- Degenerative joint disease, trauma and other less intense inflammatory processes can also cause effusions. The swelling may be acute or chronic, with symptoms based on the size of the effusion and the underlying problem.

Palpation with Knee Extended (continued)

- Palpate from top to bottom, including the quadriceps tendon at its attachment to the superior pole of the patella, along the patella, the patellar tendon at the inferior pole of the patella, along the patellar tendon, and the tibial tuberosity (Figures 14-1 and 14-2). Note any tenderness.
- Palpate the medial and lateral patellar facets and note any tenderness.
- Perform a patellar grind test. With your hand pushing the patella into the trochlea, ask the patient to tighten the quadriceps muscle against this patellar resistance. A grinding sound and/or pain may indicate patellofemoral chondromalacia (details to follow). However, this test is often positive for grinding and/or pain in patients with normal knees or patellofemoral osteoarthritis.

Findings and Their Meaning: Patellofemoral Syndrome (Figure 14-6)

- Problems can occur with the articulation and tracking of the patella along the femur during flexion and extension.
- As a result, cartilage lining the undersurface of the patella can become irritated and worn down.

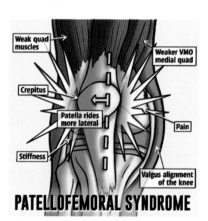

FIGURE 14-6 · **Pathophysiology of patellofemoral syndrome.** VMO, vastus medialis oblique. (Reproduced with permission from Cathy Cichon, MD.)

- Known as chondromalacia, this process causes anterior knee pain with activity and often after prolonged sitting. A large Q angle, a measurement of the angle formed by the intersection of a line drawn from the anterosuperior iliac spine to the midpoint of the patella and the proximal extension of a line drawn from the tibial tubercle to the midpoint of the patella (**Figure 14-7**), can be associated with an increased risk of having patellofemoral syndrome. Other positive findings include crepitus, patellar facet tenderness, and a positive patellar grind test.

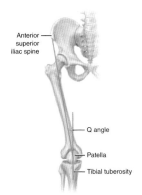

FIGURE 14-7 · **The Q angle.** (Reproduced with permission from Parks E. *Practical Office Orthopedics.* New York: McGraw Hill; 2017.)

RANGE OF MOTION AND STRENGTH

- Active ROM: Ask the patient to bend the knee, gauging whether they can fully extend and flex. This is referred to as their active ROM. Full extension is 0 degrees; full flexion is approximately 135 degrees.
- Passive ROM: This is done if the patient does not have full active ROM. Put one hand on the patella and grasp the ankle or calf with your other hand and gently flex the knee.
  - Note the extent to which you can flex and extend the knee, referred to as passive ROM.
  - Placing the hand on the patella, feel for crepitus while you flex/extend the knee. This is a cracking/grinding sensation that occurs with movement that may suggest degenerative joint disease (**Figure 14-8**) or patellofemoral syndrome. It reflects a loss of the normal smooth movement between the articulating structures (femur, tibia, and patella).

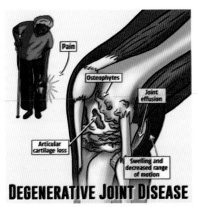

FIGURE 14-8 · **Clinical findings in degenerative joint disease.** (Reproduced with permission from Cathy Cichon, MD.)

- If passive ROM elicits pain, stop and note at what point in the ROM this occurs. It is important to note that many patients report noises (eg, creaking, popping, cracking) associated with joint movement. The vast majority of these sounds are not clinically significant. Rather, pain and functional limitation are the subjective complaints that carry clinical relevance.
- Strength testing is done by having the patient extend the knee while the examiner resists this motion (quadriceps strength) and by flexing the knee while the examiner resists this motion (hamstring strength).

Findings and Their Meaning: Limitations in ROM

There are many causes of loss of range of motion of the knee, including:

- Acute knee injury to an internal structure (eg, ligament, meniscus) or a fracture, causing an effusion (sometimes related to blood in the knee joint)
- Lack of appropriate rehabilitation after surgery
- Stiffness due to degenerative joint disease
- Patellofemoral disorders such as patellofemoral syndrome, patellar instability or patellar tendinitis
- Infection (septic arthritis) with an effusion

PALPATION WITH KNEE FLEXED 90 DEGREES

- On the medial aspect of the knee, palpate along the medial joint line and the MCL. Feel for tenderness or evidence of bony prominences (osteophytes) (**Figure 14-9**).

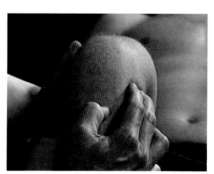

FIGURE 14-9 · **Palpating the medial joint line.** (Reproduced with permission from Lawry GV. *Systematic Musculoskeletal Examinations*. New York: McGraw Hill; 2012, Figure 5-61.)

- Below the joint line, on the proximal medial tibia, palpate over the pes anserine bursa. This is the site where the sartorius, gracilis, and semitendinosus tendons attach (**Figure 14-10**, photo on left).
- Palpate along the lateral joint line and LCL, noting any tenderness or bony prominences.
- On the lateral aspect of the thigh and knee, palpate the iliotibial band (ITB) and its insertion along the lateral tibia at Gerdy's tubercle (Figure 14-10A and B, drawing on right). Note any tenderness.
- Palpate the ITB as you flex/extend the knee. Popping of the ITB over the lateral femoral condyle can occur with knee ROM. Palpation over the ITB during this maneuver typically will reproduce pain.

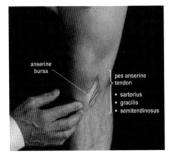 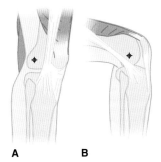

A   B

FIGURE 14-10 · Palpating the pes anserine bursa and iliotibial band. (Left photo: Reproduced with permission from Lawry GV. *Systematic Musculoskeletal Examinations*. New York: McGraw Hill; 2012, Figure 5-69A. Right illustration: Reproduced with permission from Simon RR, Sherman SC, Koenigsknecht SJ. *Emergency Orthopedics: The Extremities*. 5th ed. New York: McGraw Hill; 2007.)

Findings and Their Meaning: Medial and Lateral Knee Pain

- Joint line tenderness may occur with osteoarthritis, meniscal tears, and MCL/LCL injuries if tenderness is over the ligament.
- Patients who limp or have tight hamstrings can develop pain over the pes anserine bursa (bursitis).
- ITB tenderness or popping can indicate ITB syndrome, which is a common knee overuse injury caused by inflammation of the distal portion of the ITB, resulting in lateral knee pain.

LIGAMENT EXAM

Provocative Tests to Assessment Integrity of Ligaments (details to follow):

- Anterior/posterior drawer (ACL/PCL), 90 degrees
- Lachman (ACL), 30 degrees
- Varus stress (LCL)
- Valgus stress (MCL)

Normal Anatomy and Function

- The ligaments are strong tissues that connect bone to bone. In the knee, they assure stability and correct alignment. The 4 main ligaments in the knee are the ACL, PCL, MCL, and LCL (Figures 14-1 and 14-2).
- The MCL and LCL provide stability in response to medial and lateral joint stress.
- The cruciate ligaments limit anterior (ACL) and posterior (PCL) movement of the femur on the tibia and limit the degree to which the knee can rotate.

Common Mechanisms of Injury and Clinical Clues for Each of the Major Ligaments (Figure 14-11)

- Injury usually requires significant force.
- Following a ligamentous injury, there is generally acute pain and swelling, and the injured person will often report hearing a "pop" (the sound of the ligament tearing).
- After the acute swelling and pain have subsided, the patient may report pain and instability (sensation of the knee giving out) during any maneuver that would expose the deficiency created by the damaged ligament (eg, rotation, during which there is nothing to "check" the movement of the femur on the tibia in the setting of ACL disruption).

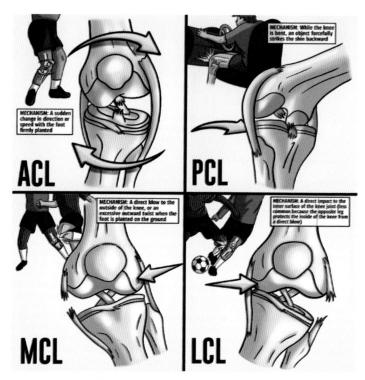

FIGURE 14-11 · **Mechanism of ligament injuries.** ACL, anterior cruciate ligament; LCL, lateral collateral ligament; MCL, medical collateral ligament; PCL, posterior cruciate ligament. (Reproduced with permission from Cathy Cichon, MD.)

- ACL injury: Most commonly injured when the foot is planted while extreme rotational force is applied (eg, a cleated foot caught in the turf while an athlete attempts to rotate toward that side). The ACL may also be injured from a direct force on the lateral knee while the foot is planted.
- PCL injury: Much less commonly injured than the ACL. Posterior force on the tibia (eg, the tibia striking against the dashboard in a motor vehicle accident) can lead to disruption.
- LCL injury: Direct force on the medial aspect of the knee while the foot is planted.
- MCL injury: Direct force on the lateral aspect of the knee while the foot is planted.
- Given the forces required to tear a ligament, menisci are often damaged at the same time. It is also possible to tear more than one ligament at once.

When Testing Any Ligament, Remember to Do the Following

- Begin your exam with the asymptomatic knee. This gives you some sense of the individual's normal degree of laxity. That is, the "tightness" of everyone's ligaments varies somewhat. By working on their unaffected side, you will define "normal." It also helps to generate a sense of trust between you and the patient.
- If you are unsure as to whether there really is an abnormality, check back and forth between the normal and abnormal sides. This will enhance your ability to identify differences.
- Detecting subtle findings takes lots of practice, particularly if you do not have a great sense for the range of normal.
- It can be extremely difficult to examine the acutely injured knee because swelling and movement often causes significant pain. The patient is understandably apprehensive and

will use surrounding muscles to prevent movement. It may be necessary to wait until the acute inflammation resolves (with rest, elevation, anti-inflammatory medications, and time) before being able to perform an accurate exam.

Anterior Drawer Test for Anterior Cruciate Ligament and Posterior Drawer Test for Posterior Cruciate Ligament

- As you have just completed palpating with the knee flexed at 90 degrees, the next tests to perform are the anterior and posterior drawer tests, which are done at 90 degrees of knee flexion.
- The patient is supine with the knee flexed to 90 degrees.
- Gently sit on the foot. Grasp below the knee with both hands, with your thumbs resting vertically across the medial and lateral joint line.
- Gently pull forward, gauging how much the tibia moves forward in relation to the femur. The ACL, if intact, will provide a discrete end point (**Figure 14-12**).

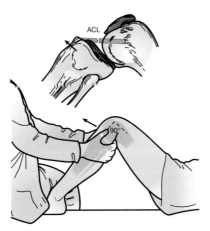

FIGURE 14-12 · **Anterior drawer test for anterior cruciate ligament.** (Reproduced with permission from Stone JH, ed. *Current Diagnosis & Treatment: Rheumatology.* 4th ed. New York: McGraw Hill; 2021.)

- Then gently push backward with the base of your hands, gauging how much the tibia moves posteriorly in relation to the femur. The intact PCL will give a discrete end point (**Figure 14-13**).

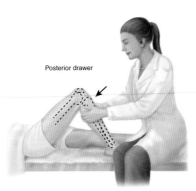

FIGURE 14-13 · **Posterior drawer test for posterior cruciate ligament.** (Reproduced with permission from Parks E. *Practical Office Orthopedics.* New York: McGraw Hill; 2017.)

- Compare both of these tests to the other knee.
- A corollary to the posterior drawer test is the posterior sag. With the knee flexed at 90 degrees, observe for the tibia falling backward (or sagging) (**Figure 14-14**).

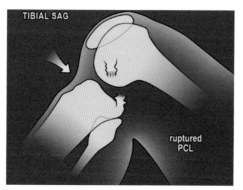

FIGURE 14-14 · **Posterior sag due to ruptured posterior cruciate ligament (PCL).** (Reproduced with permission from Lawry GV. *Systematic Musculoskeletal Examinations.* New York: McGraw Hill; 2012.)

Findings and Their Meaning: Anterior Cruciate Ligament Injury and Anterior Drawer Test

- If the ACL is completely torn, the tibia will feel relatively unrestrained in the degree to which it can move forward. This is referred to as not having a firm end or check point.

Findings and Their Meaning: Posterior Cruciate Ligament Injury and Posterior Drawer and Sag Sign

- If the PCL is completely torn, the tibia will feel relatively unrestrained in the degree to which it moves backward.
- If the PCL is completely torn, the tibia may appear to "sag" backward even before you apply any force (Figure 14-14).

Anterior Cruciate Ligament and Lachman Test

- The Lachman test is performed with the knee flexed to **30 degrees.**
- Grasp the right femur just above the knee with your left hand and the proximal tibia with your right.
- Flex the knee slightly.
- Pull up sharply (toward your belly button) with your right hand while stabilizing the femur with the left (**Figure 14-15**).
- The intact ACL will limit the amount of distraction that you can achieve. The intact ACL is described as providing a firm end point during Lachman testing.
- Compare this to the other leg, reversing your hand position.
- The patient must be able to relax their leg for this test to work. If they cannot do this, then compensatory muscles will limit the degree of motion, making it very difficult to assess the integrity of the ACL.

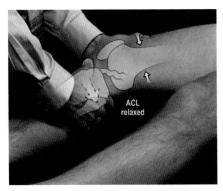

FIGURE 14-15 · **Lachman test. ACL, anterior cruciate ligament.** (Reproduced with permission from Lawry GV. *Systematic Musculoskeletal Examinations.* New York: McGraw Hill; 2012, Figure 5-43A.)

PEARL: The Lachman test has better sensitivity and specificity for diagnosing ACL tears than the anterior drawer test. This is due to the angle of knee flexion, which is 30 degrees with the Lachman as compared with 90 degrees for the anterior drawer.

Anterior Cruciate Ligament and Drop Leg Lachman Test

This test is to be performed on large or heavy legs.

- The drop leg Lachman test is physically easier to perform than the Lachman test, especially when evaluating large/heavy legs and/or if the examiner's hands are small. It is a sensitive method of demonstrating anterior laxity in an ACL-deficient knee.
- The patient is supine and the leg to be examined is abducted off the side of the table and flexed 30 degrees (**Figure 14-16**).
- The thigh is stabilized to the examining table with one of the examiner's hands, and the patient's foot is held between the examiner's knees in 30 degrees of flexion.
- The examiner's free hand provides the anteriorly directed force, as done in the Lachman test.
- Feel for anterior translation of the tibia and whether there is a good end point.

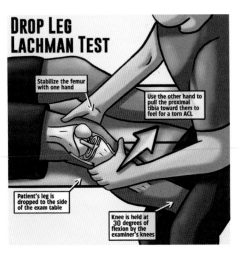

FIGURE 14-16 · **Drop leg Lachman test. ACL, anterior cruciate ligament.** (Reproduced with permission from Cathy Cichon, MD.)

Medial Collateral Ligament and Valgus Stress Test

- Slightly flex the right knee (**Figure 14-17**). 30 degrees of knee flexion isolates the MCL from the other supporting structures.

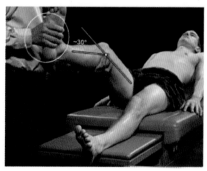

FIGURE 14-17 · Valgus stress test for medial collateral ligament. (Reproduced with permission from Lawry GV. *Systematic Musculoskeletal Examinations*. New York: McGraw Hill; 2012, Figure 5-56.)

- Place your left hand along the lateral aspect of the knee.
- Place your right hand on the ankle or calf.
- Push steadily inward with your left hand while supplying an opposite force with the right and assess for any joint opening medially (**Figure 14-18**).
- Reverse hand position to assess the left knee.

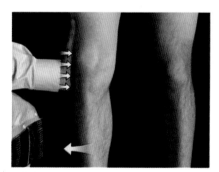

FIGURE 14-18 · Forces to apply for valgus stress test. (Reproduced with permission from Lawry GV. *Systematic Musculoskeletal Examinations*. New York: McGraw Hill; 2012, Figure 5-51.)

Lateral Collateral Ligament and Varus Stress Test

- Slightly flex the right knee. 30 degrees of knee flexion isolates the LCL from the other supporting structures.
- Place your right hand under the knee and along its medial aspect.
- Place your left hand on the ankle or calf.
- Push steadily outward with your right hand while supplying an opposite force with the left.
- Reverse hand position to assess the left knee (**Figure 14-19**).

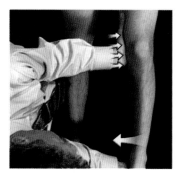

FIGURE 14-19 · **Forces to apply for varus stress test.** (Reproduced with permission from Lawry GV. *Systematic Musculoskeletal Examinations.* New York: McGraw Hill; 2012, Figure 5-57.)

Findings and Their Meaning: Medial or Lateral Collateral Ligament Injury

- If the MCL is completely torn, the joint will "open up" along the medial aspect. If the LCL is completely torn, the joint will "open up" along the lateral aspect.
- If the joint opens up with the knee at 0 degrees flexion this may indicate a combined injury of the collateral and cruciate ligaments.
- Additionally, palpation along the course of the ligament may also elicit pain if it has been injured.
- With a partial tear of the collateral ligament, the joint might open up slightly, but there will still be a good end point, limiting the joint from complete laxity.

MENISCAL EXAM

In addition to causing joint line tenderness, meniscal tears may be diagnosed with one of the following:
- McMurray test
- Thessaly test

Normal Anatomy and Function

- The menisci sit on top of the tibia and provide a cushioned articulating surface between the curved femur and the flat tibia (**Figure 14-20**).

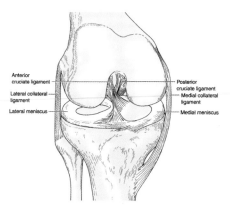

FIGURE 14-20 · **Meniscal anatomy.** (Reproduced with permission from Simon RR, Sherman SC, Koenigsknecht SJ. *Emergency Orthopedics.* 5th ed. New York: McGraw-Hill Education; 2007.)

- Symptoms occur when a torn piece of meniscus interrupts the normal smooth movement of the joint.
- Meniscal tears can cause a sensation of pain, instability ("giving out"), or locking in position. Injury may also cause swelling. If the meniscus has been injured and no longer adequately covers the tibia, damage can occur to the underlying bone, leading to degenerative arthritis (Figure 14-8).

Meniscal Evaluation and McMurray Test (Figure 14-21)

- When examining the knee, place your top hand so that your index finger is aligned along the medial joint line and your thumb is along the lateral joint line.
- Grasp the foot with your other hand and fully flex the knee.
- Gently turn the ankle so that the foot is pointed outward (everted). Then gently extend the knee with a slight valgus stress.
- Feel for a painful pop along the medial joint line under your index finger.
- Now, return the knee to the fully flexed position, and turn the foot inward (inversion). Then extend the knee with a slight varus stress.
- Feel for a painful pop along the lateral joint line under your thumb.

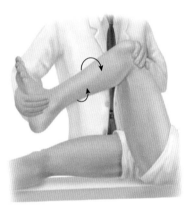

FIGURE 14-21 · **McMurray test for a torn meniscus.** (Reproduced with permission from Edward (Ted). *Parks: Practical Office Orthopedics.* New York: McGraw Hill, 2018.)

> PEARL: With the McMurray test, the patient's heel points in the direction of the meniscus you are testing. If the heel is pointing medially (foot everted or pointing laterally), you are testing the medial meniscus.

Meniscal Evaluation and Thessaly Test

The Thessaly test is a dynamic reproduction of joint loading in the knee. In a patient with a meniscal tear, this test will produce the patient's reported symptoms (**Figure 14-22**).

- The uninjured leg is tested first so that the patient can learn how to keep the knee in the flexed position while twisting.
- The patient faces the examiner with weight on one leg and holds the examiner's hands for balance.

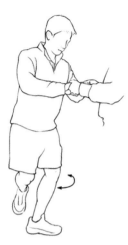

FIGURE 14-22 · **Thessaly test for meniscal pathology.** (Reproduced with permission from Toy EC, et al, eds. *Case Files: Family Medicine.* 5th ed. New York: McGraw Hill; 2021.)

- The patient flexes the standing leg approximately 20 degrees.
- Assist the patient in rotating their torso right and left while on the one, flexed leg.
- Pain or a sense of locking/catching in the knee over the medial joint line when the body pivots medially indicates a possible medial meniscal tear.
- Pain or a sense of locking/catching in the knee over the lateral joint line when the body pivots laterally indicates a possible lateral meniscal tear.

Findings and Their Meaning: Meniscal Tears (Figure 14-23)

- Joint line tenderness with a palpable click or pop felt on McMurray test or a pain associated with Thessaly test may indicate a meniscal tear.

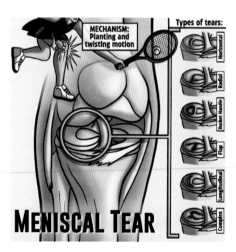

FIGURE 14-23 · Meniscal tear: mechanism of injury and types of tears. (Reproduced with permission from Cathy Cichon, MD.)

Table 14-1 provides a comparison of symptoms and findings for 3 common causes of knee pain: osteoarthritis, meniscus tear, and patellofemoral pain syndrome.

TABLE 14-1 • Diagnoses at a Glance: Common Causes of Knee Pain			
	Patellofemoral Pain Syndrome	Meniscus Tear	Osteoarthritis
Demographic	18-35 years, more in females	35-50 years, more in males	Usually >60 years, but younger if had prior trauma
Activity	Overuse injury, running or jumping	Acute twisting or degenerative from arthritis	Chronic, progressive knee pain
Swelling	Soft tissue (no effusion)	Sometimes if effusion is present; usually occurs within 24 hours of injury	Sometimes if effusion is present
Locking	May endorse but usually due to crepitus	If bucket handle tear where edge of meniscal tear folds back into joint	May occur with floating bone fragments, but usually sensation due to crepitus
Instability	Pain may lead to this sensation, especially down hills or stairs	Not usually, unless locking	Common complaint usually from other impairments such as knee pain, range of motion, and quadriceps strength

Table 14-2 provides a comparison of symptoms and findings for 4 additional common causes of knee symptoms: ACL tear, MCL tear, pes anserine bursitis, and ITB syndrome.

TABLE 14-2 • Diagnoses at a Glance: 4 Additional Common Causes of Knee Pain				
	Anterior Cruciate Ligament Tear	Medial Collateral Ligament Tear	Pes Anserine Bursitis	Iliotibial Band Syndrome
Demographic	Usually under 40	Any age	Any age	Any age
Mechanism of injury	Traumatic/twisting injury (noncontact)	Valgus force to the knee	Overuse, limping	Overuse, running
Swelling	Yes, within an hour	Yes, medially	Sometimes over anteromedial, proximal tibia	No
Locking	No, unless concomitant bucket handle meniscal tear	No	No	No
Location of pain	Nonlocalizable, possibly lateral	Medial knee	Anteromedial aspect of the proximal tibia	Lateral knee
Instability	Yes	No, unless high-grade tear	No	No

SUMMARY

- The knee exam is very important for aiding in the diagnosis of common knee conditions.
- As with all musculoskeletal exams, focus on observation, palpation, ROM, strength, and then the provocative tests.
- For videos of the knee exam, please refer to the YouTube channel SdMskProject, where there are a variety of open access physical exam and injection videos (see Bibliography for links).

🖥 TELEHEALTH TIPS

Investigating knee concerns can be done in a telehealth visit.

- Historical information can be obtained in the usual fashion.
- Adequate exposure is necessary to enable visualization of both knees. The best approach is to have the patient wear shorts. If that is not possible, do the best you can to see the areas in question.
- Position the camera so that both knees can be seen. It is unlikely that the patient will be able to give you an adequate view if they are lying down (nor will they have a table). The knees might be well visualized with the patient seated. Camera repositioning and/or assistance from a caregiver may be necessary to visualize some body parts.
- Because gait may be difficult to view by video even with the assistance of a caregiver, consider asking the patient to take a photograph or video clip and sharing it through messaging via a secure health portal.
- While the patient is sitting, note any obvious deformity, discoloration, or asymmetry as you compare the 2 knees.
- Ask the patient to point with a finger to the area(s) that hurts.
- Knee palpation (**Figure 14-24**): Ask the patient to press on the (1) superior pole of the patella, (2) inferior pole, and (3) medial and (4) lateral patellar facets and indicate if this causes pain.

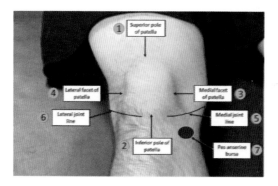

FIGURE 14-24 • **Self-palpation of the knee.** (Photo provided by Kalli Hose, MD.)

- Ask the patient to palpate along the (5) medial and (6) lateral joint line and over the (7) pes anserine bursa and ask if this causes pain.
- Active ROM can be assessed by asking the patient to fully flex and extend each knee separately, from the sitting position.
- To assess for crepitus, ask the patient to place their palm over the patella and feel for grinding or popping when they flex and extend their knee.
- Perform a squat (Ege) test: With both feet flat on the ground and from a standing position, ask the patient to squat down past 90 degrees. If they have pain or hear a pop in the knee with this motion, it may indicate a meniscal tear.
- The future of the telehealth knee exam may include the use of accelerometers, gyroscopes, camera-based motion software, and inertial sensor monitoring units.
- Those with concerning symptoms or findings usually need to be referred for in-person evaluation with appropriate urgency.

> **PEARL:** The most advantageous part of the telehealth knee exam is having the patient palpate the knee and locate the area of pain or tenderness. This helps to guide the provider toward a possible diagnosis.

✓ SUMMARY OF SKILLS CHECKLIST

❑ Clean your hands

Inspection, Noting in Particular
❑ Abnormal gait*
❑ Alignment deformity (varus, valgus, neutral)*
❑ Bony abnormalities*
❑ Quad atrophy*
❑ Erythema*

Palpation with Knee Extended, Noting in Particular
❑ Effusion
❑ Quad tendon*
❑ Patellar tendon*
❑ Tibial tubercle*
❑ Patellar facet*
❑ Patellar grind (Quad apprehension) test

ROM, Noting in Particular
❑ 0 - 135 degrees*
❑ Crepitus*

Palpation with Kneed Flexed 90 Degrees, Assessing
❑ Medial joint line tenderness*
❑ Medial collateral ligament (MCL)
❑ Pes anserine bursa*
❑ Lateral joint line*
❑ Lateral collateral ligament (LCL)

Provocative Testing
❑ Anterior drawer (ACL at 90)
❑ Posterior drawer (PCL at 90)
❑ Lachman's test (ACL at 30)
❑ Valgus stress (MCL)
❑ Varus stress (LCL)
❑ McMurray (medial and lateral meniscal compression)
❑ Thessaly
❑ Clean your hands

*indicates that this exam maneuver can be done via Telehealth

BIBLIOGRAPHY

Achar SA, Taylor KS, eds. *The 5-Minute Sports Medicine Consult.* 3rd ed. Philadephia: Lippincott Williams & Wilkins; 2019.

Adler GG, Hoekman RA, Beach DM. Drop leg Lachman test. A new test of anterior knee laxity. *Am J Sports Med.* 1995;23(3):320-323.

Chapman MW. *Chapman's Orthopaedic Surgery*. 3rd ed. Philadelphia: Lippincott; 2002:2247-2265.

El-Gabalawy HS, Duray P, Goldbach-Mansky R. Evaluating patients with arthritis of recent onset. *JAMA*. 2000;284:2368-2373.

Felson D. Osteoarthritis of the knee. *N Engl J Med*. 2006;354:841-848.

Goldberg C. Practical guide to clinical medicine: musculoskeletal exam. June 13, 2022. Accessed https://meded.ucsd.edu/clinicalmed/introduction.html.

Griffin LY. *Essentials of Musculoskeletal Care*. 3rd ed. Chicago: American Academy of Orthopedics; 2005:469-484.

Hose M, Quan A. Diagnosis driven physical exam of the knee. Accessed March 25, 2023. https://www.youtube.com/watch?v=CHjQ_0QPZXk.

Hose K, Quan A. San Diego Musculoskeletal Project (SdMskProject) knee exam part 1: anatomy. Accessed March 25, 2023. https://youtu.be/CHjQ_0QPZXk.

Hose K, Quan A. SdMskProject knee exam part 2: inspection and palpation. Accessed March 25, 2023. https://youtu.be/xqH9kroTeWs.

Hose K, Quan A. SdMskProject knee exam part 3: ROM and strength. Accessed March 25, 2023. https://youtu.be/1UryTEanPE8.

Hose K, Quan A. SdMskProject knee exam part 4: provocative tests. Accessed March 25, 2023. https://youtu.be/RW1c0CU97nQ.

Jackson JL, O'Malley PG, Kroenke K. Evaluation of acute knee pain in primary care. *Ann Intern Med*. 2003;139:575-599.

Lamplot JD, Pinnamaneni S, Swensen-Buza S, et al. The virtual shoulder and knee physical examination. *Orthop J Sports Med*. 2020;8(10):2325967120962869.

Lonner JH. A 57-year-old man with osteoarthritis of the knee. *JAMA*. 2003;289:1016-1025.

Manske RC, Davies GJ. Examination of the patellofemoral joint. *Int J Sports Phys Ther*. 2016;11(6): 831-853.

Netter FH. *Atlas of Human Anatomy*. Summit, NJ: Ciba-Geigy Corporation; 1989:395-402, 476-480.

Richie A, Francis ML. Diagnostic approach to polyarticular joint pain. *Am Fam Phys*. 2003;68: 1151-1160.

Simon RR, Koenigsknecht SJ. *Emergency Orthopedics: The Extremities*. 3rd ed. Stamford CT: Appleton and Lange; 1996:386-410, 437-460.

Smith CC. Evaluating the painful knee: a hands-on approach to acute ligamentous and meniscal injuries. *Adv Studies Med*. 2004;4:362-369.

Solomon DH, Simel DL, Bates DW. Does this patient have a torn meniscus or ligament of the knee? *JAMA*. 2001;286:1610-1620.

15

Shoulder Exam

Anna Quan, MD

INTRODUCTION

Musculoskeletal complaints account for >20% of outpatient visits and will likely increase as the population ages. Shoulder pain is the third most common musculoskeletal complaint, behind back and knee pain. An efficient shoulder examination is a useful tool to guide diagnosis and treatment, as well as appropriate referrals.

In terms of functionality, the shoulder joint can be viewed as a sideways golf ball on a tee (**Figure 15-1**). The primary benefit of the ball-and-socket alignment is that it allows the hand to be positioned precisely in space, maximizing our ability to function within an amazing 360-degree arc. The downside of this wide mobility is a trade-off with shoulder stability, which depends on both static (shoulder joint capsule) and dynamic (rotator cuff muscles) stabilizers to keep the humerus aligned in the joint.

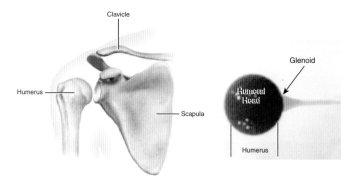

FIGURE 15-1 • **Functional anatomy of the shoulder.** (Line drawing reproduced with permission from Parks E. *Practical Office Orthopedics.* New York: McGraw Hill; 2017. Photo from *Practical Guide to Clinical Medicine: Shoulder Exam.* Available from: https://meded.ucsd.edu/clinicalmed/joints2.html.)

Because the simple elegance of shoulder anatomy allows a 360-degree arc, the shoulder examination includes testing in multiple planes, so the sheer number of exam maneuvers starts to stack up quickly. We will use a few simple acronyms to organize our shoulder exam into diagnostic categories. A little organization goes a long way toward mastering a quick and efficient diagnosis-driven shoulder evaluation. Note that this exam is typically performed only when patients have shoulder pain and/or impaired function. The core components of the exam are provided in **Table 15-1**.

TABLE 15-1 • Core Components of the Shoulder Exam	
Shoulder Exam Sections	Memory Tips
Observation/inspection	Skin/muscles/bones
Palpation	ABC'S
Range of motion/strength	SITS
Provocative tests	BIAS

A caveat: The shoulder examination presented in this chapter is geared toward the initial evaluation and diagnosis of common causes of shoulder pain. Additional tests targeting less common shoulder diagnoses can be added to your exam skills if you enter a specialty field like sports medicine or orthopedics.

SHOULDER ANATOMY

The shoulder joint is created by the confluence of 3 bony structures: the scapula, humerus, and clavicle (**Figure 15-2**). These are held together by ligaments and an intricate web of muscles. We will review shoulder anatomy as we learn the exam—namely, anatomy of pertinent bony prominences for observation/palpation and the detailed anatomy of the rotator cuff muscles for range-of-motion (ROM) and strength exams.

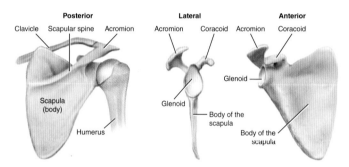

FIGURE 15-2 • **Bony anatomy of shoulder.** (Reproduced with permission from Parks E. *Practical Office Orthopedics.* New York: McGraw Hill; 2018.)

OBSERVATION

- Shoulder observation can be summarized by looking for changes in skin, muscles, and bones (**Figure 15-3**).
- Start by looking at the normal (or less painful) side. It is important to have good exposure so that you can see the key structures. This is best accomplished with the patient's shirt off.
- **Skin:** Note any obvious scars, asymmetry, or redness that may indicate inflammation.

> **PEARL:** Septic arthritis (infection within the joint) causes acute pain, redness, fever, and other findings and is an urgent situation meriting immediate additional evaluation.

- **Muscles:** The patient's dominant hand side often has more developed musculature, which is normal.

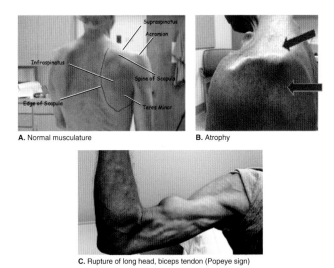

A. Normal musculature

B. Atrophy

C. Rupture of long head, biceps tendon (Popeye sign)

FIGURE 15-3 • **Anatomy and selected findings identifiable by observation. (A)** Normal musculature. **(B)** Atrophy. **(C)** Rupture of long head, biceps tendon (Popeye sign).

PEARL: Decreased shoulder muscle bulk on the dominant hand side can be considered relative atrophy.

- Note any asymmetry, biceps rupture (ie, Popeye sign), or muscle atrophy, which may indicate chronic rotator cuff tears (Figure 15-3).
- **Bones:** Bony abnormalities such as prior clavicular fracture or acromioclavicular (AC) joint separation often leave chronic changes such as bony calluses or a step off at the AC joint (**Figure 15-4**).

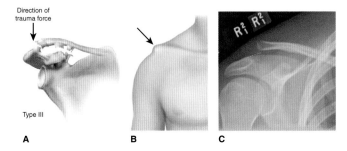

A

B

C

FIGURE 15-4 • **Normal bony anatomic landmarks and findings of acromioclavicular (AC) joint separation.** (Reproduced with permission from Parks E. *Practical Office Orthopedics*. New York: McGraw Hill; 2017.)

PALPATION

Palpation of a few key points, remembered with ABC'S, can direct you toward a shoulder pain diagnosis. Key anatomic features are shown in **Figure 15-5**.

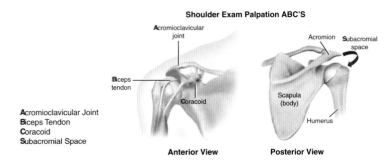

FIGURE 15-5 • Anatomy of shoulder ABC'S. (Modified with permission from Parks E. *Practical Office Orthopedics.* New York: McGraw Hill; 2018.)

ABC'S: Acromioclavicular Joint

- Follow the clavicle past its lateral bony edge to palpate the AC joint line—you need to palpate with enough pressure to feel through the thick AC ligament (**Figure 15-6**).
- Tenderness to palpation may indicate AC osteoarthritis or inflammation.

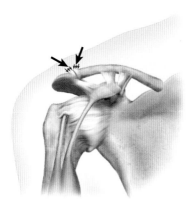

FIGURE 15-6 • Acromioclavicular joint. (Reproduced with permission from Parks E. *Practical Office Orthopedics.* New York: McGraw Hill; 2018.)

> **PEARL:** AC osteoarthritis is a common finding on shoulder x-rays, but a lack of AC joint tenderness means AC pathology is unlikely to be the cause of the shoulder pain.

ABC'S: Biceps

- Palpate the long head of the biceps tendon by placing your thumb just above the axilla and rolling it medial to lateral in the bicipital groove. Start 1 inch above the axilla, along the line where a shirt seam would lie (**Figure 15-7**).
- The biceps tendon roll is usually a little uncomfortable for all patients, but reproducible tenderness (ie, "Yes, that's the pain I've been feeling!") indicates that biceps tendonitis may be one of the causes of shoulder pain.

> **PEARL:** Patients may have more than one source of shoulder pain.

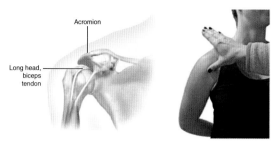

FIGURE 15-7 • Biceps anatomy and technique for palpating the long head. (Reproduced with permission from Parks E. *Practical Office Orthopedics.* New York: McGraw Hill; 2017.)

ABC'S: Coracoid

- Place 3 fingers over the AC joint, and slide inferior until you feel the bony coracoid (**Figure 15-8**) jutting out just below the clavicle. The more overlying tissue the patient has, the deeper you will need to palpate.

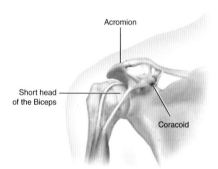

FIGURE 15-8 • Coracoid and short head of biceps anatomy. (Modified with permission from Parks E. *Practical Office Orthopedics.* New York: McGraw Hill; 2018.)

- Tenderness at the coracoid can be a clue that the attachments to this anchor point are tight and stiff, including the short head of the biceps or the ligaments connecting the coracoid to the acromion, humerus, or clavicle.

> PEARL: The coracoid can be tender in patients with biceps tendonitis or adhesive capsulitis.

ABC'S: Subacromial Space

- First, identify the acromion by walking your fingers along the spine of the scapula until you reach its lateral endpoint, which is the acromion (**Figure 15-9**).

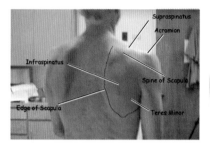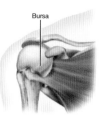

FIGURE 15-9 • **Anatomy of acromion, subacromial space, and bursa.** (Photo from *Practical Guide to Clinical Medicine: Shoulder Exam.* Available from: https://meded.ucsd.edu/clinicalmed/joints2.html. Line drawing reproduced with permission from Parks E. *Practical Office Orthopedics.* New York: McGraw Hill; 2018.)

- Then gently apply pressure under the lateral and posterior borders of the acromion to palpate the subacromial (SA) space (**Figure 15-10**).
- Tenderness at the SA space points toward a diagnosis of SA impingement (for details, see the section on impingement tests toward the end of this chapter).

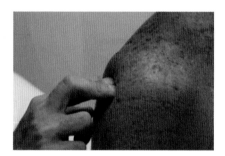

FIGURE 15-10 • **Palpating subacromial space.** (Photo from *Practical Guide to Clinical Medicine: Shoulder Exam.* Available from: https://meded.ucsd.edu/clinicalmed/joints2.html.)

- Multiple anatomic structures run through the SA space, including the SA bursa, supraspinatus tendon, and the long head of the biceps tendon before it inserts into the labrum.

> **PEARL:** Lack of tenderness at the SA bursa does not rule out impingement. Sometimes the impingement provocative maneuvers (described later in this chapter) are required to narrow the SA space enough to reproduce pain.

A summary of palpating the ABC'S is presented in **Table 15-2**.

TABLE 15-2 • Palpation Summary of the ABC'S	
Location of Tenderness	Possible Diagnosis
Acromioclavicular joint	Acromioclavicular arthritis/inflammation
Biceps tendon (long head)	Biceps tendonitis (long head)
Coracoid	Biceps tendonitis (short head)/frozen shoulder
Subacromial space	Subacromial impingement

RANGE OF MOTION AND STRENGTH: SUPRASPINATUS, INFRASPINATUS, TERES MINOR, AND SUBSCAPULARIS

- Shoulder ROM and strength tests hinge on a solid understanding of shoulder rotator cuff anatomy.
- Knowing where the supraspinatus, infraspinatus, teres minor, and subscapularis (SITS) muscles lie anatomically can help you remember each rotator cuff muscle's function (**Figure 15-11**).

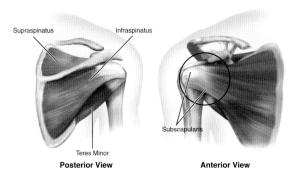

FIGURE 15-11 • SITS (supraspinatus, infraspinatus, teres minor, and subscapularis) anatomy. (Modified with permission from Parks E. *Practical Office Orthopedics.* New York: McGraw Hill; 2018.)

- The shoulder exam ROM and strength sections can be organized by examining each of the **SITS** rotator cuff muscles in 3 parameters: ROM, full tear tests, and strength tests (**Table 15-3**).

TABLE 15-3 • SITS Muscles Range of Motion and Testing			
SITS Rotator Cuff Muscles	Range of Motion	Full Tear Test	Strength Test
Supraspinatus	Abduction (0-180)	Drop arm	Empty can
Infraspinatus/Teres minor	External rotation (ER) (0-90)	ER lag	Resisted ER
Subscapularis	Internal rotation (IR) (spinous process level)	IR lag	Gerber lift-off/belly press

- Examining each SITS rotator cuff muscle in turn tests which specific muscle may have pathology along the rotator cuff injury spectrum (sprain/tendonitis > partial tear > full tear).

> **PEARL:** Performing the ROM, full tear, and strength tests together for each SITS rotator cuff muscle saves time and helps you remember which muscle you are testing.

Supraspinatus > Deltoid: Abduction (Normal Range 0 to 180 Degrees)

- The supraspinatus initiates abduction from approximately 0 to 15 degrees and then assists the deltoid up to 90 degrees, at which point, the deltoid completes the abduction arc to 180 degrees (**Figure 15-12**).
- ROM abduction: Ask the patient to lift their arms from their sides to above their head. Pain with abduction is called a painful arc.

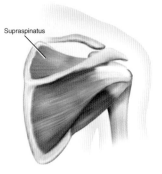

SITS Muscle:	Supraspinatus
Motion	Abduction (0–180°)
Full Tear Test	Drop Arm Test
Strength Test	Empty Can Test

FIGURE 15-12 • **Supraspinatus anatomy and function.** (Modified with permission from Parks E. *Practical Office Orthopedics.* New York: McGraw Hill; 2018.)

- If patients have limited ROM in active abduction, test passive ROM. First, have the patient relax fully while you bear the full weight of their arm. Then gently guide their arm in further abduction to see if their abduction ROM arc is truly limited (stiff endpoint) or just limited by pain.
- Full tear drop arm test: From the top of their abduction arc, ask the patient to return their arms smoothly down to their sides. Drop arm test is positive if weakness causes their arm to fall to their side under 30 degrees. A positive drop arm test raises suspicion for an acute supraspinatus full tear.
- Strength test—empty can: If drop arm test is negative, perform the empty can strength test by instructing patients to abduct their arms in the scapular plane to 45 degrees, turn thumb side down, and resist your efforts to push their arms downward (**Figure 15-13**).

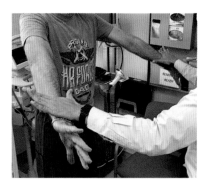

FIGURE 15-13 • **Empty can strength test.** (Photo by Anna Quan, MD.)

Findings and Their Meaning: Pain or impaired function with supraspinatus testing

- Painful arc with abduction or empty can weakness indicates supraspinatus sprain, tendonitis, inflammation, or partial tear.
- Positive drop arm may indicate an acute supraspinatus full tear. This test is only positive for a short time before other muscles compensate for abduction weakness.

PEARL: The supraspinatus is the most commonly torn rotator cuff muscle (70% of rotator cuff tears).

Infraspinatus/Teres Minor: External Rotation (Normal Range 0 to 90 Degrees)

- ROM: External rotation measurement starts with the patient's shoulders relaxed, hands straight in front, and elbows bent 90 degrees; this starting point is 0 degrees. The patient then rotates their hands outward while keeping their elbows at their sides, as you estimate the angle of external rotation. It helps to look down from the top as they rotate. If the patient can hemisect the right angle from 0 to 90 degrees at their sides, they are externally rotated 45 degrees (**Figure 15-14**).

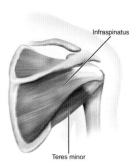

S S Muscle:	Infraspinatus Teres Minor
Motion	External Rotation (0–90°)
Full Tear Test	External Rotation Lag Sign
Strength Test	Resisted External Rotation

FIGURE 15-14 • **Infraspinatus/teres minor anatomy and function.** (Modified with permission from Parks E. *Practical Office Orthopedics.* New York: McGraw Hill; 2018.)

- If patients have limited or asymmetric external rotation ROM, test passive ROM by gently rotating their arm in further external rotation to see if ROM is truly limited (stiff endpoint) or just limited by pain.
- Full tear external rotation lag test is only done if external rotation ROM is limited or asymmetric. Test passive ROM as above and see if the patient can hold the farther passive angle. If their hand flops back forward to their active ROM limit, then the external rotation lag test is positive, which raises suspicion for an infraspinatus/teres minor full tear.
- The external rotation strength test is done by instructing patients to start at 0 degrees and then rotate externally against your resistance (**Figure 15-15**).

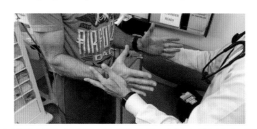

FIGURE 15-15 • **Resisted external rotation strength test.** (Photo by Anna Quan, MD.)

Findings and Their Meaning: Pain or impaired function with infraspinatus and teres minor testing

- The external lag test often remains positive in chronic infraspinatus/teres minor full tears.
- Weakness during assessment of external rotation suggests a tear or inflammation of the infraspinatus and/or teres minor.

Subscapularis: Internal Rotation (Normal Range Varies; Compare With Other Side)

- The subscapularis is responsible for internal rotation (**Figure 15-16**).

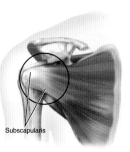

SIT**S** Muscle:	Subscapularis
Motion	Internal Rotation (highest spinous process of thumb tip)
Full Tear Test	Internal Lag Sign
Strength Test	Belly Press/Gerber Lift off

FIGURE 15-16 • **Subscapularis anatomy and function.** (Modified with permission from Parks E. *Practical Office Orthopedics.* New York: McGraw Hill; 2018.)

- ROM: Internal rotation can be measured by asking the patient to bring their hand as high as possible on their back. Charting the highest spinous level reached by the thumb tip allows you to quantify their internal rotation range to compare with prior/future visits (**Figure 15-17**).

> PEARL: The dominant hand usually is less flexible in internal rotation by 2 to 3 spinous levels as a result of greater muscle bulk. The more muscle a patient has, the less is their flexibility, but this may be normal for them. Compare with a patient's nonpainful side as their own control.

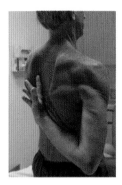

FIGURE 15-17 • **Assessing internal rotation.** (Photo from *Practical Guide to Clinical Medicine: Shoulder Exam.* Available from: "https://meded.ucsd.edu/clinicalmed/joints2.html.)

Subscapularis strength can be measured in several ways—the most common is the Gerber lift-off test.

- With the patient's hand on their back, ask them to push backward against your resistance (**Figure 15-18** B).

Alternatively, subscapularis strength can also be tested in front of the patient's torso by the belly press test.

- Stabilize the elbow while asking the patient to press their hand toward their abdomen.
- Place your hand against the patient's palm, so you can assess the level of strength as they push toward their abdomen (Figure 15-18 A).
- Measure strength compared to their nonpainful side.

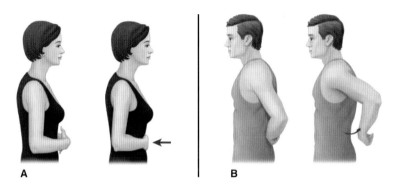

A   **B**

FIGURE 15-18 • Gerber's lift-off (B) and belly press (A) tests to assess subscapularis strength. (Reproduced with permission from Parks E. *Practical Office Orthopedics.* New York: McGraw Hill; 2018.)

Internal lag test: Assessing for a full tear of the subscapularis.

- After you complete the Gerber lift-off, gently pull the patient's hand further off their back.
- If they can maintain an air space between their hand and back, this indicates a negative internal lag test.
- If the patient's hand falls back onto their back due to weakness, this may indicate a full subscapularis tear.

Findings and Their Meaning: Pain or impaired function with subscapularis testing

- Weakness with subscapularis testing indicates a tear or inflammation.
- Full subscapularis tears are the least common rotator cuff tear.

Summary of SITS ROM and Strength Testing

- Pain or limitation on active ROM that is relieved during passive ROM suggests a structural problem with the affected SITS muscles/tendons, which cause pain with active ROM but not passive ROM (**Figure 15-19**).
- Pain or weakness of any of the SITS rotator cuff muscles can indicate pathology anywhere along the rotator cuff spectrum: sprain/strain > tendonitis > partial tear > full tear.

PEARL: If any of the SITS muscle full tear tests show positive weakness with history of recent trauma, fall, or injury, consider urgent MRI and orthopedics consult. Success rates of acute rotator cuff repair are higher within 4 to 6 weeks of the acute tear injury.

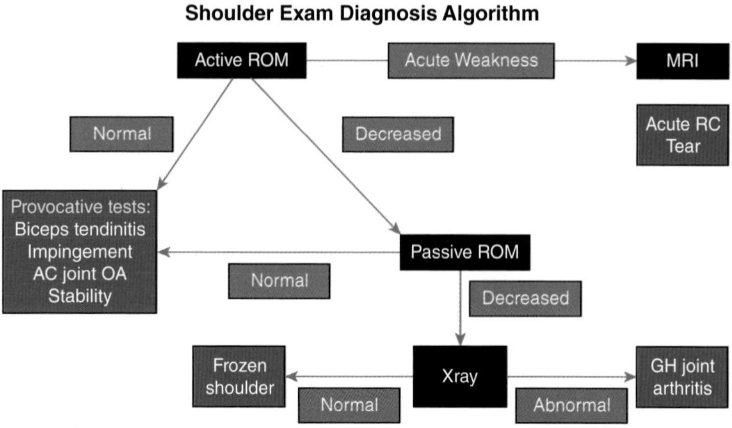

FIGURE 15-19 • Using range of motion (ROM) as a guide to shoulder diagnoses. AC, acromioclavicular; GH, glenohumeral; MRI, magnetic resonance imaging; OA, osteoarthritis; RC, rotator cuff. (Adapted from O'Kane JW, Toresdahl BG. The evidence-based shoulder evaluation. *Curr Sports Med Rep.* 2014;13(5):307-313.)

> **PEARL:** If active *and* passive ROM is decreased in all SITS muscles, your exam has essentially narrowed your diagnosis down to either glenohumeral arthritis or adhesive capsulitis (Figure 15-19).

> **PEARL:** If active or passive ROM is normal, then proceed to provocative testing for further consideration of other diagnoses (Figure 15-19).

History and Exam Clues: Glenohumeral Osteoarthritis

- Shoulder arthritis usually results from an injury that has disrupted the normal articulating surfaces.
- Over time, movement of the shoulder causes additional wear and tear, leading to degenerative joint disease and joint space narrowing.
- Patients experience pain and gradual limitation in movement. This is particularly noticeable on external rotation and abduction.
- Palpation of the glenohumeral joint with a hand placed on the shoulder during range of motion may reveal crepitus (palpable sensation of grinding).

History and Exam Clues: Adhesive Capsulitis

- Adhesive capsulitis, or frozen shoulder, can occur incidentally with no history of trauma, or after any shoulder pain causes a patient to stop moving their shoulder (**Figure 15-20**).
- Patients complain of their shoulder feeling stiff and tight, with pain in every direction.
- On exam, passive and active ROM is significantly reduced in every direction, but strength is intact (although painful) (Figure 15-19).

> **PEARL:** Frozen shoulder usually improves with slow progression of ROM exercises, although recovery can take up to 2 to 3 years. Patients often improve faster with formal physical therapy. If no improvement occurs with physical therapy, an orthopedics consult can be considered, although most cases improve without surgery.

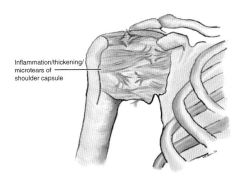

FIGURE 15-20 • **Adhesive capsulitis.** (Reproduced with permission from Mark Quan.)

PROVOCATIVE TESTING

Let's address the elephant in the room—part of the dread of the shoulder exam is elicited by the disproportionate number of eponyms attached to myriad shoulder specialty tests. Fortunately, after grouping many of the rotator cuff strength and full tear tests by SITS, we can now organize the remaining shoulder provocative tests by diagnostic categories. After you master this set of provocative tests, you can add more layers of orthopedic specialty assessments to your exam toolbox as needed. But the following will serve you well to diagnose common causes of shoulder pain.

The mnemonic **BIAS** (because orthopedic exams have a BIAS toward eponyms!) can serve as a framework of common diagnostic categories of shoulder pain (**Table 15-4**). Feel free to create your own framework if you add additional tests to this core exam.

TABLE 15-4 • BIAS and Tests Used to Assess	
Shoulder Provocative Tests: BIAS	Test Names
Biceps tests	Yergason Speed
Impingement tests	Neer Hawkins
Acromioclavicular tests	Scarf Cross arm
Stability (capsule/labrum) tests	Apprehension/relocation Load and shift O'Brien

BIAS: Biceps Tests

- The biceps muscle flexes (bends at elbow) and supinates (rotates palm upward) the forearm and assists with forward flexion (raising arm in front of body) of the shoulder (**Figure 15-21**).
- Inflammation can therefore cause pain in the anterior shoulder area with any of these movements.

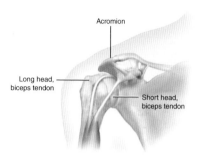

FIGURE 15-21 • **Biceps anatomy.** (Modified with permission from Parks E. *Practical Office Orthopedics.* New York: McGraw Hill; 2018.)

- You may already have a clue toward biceps tendonitis if the patient has tenderness to the biceps tendon (long head) or coracoid (short head) during your palpation exam.
- Biceps provocative tests include 2 assessments, which oppose the 2 functions of the biceps: forearm supination (Yergason) and elbow flexion (Speed) (**Figure 15-22**).

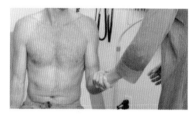 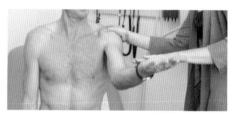

FIGURE 15-22 • **Yergason (resisted biceps supination) and Speed (resisted biceps flexion) tests for biceps tendonitis.** (Photos by Anna Quan, MD.)

Yergason Test: Resisted Biceps Supination

- Position elbow at 90 degrees of flexion and shoulder at 0 degrees (relaxed at patient's side).
- In handshake position, start with the patient's hand palm down and then direct them to turn their hand palm up (patient supinates) against your resistance.
- Pain over the biceps tendon (anterior shoulder) suggests biceps tendonitis.

Speed Maneuver: Resisted Biceps Flexion

- Position the patient's affected arm in forward flexion, palm up, and elbow at 20 degrees.
- Direct the patient to flex their arm as you provide resistance.
- In the setting of biceps tendonitis, resisted biceps flexion and supination will produce pain.

> **PEARL:** Pain anywhere other than the biceps tendon is negative for the biceps tests.

BIAS: Impingement Tests

- SA impingement is a syndrome where structures within the SA space are pinched during particular shoulder movements, causing pain (**Figure 15-23**).

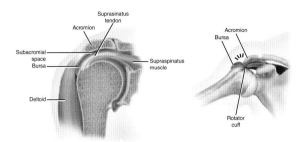

FIGURE 15-23 • **Subacromial space anatomy.** (Reproduced with permission from Parks E. *Practical Office Orthopedics.* New York: McGraw Hill; 2018.)

- SA impingement can occur from both structural and functional changes to the SA space.
- Structural factors that narrow the SA space can occur with degenerative changes (eg, AC osteophytic growth or ligament thickening or superior migration of the humeral head).
- Functional factors that narrow the SA space include imbalances in the deltoid/rotator cuff muscles or scapular rotator muscles.
- Patients with impingement may complain of pain during positions that narrow the SA space (eg, as occurs with raising the arm overhead: swimming, reaching for something on a top shelf, overhead arm positions during sleep).
- Over time, chronic repetitive impingement can lead to fraying, tears, and even complete disruption of the affected tendons.

> PEARL: Pain with SA impingement does not identify the specific anatomic pathology (ie, SA tenderness can be present from SA bursitis or anything along the SITS rotator cuff disease spectrum, including rotator cuff strain > tendonitis > partial tear > full tear).

Impingement: Neer Test

- Neer test is a passive test for the patient; you do the work while their arm is relaxed (**Figure 15-24**).
- Place one of your hands on the patient's scapula and grasp their forearm with your other. The patient's arm should be internally rotated such that the thumb is pointing downward—this positions the greater tuberosity of the humerus against the acromion as you raise their arm.

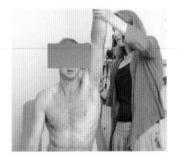
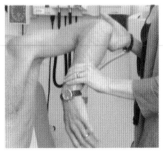

FIGURE 15-24 • **Impingement tests: Neer (left) and Hawkins (right) tests.** (Photos by Anna Quan, MD.)

- Gently raise the arm in passive forward flexion, positioning the hand over the head.
- Pain at any point of the Neer test suggests impingement, and you can stop.

Impingement: Hawkins Test

- The Hawkins test also is a passive test for the patient; the patient's arm should be relaxed (Figure 15-24).
- Raise the patient's arm to 90 degrees of abduction.
- Then rotate it internally (ie, thumb pointed down). This motion again narrows the SA space by impinging the greater tubercle of the humerus against the acromion.
- Pain with the Hawkins maneuver suggests SA impingement.

BIAS: Acromioclavicular Tests

The AC joint is minimally mobile (**Figure 15-25**). However, the AC joint sustains a lot of wear and tear with repetitive lifting and shoulder adduction, so AC inflammation and osteoarthritis are common causes of shoulder pain.

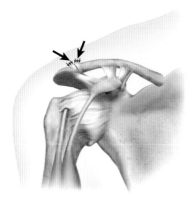

FIGURE 15-25 • **(A-C) Joint anatomy.** (Reproduced with permission from Parks E. *Practical Office Orthopedics*. New York: McGraw Hill; 2018.)

Acromioclavicular Test: Scarf (Active Adduction)

- Ask the patient to reach across and pat their other shoulder; their arm becomes like a scarf around their neck (**Figure 15-26**).

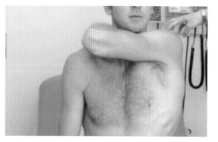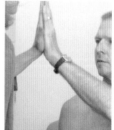

FIGURE 15-26 • **Scarf test (left) and cross arm test (right).** (Photos by Anna Quan, MD.)

- Ask the patient if they have pain at the AC joint, where the lateral end of the clavicle articulates with the acromion.
- The Scarf test is positive if the active adduction recreates pain at the AC joint.

PEARL: Patients can have a normal AC joint appearance (ie, no arthritis) on x-ray and still have AC inflammation from repetitive injury (eg, young weightlifters).

Acromioclavicular Test: Cross Arm (Resisted Adduction)
- Hold your hand up at the nonpainful side of the patient (Figure 15-26).
- Ask the patient to reach across their chest and actively push against your hand.
- The cross arm test is positive if resisted adduction elicits pain at the AC joint.

PEARL: If pain is elicited anywhere other than the AC joint, the scarf and cross arm tests are negative.

BIAS: Stability Tests
- The shoulder labrum is a tough tissue that lines and deepens the shallow cup formed by the scapular fossa that articulates with the humeral head (**Figure 15-27**).
- The shoulder capsule consists of ligaments that overlap over the outside of the glenohumeral joint to form a static stabilizer.

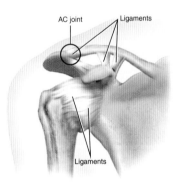

FIGURE 15-27 · Glenohumeral joint anatomy. (Reproduced with permission from Parks E. *Practical Office Orthopedics*. New York: McGraw Hill; 2018.)

- The rotator cuff muscles serve as dynamic stabilizers, contracting when needed to help stabilize the glenohumeral joint as it moves through different positions.
- Together, the labrum, capsule, and rotator cuff stabilize the glenohumeral joint, so the humerus can function within a 360-degree arc without dislocating from the shallow glenoid fossa.
- Tears of the static shoulder capsule or labrum stabilizers can generate feelings of pain, clicking, laxity, instability, or a "dead arm" sensation. The patient may have a history of trauma or recurrent dislocation, where the humerus actually pops out of joint.

PEARL: If you already have a strong suspicion for one of the common shoulder pain diagnoses based on the exam thus far, instability testing may not be necessary. But if patients have a history of dislocation or complain of a sense of laxity, instability, or clicking, stability testing may shed light on a labral or capsular cause for their pain.

Stability: Apprehension Test

- Have the patient lie on their back with the arm hanging off the bed (**Figure 15-28**).
- Grasp their elbow in your hand and abduct the humerus to 90 degrees.
- Gently externally rotate their arm in a "wind up pitching" position.
- The apprehension test is positive if the patient complains of uneasiness, discomfort, pain, or a feeling that the arm is about to pop out of joint at any point in the maneuver.

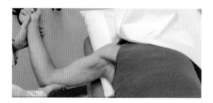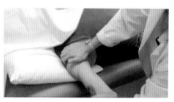

FIGURE 15-28 • Stability assessment. Apprehension (left) and relocation (right) tests. (Photos by Anna Quan, MD.)

Stability: Relocation Test

- Only perform the relocation test if the apprehension test is positive (Figure 15-28).
- Repeat the apprehension test, but this time stabilize the glenohumeral joint by firmly pressing the anterior humeral head down into the glenoid fossa while again winding the patient's arm into the pitching position.
- The relocation test is positive if you are able to relieve their pain by stabilizing the humerus at the glenohumeral joint (as described above) while you rotate them further back in the "wind up" position.

Stability: Load and Shift Test

- This test can be performed with the patient sitting or lying supine (**Figure 15-29**).
- Firmly grip the humeral head and then "load" pressure by pushing in toward the glenohumeral joint.

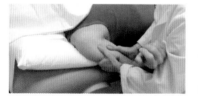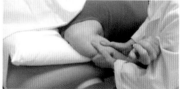

FIGURE 15-29 • Load (left) and shift (right) test. (Photos by Anna Quan, MD.)

- Then gently "shift" the humeral head anterior and posterior, feeling for laxity or clicks.
- The load and shift test is positive if the maneuver demonstrates laxity or reproduces a sense of instability.

> PEARL: Pain during the load and shift test with no laxity or instability may indicate a labral SLAP (superior labrum anterior to posterior) tear (see O'Brien test for details).

Stability: O'Brien Test for Labral Tear

- The O'Brien is a test for a SLAP tear. A SLAP tear is one of the most common types of labral tears and usually occurs where the long head of the biceps tendon inserts into the labrum (**Figure 15-30**).

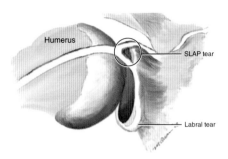

FIGURE 15-30 • **SLAP (superior labrum anterior and posterior) tear of labrum.** (Reproduced with permission from Mark Quan.)

- Position the patient with their arm at shoulder level, pointing 45 degrees across their chest (**Figure 15-31**).
- With the thumb pointing down, ask the patient to raise their arm while you resist their upward motion.

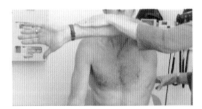 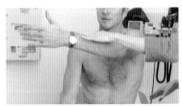

FIGURE 15-31 • **O'Brien test.** (Photos by Anna Quan, MD.)

- Now have them orient their arm so that the thumb is pointing up. Ask them to again raise their arm while you resist their upward motion.
- O'Brien test is positive (suggestive of a SLAP tear) if pain at the top of the shoulder is greater in the thumb down position.

> PEARL: Often patients with a SLAP tear have pain at the top of their shoulder during the Speed test because stressing the long head of the biceps causes traction at the long head tendon insertion into the labrum.

REFERRED PAIN TO THE SHOULDER AREA

It is important to recognize that not all shoulder pain is caused by shoulder pathology. In these instances, the history is usually revealing. A few sites can cause referred symptoms, as follows:

- Intra-abdominal inflammation can cause pain to be referred to the shoulder. In particular, inflammatory processes that occur just below the diaphragm may be referred to the shoulder (eg, splenic abscess can cause pain referred to the left shoulder).

- Intrathoracic processes can also cause referred symptoms. Heart attacks, for example, can generate pain that radiates to the left shoulder.
- Cervical spine pathology can cause irritation of the cervical nerve roots, in particular C5 and C6. This can generate a burning or tingling type of pain that is referred to the deltoid area.

🖳 TELEHEALTH TIPS

- · Historical information can be obtained in the usual fashion.
- · Adequate exposure to enable visualization of both shoulders is helpful. If possible, have the patient remove their shirt (bras can remain on) or wear a tank top to allow good visualization.
- · Observation will be much the same on video as in person. Note any obvious deformity, discoloration, or asymmetry of skin, muscles, or bones. Remember to have the patient turn around for you to see their posterior shoulder musculature to assess for atrophy.
- · For palpation, you can ask the patient to point with a finger to the area(s) that hurts.
- · The patient can also demonstrate the shoulder motion(s) that exacerbate their pain.
- · You can walk the patient through a shoulder ROM exam by standing up and asking them to mirror you as you demonstrate proper abduction, external rotation, and internal rotation.
- · Strength, full tear testing, and provocative tests are a little more difficult with video visits, but if you think your patient can follow complex instructions, your best option may be to use a public source virtual shoulder exam video tool (eg, Virtual Shoulder Exam: https://www.youtube.com/watch?v=WjCDgSSQ_ng).
  - · During the video visit, you can share your screen to stream the video for the patient to mirror as you watch their responses.
  - · Alternatively, send the video link to the patient via your telehealth chat and have them stream the link from home (for less lag).

✔ SUMMARY OF SKILLS CHECKLIST

❑ Clean your hands

Inspection
❑ Skin abnormality
❑ Bony abnormality
❑ Muscle abnormality

Palpation ABC'S
❑ **A**cromioclavicular joint
❑ **B**iceps tendon
❑ **C**oracoid
❑ **S**ubacromial space

ROM/Strength: SITS

Supraspinatus/Deltoid: Abduction scapular plane
❑ ROM active
❑ ROM passive
❑ Full tear: Drop arm test
❑ Motor: Empty can test

Infraspinatus/Teres minor: External rotation (ER)
- ❏ ROM active
- ❏ ROM passive
- ❏ Full tear: ER lag
- ❏ Motor (resisted ER)

Subscapularis: Internal rotation (IR)
- ❏ ROM active (spinous level)
- ❏ ROM passive
- ❏ Full tear: IR lag
- ❏ Motor: Gerber lift-off/belly press

Provocative Tests: BIAS

Biceps
- ❏ Yergason (resisted supination)
- ❏ Speed (resisted flexion)

Impingement
- ❏ Neer
- ❏ Hawkins

Acromioclavicular
- ❏ Scarf
- ❏ Cross arm

Stability
- ❏ Apprehension/relocation
- ❏ Load and shift
- ❏ O'Brien
- ❏ Clean your hands

BIBLIOGRAPHY

Burbank KM, Stevenson HS, Czarnecki GR, Dorfman J. Chronic shoulder pain: part I. Evaluation and diagnosis. *Am Fam Physician.* 2008;77(4):453-460.

Burbank KM, Stevenson HS, Czarnecki GR, Dorfman J. Chronic shoulder pain: part II. Treatment. *Am Fam Physician.* 2008;77(4):493-497.

Goldberg C. Practical guide to clinical medicine: musculoskeletal exam. Accessed February 7, 2023. https://meded.ucsd.edu/clinicalmed/joints.html.

Hermans J, Luime JJ, Meuffels DE, et al. Does this patient with shoulder pain have rotator cuff disease? The rational clinical examination systematic review. *JAMA.* 2013;310(8):837-847.

Moen MH, de Vos RJ, Ellenbecker TS, et al. Clinical tests in shoulder exam: how to perform them. *Br J Sports Med.* 2010;44:370-375.

Parks E. The shoulder. In: *Practical Office Orthopedics.* New York: McGraw Hill; 2017. Accessed June 28, 2022. https://accessmedicine.mhmedical.com/content.aspx?bookid=2230&sectionid=172778318.

Quan A. Shoulder musculoskeletal physical exam for virtual visits [Video]. SDMSKPROJECT YouTube Channel. Accessed June 28, 2022. https://www.youtube.com/watch?v=WjCDgSSQ_ng.

Quan A, Hose M. Diagnosis driven physical exam of the shoulder [Video]. SDMSKPROJECT YouTube Channel. Accessed June 28, 2022. https://www.youtube.com/watch?v=s1XccjP-R5E.

Quan A, Hose M. Shoulder exam part 3: provocative tests [Video]. SDMSKPROJECT YouTube Channel. Accessed June 28, 2022. https://www.youtube.com/watch?v=NOKebPctdHo.

Woodward TW, Best TM. The painful shoulder: part I. Clinical evaluation. *Am Fam Physician.* 2000;61:3079-3088.

Woodward TW, Best TM. The painful shoulder: part II. Acute and chronic disorders. *Am Fam Physician.* 2000;61(11):3291-3300.

16

Dermatologic Exam

Stacy Charat, MD and Jeremy A. Schneider, MD

INTRODUCTION

Unlike many other organ systems, the skin is one that can be examined even during casual encounters with patients. A thorough skin exam, however, requires focused attention and a systematic approach.

Getting Started

- Adequate lighting is imperative when performing an accurate skin exam. This includes bright overhead light and an additional focused light source, such as a penlight, flashlight, or phone light. The ability to adjust the direction of the light source is useful for providing tangential illumination, which may help in revealing subtle surface changes (**Figure 16-1**).

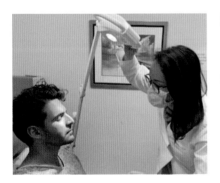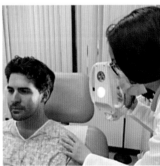

FIGURE 16-1 · **Using direct (left) and tangential lighting (right) to facilitate skin exam.** (Photos provided by Jeremy Schneider, MD.)

- For a comprehensive skin exam, the patient should change into a gown, open to the back, and leave undergarments on. Ask them to avoid wearing or to remove any makeup, jewelry, nail polish, or anything else that may obscure visualization of portions of the skin.
- The patient may either remain seated during the exam (and stand for examination of back, posterior lower extremities, and buttocks) or lie down supine for the exam, and turn to prone for exam of their back side (**Figure 16-2**).

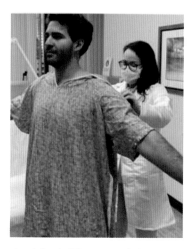

FIGURE 16 2 · **Examining a patient's back.** (Photo provided by Jeremy Schneider, MD.)

Gown Management and Appropriately and Respectfully Touching Your Patients

- Always perform hand hygiene prior to and after each exam. Doing this in the exam room, in front of the patient, is ideal.
- Keep any portions of skin that you are not actively examining covered. Uncover sensitive areas only with the patient's permission, and do not leave these areas uncovered longer than necessary to complete the exam. Bandages and dressings should be removed when feasible to evaluate the skin underneath.
- If there is a concern in the genital, rectal, or breast areas, directly ask patients if they are comfortable with an exam of these sensitive areas and arrange for a chaperone to be present for the exam. For example:
  - "Would you like me to examine the areas covered by your undergarments? If not, do you have any concerns about your skin in those areas?"
- Communicate your actions and explain the purpose of each component of the exam (eg, "I'll need to move your hair around to get a clear look at your scalp," or "Skin cancers can occur even in areas protected from the sun; I'm going to take a look at the bottoms of your feet and in between the toes for any lesions.") This can help you to keep track of what you have done and put the patient at ease.
- At all times, pay attention to your patient. If they seem to be in discomfort or distress during portions of the exam, stop and address the issue.
- If patients are not able to move or stand on their own, ask for assistance in order to position them to adequately examine their skin. Decreased mobility should not prevent an adequate examination of the skin.

Types of Skin Exams

- Integrated skin exam: The integrated skin exam is examination of the skin that occurs during other aspects of the patient encounter. It requires examiners to pay attention to the appearance of the skin while taking a history and performing a physical exam of other organ systems. While exposing the skin and inspecting during any element of the physical exam, also look at the skin for lesions that are concerning for skin cancer, are markers of other diseases, or represent risk factors for other illnesses. The observant clinician, regardless of specialty, can identify an abnormal skin finding even if it is not the primary purpose of a visit. This approach promotes early detection of skin pathology, such as a melanoma, potentially impacting patient outcomes.

- Complete skin survey: The complete skin survey is an intentional and complete examination of the entire skin, often performed to screen for skin cancer. The exam typically proceeds from "head to toe" in a systematic way.
- Symptom-driven skin exam: The symptom-driven exam is a focused exam performed in the context of specific symptoms identified by the patient with a goal of developing a differential diagnosis. The details of the exam will vary depending on the complaint but will focus on the area of concern and any other related areas or organ systems. Depending on the concern and the examiner's differential diagnosis, additional elements of the physical exam may be indicated. See the example in the "Putting It All Together" section, presented towards the end of this chapter.

HISTORY

As with any organ system, a good medical history will inform your exam. It is important to recognize that dermatologic symptoms and findings can reflect processes limited to the skin or may be manifestations of systemic disorders. As a result, historical information can provide critical insights about risk factors for specific conditions or other important clues. The general approach to history taking is described in Chapter 1. Considerations specific to dermatology include the following.

Rashes

- Timeline
- Progression in distribution (ie, did it start centrally and spread outward or did it start distally and spread centrally)
- Associated cutaneous symptoms (eg, itching, pain, burning, ulceration, bleeding, stinging, dysesthesia, hyperalgesia, anesthesia)
- Constitutional/systemic symptoms (eg, fevers, chills, myalgias, weight loss)
- Personal history of skin disease, allergic disease, or autoimmune disease
- New exposures (eg, systemic medications including over-the-counter drugs, new topical contactants, sick contacts, travel)
- Family history of skin or autoimmune diseases (eg, psoriasis, atopic dermatitis, systemic or cutaneous lupus erythematosus)
- Attempted treatments or known alleviating or aggravating factors

Growths

- How long the lesion has been present
- Any change in size, color, or shape
- Associated symptoms (eg, itching, bleeding, ulceration, pain)
- Personal or family history of skin cancer; if yes, what type(s)

> PEARL: In the case of a growth, pay attention to its location, size, color, borders (well-demarcated or poorly-defined), and symmetry (or lack thereof).

Findings and Their Meaning

Common skin cancers are listed in **Table 16-1**.

TABLE 16-1 • Diagnoses at a Glance: Common Skin Cancers

Skin Cancer	Typical Description	Image
Basal cell cancer	Pink papule or nodule with pearly appearance and peripheral dilated blood vessels	(From Usatine RP, Smith MA, Mayeaux EJ Jr, Chumley HS. *The Color Atlas and Synopsis of Family Medicine.* 3rd ed. New York: McGraw Hill; 2019, Figure 177-2. Reproduced with permission from Richard P. Usatine, MD.)
Squamous cell cancer	Pink or red papule often with scale or crust, nonhealing ulceration	(From Usatine RP, Smith MA, Mayeaux EJ Jr, Chumley HS. *The Color Atlas and Synopsis of Family Medicine.* 3rd ed. New York, McGraw Hill; 2019, Figure 178-6. Reproduced with permission from Jonthan B. Karnes, MD.)
Melanoma	Pigmented lesion with irregular color or borders or increase in size	(Reproduced with permission from Taylor SC, Kelly AP, Lim HW, Serrano AMA, eds. *Taylor and Kelly's Dermatology for Skin of Color.* 2nd ed. New York: McGraw Hill; 2016, Figure 44-2A.)

SKIN EXAM

Keys to a Thorough Exam

Whichever sequence you choose to examine the skin, maintaining internal consistency (performing the exam in the same order every time) will help ensure that you do not forget key components. The 2 key elements of the skin exam are inspection and palpation.

Skin Anatomy

When considering processes that affect the skin, it is important to understand skin anatomy and histology, which is helpful when identifying the site of any pathologic process (**Figure 16-3**). The main layers of the skin are the epidermis (outermost layer), dermis, and subcutaneous tissue. Beneath is fascia and muscle.

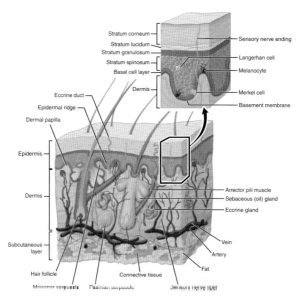

FIGURE 16-3 · **Layers of the skin.** (Reproduced with permission from Soutor C, Hordinsky MK. *Clinical Dermatology: Diagnosis and Management of Common Disorders*. 2nd ed. New York: McGraw Hill; 2022.)

Inspection

If performing a comprehensive skin exam, starting from the top (scalp) and ending with the toes will help ensure that no areas are missed.

- Beginning with the scalp, use fingers or a cotton-tipped applicator to separate/part the hair to evaluate it along with the underlying scalp, including behind the ears.
- Next, evaluate the face and anterior, lateral, and posterior aspects of the neck. Evaluate the eyelids, the creases of the nasal alae, the external ears, and the oral mucosa.
- Evaluate the upper extremities, being sure to examine the axillae, the fingernails, and the dorsal *and* palmar surfaces of the hands and fingers.
- Examine the chest. In patients with breasts, ask permission before exposing and examining the skin of the chest.
- Examine the abdomen. If the patient is in a gown, apply a second gown, drape, or sheet over the groin before lifting the gown to examine the abdomen.
- As described earlier, ask permission prior to examining the genital area and buttocks. If performing a comprehensive skin exam, this would also include evaluating the intergluteal and perianal areas. To examine the buttocks and posterior aspects of the lower extremities, you can have the patient either stand or lie prone.
- Examine the lower extremities. Include examination of the feet without socks, including the toenails, the dorsal and plantar surfaces of the feet and toes, and the interdigital web spaces.

Skin Phototype

Take note of the patient's skin phototype, which is most directly dependent on the amount of melanin pigment in the skin. The most commonly employed scale is the Fitzpatrick phototype scale, which classifies the skin based on its reaction to sunlight exposure (**Table 16-2**). It is worth noting that while commonly employed, there is ongoing dialogue about the Fitzpatrick classification system due to its subjective nature and potential misuse as a proxy for race and ethnicity.

TABLE 16-2 • Fitzpatrick Classification of Skin Types		
Skin Phototype	Burning and Tanning Reactions Upon Sun Exposure	Color of Unexposed Skin
I	Always burns, never tans	Pale white
II	Always burns, then tans	White
III	Sometimes burns, can tan without prior burn	White
IV	Usually does not burn, tans easily and deeply	White to light brown
V	Rarely burns, tans easily	Brown; moderately pigmented
VI	Burns only with very high ultraviolet radiation doses, tans	Dark brown to black; darkly pigmented

Source: Reproduced with permission from Kang S, Amagai M, Bruckner AL, et al, eds. Fitzpatrick's Dermatology. 9th ed. New York: McGraw Hill; 2019.

Additional Clinical Implications Related to Phototypes

- Skin changes such as erythema may have a subtler appearance in darker skin types (**Figure 16-4**).
- Trauma (including iatrogenic injuries from surgical or destructive procedures) is more likely to lead to postinflammatory pigment changes in darker skin.

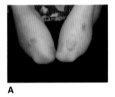 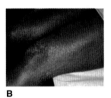 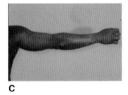 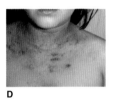

A   B   C   D

FIGURE 16-4 • **(A-D) Eczematous changes in different skin types.** (Part A: From Usatine RP, Smith MA, Mayeaux EJ Jr, Chumley HS. *The Color Atlas and Synopsis of Family Medicine*. 3rd ed. New York: McGraw Hill; 2019, Figure 154-6. Reproduced with permission from Richard P. Usatine, MD. Part B: Reproduced with permission from Burgin S, ed. *Guidebook to Dermatologic Diagnosis*. New York: McGraw Hill; 2021, Figure 8-3. Parts C and D: Reproduced with permission from Taylor SC, Kelly AP, Lim HW, Serrano AMA, eds. *Taylor and Kelly's Dermatology for Skin of Color*. 2nd ed. New York: McGraw Hill; 2016, Figure 27-1A, B.)

- Certain therapies (especially phototherapy and laser treatments) require adjustments of settings depending on phototype in order to minimize unintended injury to the skin.
- Lighter skin is more prone to photodamage and skin cancers related to ultraviolet (UV) exposure, such as squamous cell carcinoma, basal cell carcinoma, and melanoma.
- Dermatofibrosarcoma protuberans is a skin cancer unrelated to UV exposure that occurs almost twice as often in black patients as white patients.

> **PEARL:** Reviewing the appearance of various diagnoses in multiple skin types (via atlases and online resources that include skin of every color) will improve your skills.

Palpation

Palpation is often necessary to accurately describe a skin finding. For example, you may only be able to identify subtle textural change, subcutaneous masses, induration, and edema by laying hands on the patient. Distinguishing between blanchable and nonblanchable lesions also requires application of pressure to the skin.

- The tips of your fingers are the most sensitive for assessing surface changes on the skin. Passing a fingertip (or multiple fingertips) lightly over the surface of lesions can help identify scale, atrophy, induration (firmness), and perspiration.
- When assessing whether or not a lesion is blanchable, use fingertips to apply firm pressure to the area of interest for a few seconds, and then release quickly and observe whether or not there is a change in the baseline color. A lesion that blanches, meaning the pink or red color is reduced or eliminated with the application of pressure, indicates that the erythema is caused by blood that is within blood vessels that are dilated or closer to the skin surface. A lesion that does not blanch, meaning it appears the same with the application of pressure, indicates that the pink or red color is caused by blood that is outside the blood vessels.
- When assessing for the presence and character of tissue edema, use fingertips to apply firm pressure to the area of interest, and then release, observe, and palpate to determine whether and how long a depression is present.
- If there is concern for disorders that can lead to epidermal detachment (eg, pemphigus vulgaris or Stevens-Johnson syndrome), use the fingertips to apply a shearing force against the skin to determine if the top layers slough off (Nikolsky sign).
- If there is concern for dermatographism, a type of urticaria caused by pressure on the skin, rubbing or stroking the skin with the fingertips, hand, or a cotton-tipped applicator may be used to elicit the response.
- For subcutaneous lesions, the fingertips can be used in a pincer grip to assess the mobility and consistency of the lesion.
- When assessing for temperature variations, feel the surfaces with the back and/or front of your hands. When there is a laterality to the skin issue, compare the unaffected and affected sides.

> **PEARL:** Many physicians find that the thermosensitivity of the backs of their hands is better at detecting subtle temperature variations than the palms of their hands.

> **PEARL:** If you are concerned that a skin finding may indicate a communicable disease (eg, syphilis), wear gloves when palpating lesions. If you are certain that lesions are not communicable, palpation without gloves can reassure a patient that they are not contagious and reduce feelings of isolation and fear of infecting others.

Lesion Appearance

- Accurately and precisely describing the appearance of exam findings is a cornerstone of dermatologic evaluation and diagnosis. Learning this language will help in building your differential diagnosis and knowing where to look within reference texts to help guide next steps in management.
- Descriptions include identification of both primary lesions (the initial lesion of concern; **Figure 16-5**) and secondary changes (due to outside influence or the body's response to a primary lesion; **Table 16-3**).
- In the case of a rash, determining the primary morphology (and secondary changes if present), pattern, and distribution will help in constructing a focused differential diagnosis.

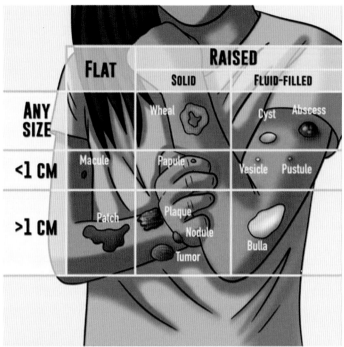

- Macule and Patch: Flat lesion; only color change is appreciated
- Papule and Plaque: Raised, palpable change in surface (when subtle, accurately distinguishing a macule from a papule may only be possible with palpation and/or tangential lighting
- Nodule: Raised lesion typically with rounded surface, which is seated below the epidermis (typically used to denote a proliferation or infiltrate in the mid-to-deep dermis or the subcutis)
- Tumor: Solid, firm lesion can be exophytic (outward proliferation above the epithelial surface), endophytic (inward proliferation below the epithelial surface), or level with the skin (depending on the location of the proliferation or infiltrate)
- Vesicle or Bulla: Serous fluid-filled space within epidermis or basement membrane zone
- Pustule: Vesicle filled with pus (leukocytes)
- Furuncle or Abscess: Similar to pustule but typically larger and/or deeper
- Wheal: Edematous papule or plaque; usually transient and well-circumscribed. Larger wheals often have an erythematous border and pale center
- Cyst: Sac-like nodule with an epithelial lining which contains fluid or other debris (typically by-products of the epithelial lining)

FIGURE 16-5 · Descriptions of primary lesions. (Reproduced with permission from Dr. Cathy Cichon, MD.)

TABLE 16-3 • Descriptions of Secondary Lesions

Secondary Change	Description	Example Diagnosis and Image
Erythema	Pink or deep red hue in the skin secondary to vasodilation; color is blanchable	**Cellulitis** (From Knoop KJ, Stack LB, Storrow AB, Thurman RJ, eds. *The Atlas of Emergency Medicine.* 5th ed. New York: McGraw-Hill; 2021, Figure 12-1. Reproduced with permission from photo contributor: Frank Birinyi, MD.)

(Continued)

TABLE 16-3 • Descriptions of Secondary Lesions (Continued)

Secondary Change	Description	Example Diagnosis and Image	
Scale	Flakes or plates of compacted, desquamated layers of stratum corneum	**Psoriasis**	(Reproduced with permission from Burgin S, ed. *Guidebook to Dermatologic Diagnosis.* New York: McGraw Hill; 2021, Figure 2-4.)
Crust	"Scab," dry plasma or exudate on the skin; can be hemorrhagic, serous, or purulent	**Pemphigus vulgaris**	(Reproduced with permission from Soutor C, Hordinsky MK. *Clinical Dermatology: Diagnosis and Management of Common Disorders.* 2nd ed. New York: McGraw Hill; 2022, Figure 2-9.)
Erosion	Loss of part of the epidermis (basement membrane intact)	**Lichenoid drug rash**	(Reproduced with permission from Soutor C, Hordinsky MK. *Clinical Dermatology: Diagnosis and Management of Common Disorders.* 2nd ed. New York: McGraw Hill; 2022, Figure 2-12.)
Ulcer	Complete loss of epidermis (including basement membrane), may include loss of part or all of dermis	**Venous stasis ulcer**	(Reproduced with permission from Soutor C, Hordinsky MK. *Clinical Dermatology: Diagnosis and Management of Common Disorders.* 2nd ed. New York: McGraw Hill; 2022, Figure 2-13.)

(Continued)

TABLE 16-3 • Descriptions of Secondary Lesions (Continued)

Secondary Change	Description	Example Diagnosis and Image
Fissure	Cleavage of the skin extending into the dermis	**Callous with fissure** (Reproduced with permission from Soutor C, Hordinsky MK. *Clinical Dermatology: Diagnosis and Management of Common Disorders.* 2nd ed. New York: McGraw Hill; 2022, Figure 2-11.)
Excoriation	Areas of trauma to the skin that result from rubbing or scratching; angulated borders and oddly geometric shapes can provide hints of "outside influence"	**Excoriations secondary to psoriasis** (From Usatine RP, Smith MA, Mayeaux EJ Jr, Chumley HS. *The Color Atlas and Synopsis of Family Medicine.* 3rd ed. New York: McGraw Hill; 2019, Figure 110-13. Reproduced with permission from Richard P. Usatine, MD.)
Atrophy	Thinning of the epidermis, dermis, or subcutaneous fat	**Lichen sclerosis** (Reproduced with permission from Soutor C, Hordinsky MK. *Clinical Dermatology: Diagnosis and Management of Common Disorders.* 2nd ed. New York: McGraw Hill; 2022, Figure 2-15.)
Lichenification	Thickening of the epidermis; exaggeration of normal skin lines; usually secondary to chronic scratching, rubbing, or friction	**Lichen simplex chronicus** (From Usatine RP, Smith MA, Mayeaux EJ Jr, Chumley HS. *The Color Atlas and Synopsis of Family Medicine.* 3rd ed. New York: McGraw Hill; 2019, Figure 110-14. Reproduced with permission from Richard P. Usatine, MD.)

(Continued)

TABLE 16-3 • Descriptions of Secondary Lesions (Continued)

Secondary Change	Description	Example Diagnosis and Image	
Scar	Permanent fibrotic change following damage to the dermis	**Scar from laceration**	(Reproduced with permission from Soutor C, Hordinsky MK. *Clinical Dermatology: Diagnosis and Management of Common Disorders.* 2nd ed. New York: McGraw Hill; 2022, Figure 20-9A.)
Keloid	Scar that extends beyond the edges of the original wound/defect	**Keloid from biopsy sites**	(Reproduced with permission from Taylor SC, Kelly AP, Lim HW, Serrano AMA, eds. *Taylor and Kelly's Dermatology for Skin of Color.* 2nd ed. New York: McGraw Hill; 2016, Figure 33-2.)
Petechiae	Pinpoint pink, red, purple, or black macules resulting from bleeding in the skin; often associated with low platelet counts and/or platelet dysfunction; do NOT blanch with pressure	**Rocky Mountain spotted fever**	(Reproduced with permission from Kaushansky K, Prchal JT, Burns LJ, Lichtman MA, Levi M, Linch DC, eds. *Williams Hematology.* 10th ed. New York: McGraw Hill; 2021, Figure 121-19.)
Purpura/ ecchymoses	Larger pink, red, purple, or black macules or papules (purpura), patches, or plaques (ecchymoses) due to bleeding in the skin; do NOT blanch with pressure	**Vasculitis**	(Reproduced with permission from Kaushansky K, Prchal JT, Burns LJ, Lichtman MA, Levi M, Linch DC, eds. *Williams Hematology.* 10th ed. New York: McGraw Hill; 2021, Figure 121-22.)

Findings and Their Meaning

Skin disorders associated with findings on palpation are listed in **Table 16-4**.

TABLE 16-4 • Skin Disorders Associated With Findings on Palpation

Palpable Finding	Example Diagnosis	Image
Fine scale	Pityriasis rosea: scaly, self-limited skin eruption, often bilateral, linked to viral infections	 (From Usatine RP, Smith MA, Mayeaux EJ Jr, Chumley HS. *The Color Atlas and Synopsis of Family Medicine.* 3rd ed. New York: McGraw Hill; 2019, Figure 159-3. Reproduced with permission from Richard P. Usatine, MD.)
Thick scale	Psoriasis: well-demarcated, pink-to-red plaques with white or silver scale; frequently involves scalp and extensor surfaces, although can occur in any location, including intertriginous/ "inverse" distribution	 (Reproduced with permission from Burgin S, ed. *Guidebook to Dermatologic Diagnosis.* New York: McGraw Hill; 2021, Figure 2-4.)
Atrophy	Lichen sclerosus: white, sclerotic, and atrophic plaques with surrounding red-to-violaceous border; commonly affects anogenital region, although extragenital lesions can also occur	 (Reproduced with permission from Soutor C, Hordinsky MK. *Clinical Dermatology: Diagnosis and Management of Common Disorders.* 2nd ed. New York: McGraw Hill; 2022, Figure 32-8.)

(Continued)

TABLE 16-4 • Skin Disorders Associated With Findings on Palpation (Continued)

Palpable Finding	Example Diagnosis	Image
Blanching (color goes away when pressure applied and then returns)	Viral exanthem: wide-spread blanchable pink-to-red macules/patches and/or papules/plaques	(Reproduced with permission from Suneja M, Szot JF, LeBlond RF, Brown DD. *DeGowin's Diagnostic Examination*. 11th ed. New York: McGraw Hill; 2020, Figure 6-20.)
Nonblanching	Petechiae: pinpoint, nonblanching, red, brown, and/or vio-laceous macules; most commonly observed on the lower extremities	(Reproduced with permission from Kang S, Amagai M, Bruckner AL, et al, eds. *Fitzpatrick's Dermatology*. 9th ed. New York: McGraw Hill; 2019, Figure 1-1.)
Edema	Volume overload due to heart failure: photo shows indentation (pitting) of the skin left behind after applying fingertip pressure	(Reproduced with permission from Kemp WL, Burns DK, Brown TG. *Pathology: The Big Picture*. New York: McGraw Hill; 2008, Figure 8-3B.)
Epidermal detachment	Stevens-Johnson syndrome: severe mucocutaneous adverse reaction to medication resulting in dusky red-to-violaceous macules on the skin with subsequent develop-ment of flaccid bullae and denudation (loss of epidermal layer); mucosal involvement presents with bullae, erosions, and hemor-rhagic crusting	(Reproduced with permission from Loscalzo J, Fauci AS, Kasper DL, et al, eds. *Harrison's Principles of Internal Medicine*. 21st ed.Cutaneous Drug Reactions, New York: McGraw Hill; 2022, Figure 60-7.)

(Continued)

TABLE 16-4 • Skin Disorders Associated With Findings on Palpation (Continued)		
Palpable Finding	Example Diagnosis	Image
Dermatographism	Urticaria: well-circumscribed, pink, edematous papules or plaques (can be irregularly-shaped), frequently with a pale center; dermatographism (pictured) is a form of physical urticaria, induced by rubbing the skin	(From Usatine RP, Smith MA, Mayeaux EJ Jr, Chumley HS. *The Color Atlas and Synopsis of Family Medicine.* 3rd ed. New York: McGraw Hill; 2019, Figure 156-5. Reproduced with permission from Richard P. Usatine, MD.)
Rubbery subcutaneous nodule	Lipoma: discrete, benign tumor comprising mature fat cells (adipocytes) that feels soft and rubbery and is freely mobile; can be solitary or multiple.	(Reproduced with permission from Soutor C, Hordinsky MK. *Clinical Dermatology: Diagnosis and Management of Common Disorders.* 2nd ed. New York: McGraw Hill; 2022, Figure 20-8.)
Compressible subcutaneous nodule	Epidermal inclusion cyst: dome-shaped nodule, firm but partially compressible on palpation; sometimes a central punctum is visible	(Reproduced with permission from Soutor C, Hordinsky MK. *Clinical Dermatology: Diagnosis and Management of Common Disorders.* 2nd ed. New York: McGraw Hill; 2022, Figure 20-10.)

(Continued)

TABLE 16-4 • Skin Disorders Associated With Findings on Palpation (Continued)		
Palpable Finding	Example Diagnosis	Image
Fluctuant subcutaneous nodule	Abscess: a localized inflammatory process typified by local accumulation of white blood cells in the dermis and/or subcutaneous tissue; usually forms in response to infection and often tender and warm on palpation	(From Usatine RP, Smith MA, Mayeaux EJ Jr, Chumley HS. *The Color Atlas and Synopsis of Family Medicine.* 3rd ed. New York: McGraw Hill; 2019, Figure 127-2. Reproduced with permission from Richard P. Usatine, MD.)
Warmth and often tenderness	Cellulitis: infection of the deep dermis and subcutaneous tissue; the skin is erythematous and often swollen, warm, and painful on palpation	(From Knoop KJ, Stack LB, Storrow AB, Thurman RJ, eds. *The Atlas of Emergency Medicine.* 5th ed. New York: McGraw-Hill; 2021, Figure 12-2. Reproduced with permission from photo contributor: Robert Tubbs, MD.)

PEARL: If evaluating a pigmented lesion concerning for skin cancer, it is useful to compare the lesion to the patient's other pigmented nevi (moles) to see if it is similar or looks different. A pigmented lesion that is distinct from the other nevi (sometimes called an "ugly duckling") is more concerning for melanoma.

Findings and Their Meaning: Patterns and Shapes

Some cutaneous processes display specific shapes and patterns that aid in diagnosis. Common patterns are shown in **Table 16-5**.

Findings and Their Meaning: Distributions

- Lesions may be generalized (occurring over the entire body) or focal (in one location).
- Lesions that are discrete or separated from one another and then begin to merge into one another are referred to as coalescing or coalescent.

TABLE 16-5 • Common Patterns and Shapes

Pattern or Shape	Description	Example Diagnoses	Example Image
Linear	Lesions arranged in a linear pattern may indicate an "outside job" or occur within sites of trauma	Allergic contact dermatitis, psoriasis, lichen planus, warts	**Allergic contact dermatitis** (Reproduced with permission from Soutor C, Hordinsky MK. *Clinical Dermatology: Diagnosis and Management of Common Disorders*. 2nd ed. New York: McGraw Hill; 2022, Figure 2-25.)
Grouped/ clustered	Grouping or clustering of lesions	Herpetic infections and arthropod bites	**Herpes simplex** (Reproduced with permission from Soutor C, Hordinsky MK. *Clinical Dermatology: Diagnosis and Management of Common Disorders*. 2nd ed. New York: McGraw Hill; 2022, Figure 2-23.)
Annular	Ring-shaped lesions	Tinea corporis, secondary syphilis, subacute cutaneous lupus, granuloma annulare, and erythema annulare centrifigum	**Tinea corporis** (Reproduced with permission from Soutor C, Hordinsky MK. *Clinical Dermatology: Diagnosis and Management of Common Disorders*. 2nd ed. New York: McGraw Hill; 2022, Figure 2-20.)

(Continued)

TABLE 16-5 • Common Patterns and Shapes (Continued)			
Pattern or Shape	Description	Example Diagnoses	Example Image
Nummular/ discoid/round	Coin-shaped lesions	Discoid lupus and nummular eczema	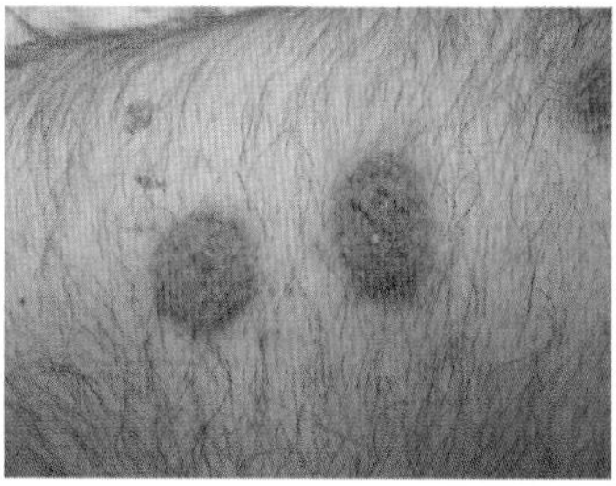 (Reproduced with permission from Soutor C, Hordinsky MK. *Clinical Dermatology: Diagnosis and Management of Common Disorders.* 2nd ed. New York: McGraw Hill; 2022, Figure 8-16.)
Geographic pattern, serpiginous (urticaria)	Consisting of multiple different serpiginous or ring shapes	Urticaria, paraneoplastic phenomena, mycosis fungoides	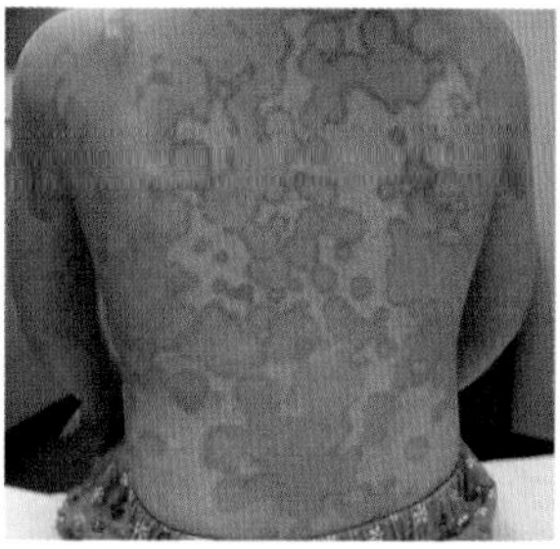 **Erythema marginatum** (Reproduced with permission from Milgrom EC, Usatine RP, Tan RA, et al: Practical Allergy. Philadelphia, PA: Elsevier; 2003. *The Color Atlas and Synopsis of Family Medicine*, 3e. New York: McGraw Hill; 2019, FIGURE 156-11, ISBN 9781259862045. Photo contributor: Daniel Stulberg, MD.)
Retiform/ reticulate	Net-like pattern that indicates vascular etiology	Retiform purpura and other vasculopathies/ vasculitides	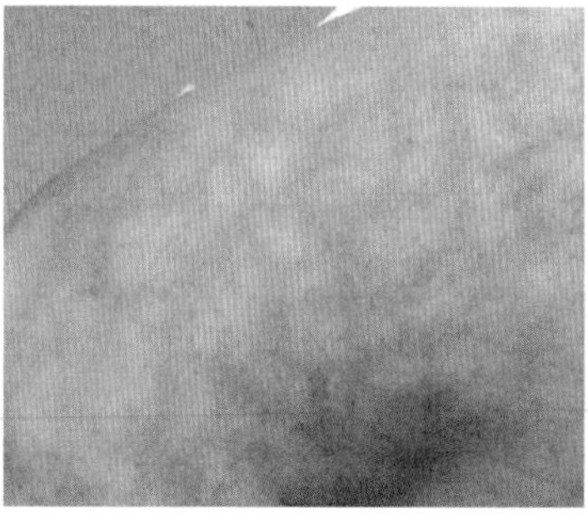 **Livedo reticularis** (Reproduced with permission from Soutor C, Hordinsky MK. *Clinical Dermatology: Diagnosis and Management of Common Disorders.* 2nd ed. New York: McGraw Hill; 2022, Figure 2-28.)

(Continued)

TABLE 16-5 • Common Patterns and Shapes (Continued)

Pattern or Shape	Description	Example Diagnoses	Example Image
Umbilicated	Centrally indented	Molluscum contagiosum and, more rarely, fungal infections (eg, histoplasmosis, talaromycosis)	**Molluscum contagiosum** (From Usatine RP, Smith MA, Mayeaux EJ Jr, Chumley HS. *The Color Atlas and Synopsis of Family Medicine.* 3rd ed. New York: McGraw Hill; 2019, Figure 136-4. Reproduced with permission from Richard P. Usatine, MD.)
Targetoid	Describes a macule, papule, patch, or plaque with concentric rings of varying colors	Erythema multiforme, erythema chronicum migrans	**Erythema multiforme** (Reproduced with permission from Soutor C, Hordinsky MK. *Clinical Dermatology: Diagnosis and Management of Common Disorders.* 2nd ed. New York: McGraw Hill; 2022, Figure 2-22.)

HAIR EXAM

- During examination of the head, assess the health of the scalp skin and note any alterations in hair density or the hairs themselves. Hair issues may occur in isolation or as manifestations of systemic problems.
- As with the nail exam, a dermatologist may use a dermatoscope to further evaluate abnormalities in the follicular openings, perifollicular skin, vascular structures, and hair shafts.

Findings and Their Meaning: Hair Loss

When evaluating a patient with hair loss, the following historical and exam features can provide clues that help determine the cause:

- Timing of the loss:
  - Sudden hair loss is more likely to be due to acute inflammatory processes (eg, alopecia areata), acute toxic injury, or metabolic disturbances (as in anagen effluvium related to chemotherapy or telogen effluvium in the setting of crash dieting or acute illness) (**Figure 16-6**).

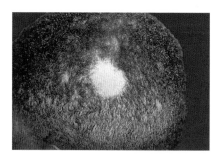

FIGURE 16-6 · **Alopecia areata.** (Reproduced with permission from Soutor C, Hordinsky MK. *Clinical Dermatology: Diagnosis and Management of Common Disorders.* 2nd ed. New York: McGraw Hill; 2022, Figure 30-5A.)

  - Gradual hair loss is more typical of hormonally-driven processes (androgenetic alopecia) or related to chronic diseases (eg, iron deficiency, hypothyroidism, systemic lupus erythematosus) (**Figure 16-7**). Additionally, certain inflammatory processes may progress more slowly in some patients, including some presentations of discoid lupus, lichen planopilaris, or other scarring alopecias.

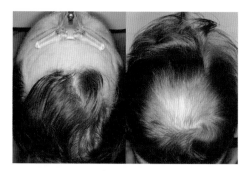

FIGURE 16-7 · **Androgenetic alopecia.** (Reproduced with permission from Kang S, Amagai M, Bruckner AL, et al, eds. *Fitzpatrick's Dermatology.* 9th ed. New York: McGraw Hill; 2019, Figure 85-2.)

- Pattern and distribution of loss:
  - Examples of causes of localized or patterned hair loss include alopecia areata (usually round patches, although there are other, less common patterns), androgenetic alopecia (pattern and sequence of progression differ according to biologic sex), central centrifugal cicatricial alopecia, frontal fibrosing alopecia, syphilitic alopecia (often described as "moth-eaten" in appearance), traction alopecia, and trichotillomania (patients chronically pulling on their own hair).

- Examples of causes of diffuse hair loss include telogen effluvium or anagen effluvium and the totalis and universalis variants of alopecia areata (**Figure 16-8**).

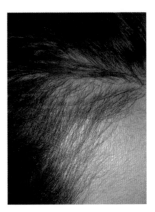

FIGURE 16-8 · **Telogen effluvium.** (From Usatine RP, Smith MA, Mayeaux EJ Jr, Chumley HS. *The Color Atlas and Synopsis of Family Medicine.* 3rd ed. New York: McGraw Hill; 2019, Figure 76-5. Reproduced with permission from Richard P. Usatine, MD.)

- Whether hairs are shedding or breaking:
  - Shedding from the root defines true hair loss.
  - Breaking along the shaft is caused by weakening of the internal structures of the hair and is most often caused by external factors, including bleaching, coloring, permanent and other chemical treatments, thermal damage from heated styling devices, or excessive brushing/combing (**Figure 16-9**). Hair breakage can also hint at genetic conditions that increase hair fragility (eg, ectodermal dysplasia and Menkes disease).

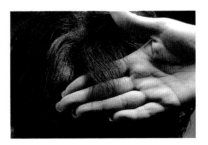

FIGURE 16-9 · **Hair breakage from styling tools.** (Reproduced with permission from Taylor SC, Kelly AP, Lim HW, Serrano AMA, eds. *Taylor and Kelly's Dermatology for Skin of Color.* 2nd ed. New York: McGraw Hill; 2016, Figure 6-12.)

- Ask about association with other health status changes or medications or physiologic or emotional stressors.
- Ask about associated scalp symptoms such as itching, burning, scaling, flaking, or discoloration.
  - These may be a sign of scalp pathology such as psoriasis or seborrheic dermatitis (dandruff).

- Look for signs of scarring/fibrosis.
  - You may see reduced hair density at follicles or multiple hairs appearing to emerge from the same follicular opening (polytrichia).
  - These changes imply a scarring process such as central centrifugal cicatricial alopecia, discoid lupus, lichen planopilaris, folliculitis decalvans, or dissecting cellulitis.

NAIL EXAM

A thorough nail exam can aid in the diagnosis of infectious, inflammatory, neoplastic, metabolic, genetic, drug-induced, and external processes. As noted earlier, nail findings can reflect local disorders or may be manifestations of systemic processes. Understanding the normal functioning and anatomy of the nail unit will help in diagnosing and treating disorders of the nail.

Nail Anatomy (Figure 16-10)

From proximal to distal, the normal nail unit consists of:
- Proximal nailfold (including the dorsal and ventral aspects), which covers the proximal portion of the nail matrix, responsible for forming the dorsal nail plate.
- Eponychium and cuticle, which overlap the proximal portion of the nail plate.
- Lunula, which is the visible portion of the distal nail matrix (responsible for forming the ventral nail plate) extending beyond the proximal nailfold.
- Nail plate, which is attached to the underlying nail bed.
- Onychodermal band, which marks the transition of the nail bed to the hyponychium.
- Free edge of the nail plate and the distal boundary of the tight seal, which keeps out pathogens and allergens.

The nail plate itself is made up of keratin. Melanocytes within the nail matrix synthesize melanin and can lead to pigmentation of portions of the nails.

> PEARL: Normal fingernail growth is approximately 3 mm per month, and normal toenail growth is approximately 1 mm per month.

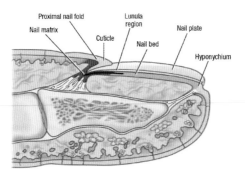

FIGURE 16-10 · **Nail anatomy.** (Reproduced with permission from Taylor SC, Kelly AP, Lim HW, Serrano AMA, eds. *Taylor and Kelly's Dermatology for Skin of Color.* 2nd ed. New York: McGraw Hill; 2016.)

Inspection

Assess the general shape, texture, and color of each fingernail and toenail and the skin surrounding the nails as well. When indicated, a dermatologist may use specialized tools (eg, a dermatoscope or capillaroscope) to assess the nailfold capillaries. Common nail pathologies are listed in **Table 16-6**.

TABLE 16-6 • Diagnoses at a Glance: Common Nail Pathology		
Name of Process	Description	Image
Paronychia	Acute, painful inflammation of the nailfolds caused by infection (usually staphylococcal or streptococcal species)	(Reproduced with permission from Arturo P. Saavedra, Ellen K. Roh, Anar Mikailov *Fitzpatrick's Color Atlas and Synopsis of Clinical Dermatology,* 9e. New York: McGraw Hill; 2023.)
Onychocryptosis (ingrown nail)	Penetration of the nail plate into the adjacent nailfold skin; can occur due to improper trimming of the nail, trauma, or anatomic abnormality; may be complicated by secondary infection	(From Usatine RP, Smith MA, Mayeaux EJ Jr, Chumley HS. *The Color Atlas and Synopsis of Family Medicine.* 3rd ed. New York: McGraw Hill; 2019, Figure 200-1. Reproduced with permission from Richard P. Usatine, MD.)
Onycholysis	Distal separation of the nail plate from the nail bed, caused by trauma or infections	(Reproduced with permission from Kang S, Amagai M, Bruckner AL, et al, eds. *Fitzpatrick's Dermatology.* 9th ed. New York: McGraw Hill; 2019, Figure 97-2.)

(Continued)

TABLE 16-6 • Diagnoses at a Glance: Common Nail Pathology (Continued)

Name of Process	Description	Image
Beau's lines	Transverse depressions in the nail plate that can be seen with trauma, severe illness, chemotherapy, malnutrition, or other processes that disrupt growth	 (Reproduced with permission from Soutor C, Hordinsky MK. *Clinical Dermatology: Diagnosis and Management of Common Disorders.* 2nd ed. New York: McGraw Hill; 2022, Figure 31-9.)
Pitting	Pit-like depressions in the nail plate associated with psoriasis, alopecia areata, eczema, and other disorders	 (Reproduced with permission from Soutor C, Hordinsky MK. *Clinical Dermatology: Diagnosis and Management of Common Disorders.* 2nd ed. New York: McGraw Hill; 2022, Figure 31-11.)
Koilonychia	Spoon-like curvature of the nail plate, associated with iron deficiency, lupus, hypothyroidism, hemochromatosis, and other disorders	 (Reproduced with permission from Wolff K, Johnson RA, Saavedra AP, Roh EK. *Fitzpatrick's Color Atlas and Synopsis of Clinical Dermatology.* 8th ed. New York: McGraw Hill; 2017, Figure 32-31.)
Melanonychia	Brown discoloration, typically in the form of a longitudinal band; can be due to malignant (acral lentiginous melanoma) or benign melanocytic tumors (nevi); when multiple nails are involved, can be a normal variant or can be due to medications, infections, endocrinopathy (eg, Addison's disease), inflammatory conditions	 (Reproduced with permission from Taylor SC, Kelly AP, Lim HW, Serrano AMA, eds. *Taylor and Kelly's Dermatology for Skin of Color.* 2nd ed. New York: McGraw Hill; 2016, Figure 40-2.)

(Continued)

TABLE 16-6 • Diagnoses at a Glance: Common Nail Pathology (Continued)		
Name of Process	Description	Image
Subungual hematoma	A subungual hematoma presenting as a bluish mass underneath the third fingernail	(Reproduced with permission from Burgin S, ed. *Guidebook to Dermatologic Diagnosis*. New York: McGraw Hill; 2021, Figure 13-25.)
Onychauxis	Thickening of the nail most commonly due to fungal infection, psoriasis, or trauma; can be accompanied by yellow discoloration and onycholysis	(From Richard P. Usatine, Mindy A. Smith, E.J. Mayeaux, Jr., Heidi S. Chumley *The Color Atlas and Synopsis of Family Medicine*, 3e. New York: McGraw Hill; 2019, FIGURE 198-4 ,ISBN 9781259862045. Reproduced with permission from Richard P. Usatine, MD.)

DIAGNOSTIC TESTS

A number of in-office tests can aid in diagnosis. The specifics of these studies are beyond the scope of this chapter, but they are briefly summarized in **Table 16-7**.

TABLE 16-7 • Common Diagnostic Tests and Procedures Used for Dermatologic Assessments	
Procedure	Purpose
Shave biopsy	Used to assist in diagnosis of lesions involving the epidermis and/or superficial dermis (most epidermal tumors are sampled using the shave technique)
Punch biopsy	Used to assist in diagnosis of inflammatory conditions or proliferations thought to involve the mid to deep dermis and/or subcutis
Incisional biopsy	Used to assist in diagnosis of deeper processes involving structures that may not be adequately sampled by the above techniques (eg, panniculitis, calciphylaxis)
Excisional biopsy	Used when the clinician anticipates that the entirety of a lesion will be necessary to achieve definitive diagnosis or if partial sampling is likely to lead to recurrence of the lesion (eg, cystic neoplasms)

(Continued)

TABLE 16-7 • Common Diagnostic Tests and Procedures Used for Dermatologic Assessments (Continued)

Procedure	Purpose
Skin scraping	Used in conjunction with potassium hydroxide preparation and microscopic evaluation for dermatophytes and other fungal infections; used with mineral oil preparation and microscopic evaluation for scabies or other ectoparasite infestations
Skin swab cultures or polymerase chain reaction/nucleic acid amplification test	Used for speciation and to identify antimicrobial susceptibilities in cases of superficial bacterial, fungal, viral, or mycobacterial infections
Ultraviolet blacklight (Wood's lamp) exam	Used to assess for pigmentary disorders (eg, vitiligo), define borders of melanocytic lesions, detect porphyrin deposition in the skin or teeth, or identify infection/colonization with infectious organisms
Magnifying lens or loupes	Used for magnification of lesions when additional detail is helpful for diagnosis
Dermatoscopy (also called dermoscopy)	Used for magnification and used to perform epiluminescence microscopy (a noninvasive means to evaluate pigmented lesions)

PUTTING IT ALL TOGETHER

- Once you have evaluated the patient, categorizing the process(es) you have observed based on morphology will help in constructing your differential diagnosis and management plan:
  - If evaluating a growth or neoplastic lesion, does it appear to be an epidermal process (eg, a scaly papule or plaque), a melanocytic process (eg, a pigmented macule or patch), or a dermal or subcutaneous process (eg, a nodule or tumor)?
  - If evaluating a rash, does there appear to be epidermal involvement/change (eg, are there papules, vesicles, or pustules or pigmentary changes visible)? Are there secondary change such as scale, crust, erosions, or ulcerations? Or does the process seem to spare the epidermis (eg, blanchable erythema or nonblanchable purpura, edema, or induration without surface change)?
- When you feel that you have accurately determined the morphology, pattern, and distribution of the condition, think through broad etiologic categories (eg, neoplastic, infectious, inflammatory, including autoimmune/autoinflammatory disease, medication/drug-induced, metabolic/endocrine, genetic, vascular, toxic/environmental exposure) to organize your differential diagnosis.

Case Example 1

A 23-year-old man with no significant past medical history presents for itchy lesions on the upper back and posterior neck, ongoing for 6 months. The rash is more noticeable after sun exposure. He has tried using an over-the-counter topical steroid (hydrocortisone 1% cream), which he applied twice daily for 2 weeks without improvement. He takes no oral medications, prescription or over-the-counter. Other than the recent use of the hydrocortisone, he denies any new soaps, lotions, detergents, or other changes to his skin care routine. He denies history of skin cancer or other dermatologic disease in himself or his family. On examination of his upper back and posterior neck, you see the lesions shown in **Figure 16-11**.

The lesions can be described as hyperpigmented, circular and oval, thin papules with subtle, fine scale. The secondary scale becomes much more noticeable with gentle stretching or light scratching of the lesions. This finding is termed inducible scale and is depicted in **Figure 16-12**.

Recall that erythema may be less obvious and can appear as dyspigmentation in patients with darker skin phototypes. With this in mind, you consider processes that can present with multiple erythematous or hyperpigmented, round-to-oval, thin, scaly papules on the trunk. You come up with the following focused differential diagnosis, organized by etiology:

- Infectious: tinea versicolor, tinea corporis, secondary syphilis
- Inflammatory: pityriasis rosea, guttate psoriasis, nummular eczema
- Medication/drug-induced: not relevant to this case due to the history you have obtained, but if a new drug had been started, you could consider psoriasiform drug reaction
- Toxic/environmental exposure: allergic contact dermatitis
- Neoplastic: mycosis fungoides/cutaneous T-cell lymphoma (CTCL)

To help delineate between these diagnoses, you obtain a skin scraping from a representative lesion, place it onto a glass slide, and perform a potassium hydroxide (KOH) preparation. On microscopic analysis, you see the findings shown in **Figure 16-13**.

The presence of multiple short hyphae (the filamentous structures) and spores (the rounded structures) is sometimes termed "spaghetti and meatballs." These findings are typical for species from the genus *Malassezia* (formerly *Pityrosporum*), and this KOH preparation establishes a diagnosis of tinea versicolor.

The patient's itchy rash improves with topical application of ketoconazole 2% (antifungal) shampoo/wash.

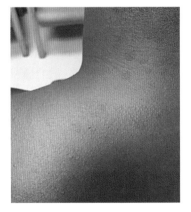

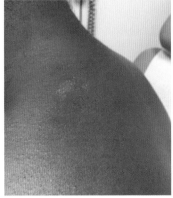

FIGURE 16-11 · **Appearance of skin lesions.** (Photo provided by Jeremy Schneider, MD.)

FIGURE 16-12 · **Secondary scale on lesion.** (Photo provided by Jeremy Schneider, MD.)

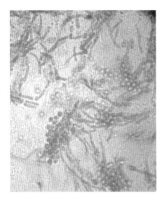

FIGURE 16-13 · **Skin scraping viewed under microscope after application of KOH.** (Reproduced with the permission from Carol Soutor, Maria K. Hordinsky *Clinical Dermatology: Diagnosis and Management of Common Disorders*, 2e New York: McGraw Hill; 2022.)

Case Example 2

Another example of using the categorization of dermatologic findings coupled with descriptors to make a diagnosis (eczema) is presented in **Figure 16-14**.

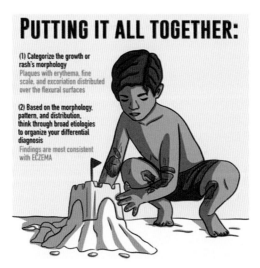

FIGURE 16-14 · **Putting it all together: eczema.** (Reproduced with permission from Dr. Cathy Cichon, MD.)

TELEHEALTH TIPS

The skin exam can be particularly well-suited to telemedicine since inspection is the primary mode of examination. As in the office-based exam, there are several requirements for a successful virtual dermatology exam:

• Lighting: Patients should be in an area with bright ambient light and have a light on their device when taking photographs or video.

• Positioning: Patients may need assistance from another person to hold a device to obtain clear, focused images.

• Technical support: Both the patient and the examiner must have a device (eg, smart phone with camera, computer with camera, digital camera) and the technical infrastructure (Internet access with the ability to stream and/or download) to view images. Images must be transmitted in high resolution.

- In broadband-poor or lighting-poor conditions, for body parts that may be difficult to view by video even with the assistance of a caregiver, or if it is difficult to hold a device still, consider asking the patient to take a photograph to share through messaging via a secure health portal. Ideally, patients will use a device capable of capturing a high-resolution image.
- Patients should show 3 views of a skin lesion in still or video images:
  - A close-up view of the area to see detailed characteristics of the lesion. For the best assessment, a high-resolution image or video is needed.
  - A distanced view of the lesion on the body to view the anatomic location, for context.
  - A view with another body part (eg, finger pointing) or item (coin or ruler nearby for reference) to demonstrate the size and scale of the lesion(s).
- Types of telehealth dermatology visits
  - Asynchronous exam: An asynchronous skin exam is when a patient sends images to a provider for interpretation at a later time or when images are captured by a technician at a medical facility and sent to a secure data storage location for interpretation by a remote provider at a later time.
  - Synchronous exam: A synchronous exam is when a patient sends still or video images to be interpreted while speaking to a provider or has a live video encounter with a provider to show the area of concern.
- There are times when a telemedicine skin exam may be insufficient to determine the etiology of a skin concern and in-person evaluation is required. This is particularly important when skin cancer or other "do not miss" diagnoses are on the differential.

✅ SUMMARY OF SKILLS CHECKLIST

- ❑ Clean your hands
- ❑ Ensure bright ambient and focused lighting
- ❑ Gown and drape appropriately
- ❑ Begin at the scalp and move systematically down to the toes, inspecting thoroughly, including the hair and nails
- ❑ Take note of skin phototype
- ❑ Identify the primary type of lesion, including size and if flat or raised
- ❑ Identify any secondary changes (due to outside influence) that have occurred
- ❑ Observe the shape or configuration of any lesions
- ❑ Note the distribution of any lesions
- ❑ Palpate any rashes or growths for blanching and to determine texture and depth of lesion
- ❑ Clean your hands

BIBLIOGRAPHY

American Academy of Dermatology learning modules. Accessed March 18, 2023. https://www.aad.org/education/basic-derm-curriculum.

Bolognia JL, Jorizzo JL, Rapini RP. *Dermatology*. St. Louis, MO: Mosby; 2007.

Boston University School of Medicine, Department of Dermatology. Integrated Skin Exam. Accessed August 11, 2023. https://www.youtube.com/watch?v=3RGTsl_zi2E.

Cox NH. Palpation of the skin–an important issue. *J R Soc Med*. 2006;99(12):598-600.

Filingeri D, Zhang H, Arens EA. Thermosensory micromapping of warm and cold sensitivity across glabrous and hairy skin of male and female hands and feet. *J Appl Physiol*. 2018;125(3):723-736.

James WD, Elston D, Mcmahon PJ. *Andrews' Diseases of the Skin Clinical Atlas E-Book: Expert Consult.* New York: Elsevier Health Sciences; 2016.

Marks JG, Miller JJ. *Lookingbill and Marks' Principles of Dermatology.* 5th ed. Rotterdam: Saunders Elsevier; 2013.

Rünger TM. Cutaneous photobiology. In: Kang S, Amagai M, Bruckner AL, et al, eds. *Fitzpatrick's Dermatology.* 9th ed. New York: McGraw Hill; 2019.

Taylor SC. Skin of color: biology, structure, function, and implications for dermatologic disease. *J Am Acad Dermatol.* 2002;46(2):S41-S62.

Ware OR, Dawson JE, Shinohara MM, Taylor SC. Racial limitations of Fitzpatrick skin type. *Cutis.* 2020;105(2):77-80.

Wolff K, Johnson RC, Saavedra A, Roh EK. *Fitzpatrick's Color Atlas and Synopsis of Clinical Dermatology.* 8th ed. New York: McGraw Hill; 2017.

17

Geriatric Exam

Roopali Gupta, MD and Jean Guan, MD

INTRODUCTION

The number of adults age 65 years and older in the United States is growing rapidly. For the first time in US history, older adults are projected to outnumber children by 2034, with nearly 1 in 4 Americans aged over 65 years old by 2060. This chapter focuses on the assessment of older adults, a population that holds a unique set of healthcare needs due to several factors:

- Higher presence of multiple chronic conditions
- Larger number of medications used
- Increased frequency of certain syndromes
- Wide variation in the level of function
- Particular focus on providing goal-aligned care

Geriatrics care benefits older adults based on their needs rather than when they reach a specific age. Geriatrics specialty care is generally most valuable when an older adult:

- Experiences conditions that cause considerable impairment or frailty (this tends to happen after age 75 or when someone starts managing a number of health conditions)
- Has family, friends, or other caregivers who start feeling considerable stress related to care
- Themselves or their family start having trouble following complex treatments or working with many different healthcare professionals for multiple health needs

The Age-Friendly Health Systems (AFHS) movement, known as 4 Ms care, is one framework that addresses the core domains of high-quality geriatrics care (**Figure 17-1**). All older adults benefit from age-friendly healthcare. The 4 Ms are:

- What *M*atters
- *M*edications
- *M*entation
- *M*obility

In this chapter, we review elements of history taking and the physical exam that are unique to older adults as well as strategies for incorporating the 4 Ms of age-friendly healthcare.

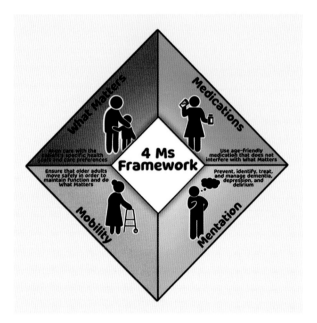

FIGURE 17-1 • **The 4 Ms framework for high-quality geriatrics care.** (Reproduced with permission from Cathy Cichon, MD.)

HISTORY TAKING IN THE OLDER PATIENT

This is done in the same fashion as with other patients and includes the history of present illness (HPI), past medical history, past surgical history, review of systems (ROS), social history, family history, and medication review (see dedicated chapters on HPI [Chapter 1] and ROS [Chapter 2] for details). We highlight the following areas that require a distinctive approach for the older adult:

- Consideration of sensory impairments
- Involvement of family members or caregivers when appropriate
- Eliciting *what matters* most for the patient
- Asking about functional status and *mobility*
- Asking about cognition and *mentation*
- Consideration of common geriatric syndromes
- Recognizing the complexity of *medication* review for older adults

Consideration of Sensory Impairments

Sensory impairments, such as with vision and hearing, are common in the older adult population. The potential barriers in communication from sensory impairments can be minimized by the following measures:

- Ensuring that the patient is wearing glasses and hearing aids if they use these assistive devices
- Using a well-lit, quiet room (eg, turning off the TV if evaluating a hospitalized patient)
- Facing the patient and sitting at eye level, which allows them to see your lips
- Speaking in a slow, even tone
- Being prepared to write questions out in large block print and/or finding out if a pocket amplifier is available in your clinical setting, if necessary.

> PEARL: An improvised pocket amplifier can be made by placing the earpieces of a stethoscope in the patient's ear and speaking into the bell.

Involvement of Family Members or Caregivers When Appropriate

Other people who support the older adult in life, such as family members or caregivers, are commonly present during healthcare encounters and can be a valuable resource when assessing the patient. However, it is critical to ask all persons in the room to identify themselves and elicit direct permission from the patient for the additional persons to be included in the visit. Make note of who is present during the visit in your documentation.

Eliciting What Matters Most for the Patient

"What matters" is one of the core domains of age-friendly healthcare. All older adults should be asked about what matters to them for person-centered care. This allows healthcare assessment and plans to align with each older adult's specific health outcome goals and care preferences, including, but not limited to, end-of-life care. The conversation typically occurs early in the encounter and includes:

- Exploration of the older adult's life context, priorities, and preferences to connect them to the impacts of care decisions and self-management
- Connection with a tangible health or care event in an older adult's life

> PEARL: Ask a question that helps understand life context and priorities. For example, "What brings you joy?" or "What are some goals you hope to achieve before your next birthday?"

- Many older adults have never been part of a discussion with a care team member beyond specific medical problems and may not be ready to engage in a "what matters" conversation. Inviting the older adult into the conversation can help frame the discussion and prepare them for these questions.

> PEARL: Ask a question to invite a conversation on what matters most to the patient. For example, "In order to align your healthcare plans on what matters most to you in your life, may I ask a few questions about your life outside of your medical concerns?"

Asking About Functional Status and Mobility

Mobility is another of the core domains of age-friendly healthcare. All older adults should be asked about their level of independence with activities of daily living (ADLs) and if there have been any recent changes (**Figure 17-2**). These are commonly asked within the HPI. Impairment in being able to complete ADLs correlates with increased risk for nursing home placement, emergency care visits, and overall mortality among community-dwelling older adults. A new change in functional status may indicate an unrecognized medical problem or cognitive impairment, both of which require additional assessment.

This assessment also includes inquiring about an older adult's ability to safely move within their life space in order to do "what matters." Life space refers to the area in which individuals move in their everyday lives. This is varied and can range from assessing ability to transfer out of bed to the ability to use transportation.

> PEARL: Ask a question about life space. For example, "During the past 4 weeks, have you been to places outside of your neighborhood?" Ask a question about falls. For example, "Have you had any falls within the last year?" or "Are you worried about falling?"

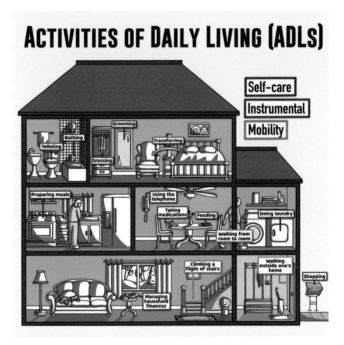

FIGURE 17-2 • Summary of activities of daily living (ADLs). These are commonly separated into instrumental activities (referred to as IADLs) and basic activities (includes self-care and mobility). (Reproduced with permission from Cathy Cichon, MD.)

Fall History

If a patient identifies that they have had any difficulty with mobility or identifies that they have fallen, a more detailed fall history should be taken and risk factors (**Figure 17-3**) identified. The history should include the following:

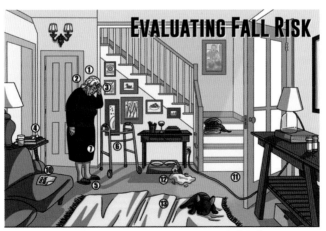

FIGURE 17-3 • **Evaluating fall risk.** (Reproduced with permission from Cathy Cichon, MD.)

- Patient activity during fall (positional change, risk-taking behavior)
- Location of fall
- Prodromal or associated symptoms
- Assessment of patient risk factors: older age, female gender, cognitive impairment, sensory changes, foot disorders, balance problems, pain/arthritis, movement disorders, history of stroke, history of falls, and vitamin D deficiency
- Assessment for environmental factors: terrain, situational hazards/obstacles (eg, low-lying furniture, loose rugs or other objects on the floor), footwear, assistive devices, and presence of grab bars
- Review of medications, especially looking out for psychoactive or anticholinergic agents
- Examples of fall histories:
  - Suboptimal history taking: Ms. Smith tripped and fell at home. She did not hit her head. She did not have any associated symptoms. She has a cane.
  - Optimal history taking: Ms. Smith turned suddenly to reach for her glasses on the coffee table. She caught the edge of her slippers on the rug, lost her balance, and stumbled forward. She was able to reach out with her hands and catch herself, so she did not hit her head. Ms. Smith did not have any preceding lightheadedness, vertigo, vision changes, chest pain, palpitations, or shortness of breath. She has been experiencing increased knee arthritis pain recently and has been using a cane for support when she is out of the house.

Asking About Cognition

Mentation is one of the core domains of age-friendly healthcare. In the outpatient setting, this typically refers to assessing for dementia and depression. Cognitive testing should be performed for all patients with memory concerns that are noted by themselves, a caregiver, or a clinician (see "Additional Assessments" later in this chapter; see also Chapter 13, Mental Status Exam, for more details). In addition, many guidelines recommend screening for cognitive impairment in the older adult, even if no concern is noted. Many patients with dementia are unrecognized in the primary care setting.

- Obtain a detailed history from the patient and a family member or somebody who knows the patient well, including:
  - Concerns about memory, including documentation of specific examples, such as missing appointments or losing keys
  - Other changes in mentation such as a change in behavior or mood
  - Length of time there has been a concern
  - Progression or change of symptoms
  - Effect of cognitive concerns on function such as the ability to drive safely

Consideration of Common Geriatric Syndromes

Geriatric syndrome is a term that refers to common health conditions in older adults that do not fit into distinct organ-based disease categories and are often the result of multifactorial etiologies. Examples include the following:

- Pressure ulcers (ask about any changes in the skin and prolonged lying in one position)
- Urinary incontinence (ask about any trouble making it to the bathroom, leaking urine, or use of pads)

- Frailty (ask about weight loss, exhaustion, slowness, or weakness)
- Malnutrition (ask about weight loss, changes in appetite, and access to food or food insecurity)

Geriatric syndromes may be addressed as part of the standard history of present illness or specifically elicited in the review of systems.

Recognizing the Complexity of Medication Review for Older Adults

Medication assessment is one of the core domains of age-friendly healthcare. A thorough medication review should be performed in patient of all ages; however, there are additional challenges associated with the use of medications in older patients, including:

- Increased number of pills (the average older adult takes 4-5 pills)
- Greater likelihood of adverse reactions related to altered drug metabolism (absorption, distribution, and clearance are less predictable), drug–drug interactions, and drug–disease interactions
- Higher risk of perpetuating a "prescribing cascade," a phenomenon that occurs when an adverse drug event is misinterpreted as a new medical condition and additional drug therapy is prescribed to treat that condition

Particular attention should be paid to obtaining an accurate medication list and assessing medication adherence. A medication list should include both prescription and over-the-counter medications and supplements. It is also important to recognize that multiple clinicians, sometimes from different health systems, may be prescribing medications. To gain clarity, it can be helpful to do the following:

- Ask the patient to bring all pill bottles and a medication list to their appointments.
- Obtain collateral information from the clinic pharmacist, patient's pharmacy, and/or patient's caregivers.

Elements to consider when assessing medication adherence include the following:

- Whether directions for administration are being followed and if those directions are practical
- Timing of doses and potential for missed doses
- Frequency of as-needed medication use
- Affordability of medication and whether there is a more cost-effective alternative

Polypharmacy is defined as the use of multiple medications (both prescription and over the counter) by an individual patient. The definition of the minimum number of medications varies, although generally, it ranges between 5 and 10. Identifying polypharmacy on the medication review should prompt a more detailed assessment for adverse outcomes associated with it, such as:

- Increased adverse drug events, falls, cognitive deficits, hospitalizations, and long-term care placement
- Decreased functional status, quality of life, and medications adherence (especially if compounded by sensory impairment)
- Perpetuation of a prescribing cascade
- Use of potentially inappropriate medications. The American Geriatrics Society Beers Criteria is a helpful resource with general guidelines (**Table 17-1**).

TABLE 17-1 • Key Principles from the American Geriatric Society Beers Criteria for Potentially Inappropriate Medication Use in Older Adults[a]	
Criterion	Rationale
First-generation antihistamines (eg, diphenhydramine, hydroxyzine)	Highly anticholinergic; risk of confusion, dry mouth, constipation, and other anticholinergic effects
Digoxin >0.125 mg/d	In heart failure, higher dosages are associated with no additional benefit and may increase risk of toxicity; slow renal clearance may increase risk of toxic effects
Tertiary tricyclic antidepressants (eg, amitriptyline)	Highly anticholinergic, sedating, and cause orthostatic hypotension
Antipsychotics for behavioral problems of dementia unless nonpharmacologic options have failed and patient is a threat to self or others	Increased risk of cerebrovascular accident (stroke) and mortality in persons with dementia
Benzodiazepines	Older adults have increased sensitivity to benzodiazepines and slower metabolism of long-acting agents; in general, all benzodiazepines increase risk of cognitive impairment, delirium, falls, fractures, and motor vehicle accidents in older adults
Nonbenzodiazepine, benzodiazepine receptor sedative-hypnotics (eg, the "Z drugs" such as zolpidem, eszopiclone)	Adverse events similar to those of benzodiazepines in older adults (eg, delirium, falls, fractures); minimal improvement in sleep latency and duration
Male androgens unless indicated for moderate to severe hypogonadism	Potential for cardiac problems and contraindicated in men with prostate cancer
Long-acting sulfonylureas (eg, glyburide, chlorpropamide)	Risk of severe prolonged hypoglycemia
Meperidine	Not an effective oral analgesic in dosages commonly used; can cause neurotoxicity
Non–cyclooxygenase-selective NSAIDs; avoid chronic use unless other alternatives are not effective and patient can take gastroprotective therapy (eg, proton pump inhibitor)	Increases risk of gastrointestinal bleeding and peptic ulcer disease; use of proton pump inhibitor or misoprostol reduces, but does not eliminate, risk
Skeletal muscle relaxants	Poorly tolerated by older adults because of anticholinergic adverse effects; sedation, risk of fracture

[a]For the full list of Beers criteria, see the American Geriatrics Society 2019 Updated AGS Beers Criteria® for potentially inappropriate medication use in older adults. https://onlinelibrary.wiley.com/doi/abs/10.1111/jgs.15767. Accessed March 15, 2020.
Source: Reproduced with permission from Walter LC, Chang A, Chen P, et al, eds. Current Diagnosis & Treatment Geriatrics. 3rd ed. New York: McGraw Hill; 2021.

PHYSICAL EXAM

The physical exam is done with the same basic components as with other patients and includes a systems-based assessment. Similar to history taking, it is critical to be mindful of sensory impairments that older adults may be facing while performing the physical exam such as difficulty hearing verbal instructions. We highlight the following areas that require distinctive attention for the older adult:

- Recognizing when standard physical exam maneuvers require modification
- Assessment of mentation
- Assessment of mobility

Recognizing When Standard Physical Exam Maneuvers Require Modification

Sensory impairments or difficulty with mobility or chronic pain may affect an older adult's ability to participate in a physical exam maneuver. Examples include the following:

- Hearing impairment that makes it difficult for the patient to hear instructions given during the exam (face patient and mimic the maneuver you would like them to perform while giving spoken instructions)
- Being unable to step onto the scale and balance without assistance (ask if a wheelchair scale is available)
- Hip or back pain with the traditional pelvic exam positioning. When this evaluation is indicated, consider modification of the position to avoid the use of the footrests.

ADDITIONAL ASSESSMENTS

Screening for Dementia

In addition to a detailed history about cognitive function from the patient and support person in the HPI, a validated tool for assessing cognition should be used when there is a concerning history. Evaluating cognition is part of the Medicare wellness visit, which is recommended annually.

- The Mini-Cog (**Figure 17-4**) is a validated assessment that is often preferred in the primary care setting due to a shorter administration time.
- The Mini-Cog combines free recall of 3 unrelated words presented verbally with a clock-drawing test and a score of performance.
- Caregiver input about a patient's cognitive abilities is typically also obtained using the AD8 Dementia Screening Interview, a validated tool designed for this purpose.

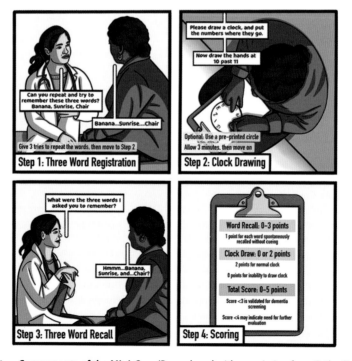

FIGURE 17-4 · Components of the Mini-Cog. (Reproduced with permission from Cathy Cichon, MD.)

Screening for Depression

Screening for depression can be done with a validated tool, such as the Patient Health Questionnaire-2 (PHQ-2), as is recommended for adults of all ages, including older adults (see Chapter 13 on Mental Status Exam for details).

Depression in older adults often goes undetected and is associated with decreased quality of life, decreased healthcare utilization, and increased morbidity and mortality. There can also be an overlap with dementia. Older adults with depression often present with a general issue such as functional change or fatigue rather than a typical complaint about mood.

Assessment of Mobility

This typically refers to evaluation of fall risk and falls, as falls are the leading cause of death from injury in older adults. A fall risk assessment should be performed at least once yearly for all older adults.

If a patient has not fallen, several examination techniques may be used to further determine their fall risk. These include the following:

- Timed Get Up and Go Test (**Figure 17-5**)
  - To assess, measure how long it takes the patient to stand without using their arms, walk 10 ft, turn around, walk back to the chair, and sit back down.
  - > or = 12 seconds to complete the TUG indicates increased risk for falls.

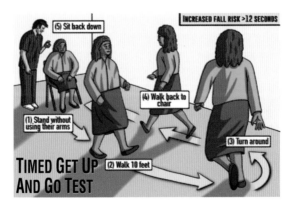

FIGURE 17-5 • **Timed Get Up and Go Test.** (Reproduced with permission from Cathy Cichon, MD.)

- 30-Second Chair Stand
  - Count the number of times a patient can stand and sit from a chair without using their arms in 30 seconds.
  - Normal ranges vary by age and gender. A below average score indicates increased risk for falls (**Table 17-2**).

TABLE 17-2 • Below Average Scores by Age for Chair Stand Test (CDC STEADI)		
Age	Men	Women
60-64	<14	<12
65-69	<12	<11
70-74	<12	<10
75-79	<11	<10
80-84	<10	<9
85-89	<8	<8
90-94	<7	<4

Source: Centers for Disease Control and Prevention. Accessed January 9, 2024. https://www.cdc.gov/steadi/pdf/steadi-assessment-30sec-508.pdf.

If a patient has fallen or expresses fear of falling, the physical exam should include the following elements. Full descriptions of these exam components can be found in the chapters on Vital Signs (Chapter 3), Cardiovascular (Chapter 7), Musculoskeletal, and Neurological (Chapter 12) evaluations:

- Orthostatic vital signs
- Gait assessment
- Evaluation for neurologic deficits (eg, muscle strength, sensation/proprioception, vision)
- Examination of feet, with particular attention paid to callouses or deformities and appropriateness of footwear

PEARL: The height of the cane or walker should be determined by the distance from the floor to the wrist joint when the patient is standing upright. With the arm hanging straight down at the side, the top of the cane should line up with the crease in the wrist.

TELEHEALTH TIPS

Functional and mobility challenges can make it difficult for an older adult to leave their home for an in-person appointment. Telemedicine visits can be an effective alternative in these situations. However, older adults may experience unique challenges with telemedicine visits related to unfamiliarity with technology and sensory impairment. There are several ways to help mitigate these challenges:

- Unfamiliarity with technology:
  - Arrange for the clinic staff to call the patient well in advance of their visit to walk them through the steps of setup. In certain situations, it may be appropriate to conduct a "practice visit" prior to the appointment to ensure familiarity with technology.
  - If the patient has provided consent, enlist the help of caregivers (eg, family, friends, home health provider, facility staff) to assist with setting up technology for the visit.
- Sensory impairment:
  - Look directly at the camera, ensure that your face is in full view, and have appropriate lighting. Ideally, make your background blank.
  - Explicitly ask if the patient can see and hear you.
  - Exaggerate your lip movements while speaking. This enhances the patient's ability to lip-read.
  - Write instructions down and hold them to the camera for the patient to read.
  - Have the patient use headsets or headphones in addition to hearing aids.

Telemedicine also affords the unique opportunity to learn more about a patient's living situation. If feasible and/or appropriate, ask the patient or caregiver to provide a tour of the home to better understand their living situation and assess for any safety issues.

✓ SUMMARY OF SKILLS CHECKLIST

History
- ❏ Consider any sensory impairments
- ❏ Consider involving family members or caregivers if appropriate
- ❏ Ask about "what matters most" to your patient
- ❏ Ask about current functional status (ADLs/Instrumental ADLs)
- ❏ Ask about falls and fear of falls
- ❏ Ask about memory and mood
- ❏ Ask about every medication used, including over the counter
- ❏ Remainder of history taking should be obtained as noted in Chapter 1, History of Present Illness

Exam
- ❏ Clean your hands
- ❏ Use any elements, as clinically appropriate, of the typical adult exam described in other chapters of this book
- ❏ Consider any sensory impairments
- ❏ Administer a validated cognitive assessment
- ❏ Administer a validated depression assessment
- ❏ Complete a gait and balance evaluation
- ❏ Clean your hands

BIBLIOGRAPHY

American Geriatrics Society. About geriatrics. Accessed March 5, 2023. https://www.americangeriatrics.org/geriatrics-profession/about-geriatrics.

Centers for Disease Control and Prevention. Stopping Elderly Accidents, Deaths, and Injuries (STEADI). Older adult fall prevention. Accessed March 5, 2023. https://www.cdc.gov/steadi/index.html.

Charlesworth CJ, Smit E, Lee DSH, Alramadhan F, Odden MC. Polypharmacy among adults aged 65 years and older in the United States: 1988-2010. *J Gerontolog A Biol Sci Med Sci.* 2015;70(8):989-995.

Gallo J, Rabins P, Lyketsos C, Tien A, Anthony J. Depression without sadness: functional outcomes of non-dysphoric depression in later life. *J Am Geriatr Soc.* 2015;45(5):570-578.

Galvin JE, Roe CM, Powlishta KK, et al. The AD8, a brief informant interview to detect dementia. *Neurology.* 2005;65:559-564.

Halli-Tierney A, Scarbrough C, Carroll D. Polypharmacy: evaluating risks and deprescribing. *Am Fam Phys.* 2019;100(1):32-38.

Institute for Healthcare Improvement. Age friendly health systems: what is an age-friendly health system? Accessed March 5, 2023. https://www.ihi.org/Engage/Initiatives/Age-Friendly-Health-Systems/Pages/default.aspx#:~:text=Age%2DFriendly%20Health%20Systems%20aim,adult%20and%20their%20family%20caregivers.

Institute for Healthcare Improvement. What matters to adults? A toolkit for health systems to design better care with older adults. Accessed March 5, 2023. https://www.ihi.org/Engage/Initiatives/Age-Friendly-Health-Systems/Documents/IHI_Age_Friendly_What_Matters_to_Older_Adults_Toolkit.pdf.

Johnson J, Rodriguez M, Snih S. Life-space mobility in the elderly: current perspectives. *Clin Interv Aging*. 2020;15:1665-1674.

Mayo Clinic. Healthy lifestyle, healthy aging. Accessed January 9, 2024. https://www.mayoclinic.org/healthy-lifestyle/healthy-aging/multimedia/canes/sls-20077060?s=3#:~:text=Check%20your%20wrist%20height.,the%20crease%20in%20your%20wrist.

Mini-Cog. Mini-Cog© – Quick Screening for Early Dementia Detection. Accessed January 9, 2024. https://mini-cog.com/.

US Census. Accessed March 4, 2023. https://www.census.gov/.

US Department of Health and Human Services. Telehealth and older patients. Accessed March 5, 2023. https://telehealth.hhs.gov/providers/health-equity-in-telehealth/telehealth-and-older-patients/.

US Preventive Services Task Forces. Recommendations for screening tests. Accessed March 4, 2023. https://www.uspreventiveservicestaskforce.org/uspstf/.

18

LGBTQ+ Healthcare

Jill Blumenthal, MD, MAS

INTRODUCTION

The lesbian, gay, bisexual, transgender, queer/questioning, intersex, asexual/aromantic/ agender, and two-spirit (LGBTQIA2S+; henceforth to be referred to as LGBTQ+) community as a whole experiences many health disparities that are associated with stigma, discrimination, and denial of basic civil and human rights. While many LGBTQ+ young adults thrive during adolescence, these factors and others put them at increased risk for negative short- and long-term health outcomes. It is critical for providers to be aware of existing health disparities in order to provide more inclusive, evidence-based, and compassionate medical care to LGBTQ+ individuals. For transgender and nonbinary (TGNB) individuals in particular, institutional and interpersonal gender discrimination can impact their experiences in the medical system. Healthcare providers can foster significant improvements in the health and well-being of the LGBTQ+ community.

> **PEARL:** Clinicians should be aware of existing health disparities to provide more inclusive, evidence-based, and compassionate medical care to LGBTQ+ individuals.

KEY TERMS AND DEFINITIONS

Table 18-1 provides definitions for commonly used LGBTQ+-related terms but is by no means exhaustive. Remember that the language used by and describing LGBTQ+ individuals may change over time, so what is recommended now may be different in the future.

TABLE 18-1 • Key Terms and Definitions	
Term	Definition
Agender	An individual who does not identify with any socially recognized gender.
Asexual	An individual who does not experience sexual attraction to others and/or has little or no desire to engage in sexual activity. Shorthand: "ace."
Bisexual	An individual who experiences sexual/affectional attraction to more than one gender identity. Some may use the term to connote the experience of attraction to all individuals regardless of gender. Shorthand: "bi."
Cisgender	An individual whose gender identity is congruent with their sex assigned at birth. Shorthand: "cis" or "cis-."

(Continued)

TABLE 18-1 • Key Terms and Definitions (Continued)

Term	Definition
Demi-sexual	An individual who only experiences sexual/affectional attraction with people who they know very well.
Gay	An individual who experiences sexual/affectional attraction to others of the same gender.
Gender	A construct drawing from social expectations, an individual's internal feelings, and expressed behaviors. Commonly confused with "sex" or "biological sex," gender is an internal construct and not determined by physical features or expression.
Gender identity	How an individual perceives themselves and/or how they feel they align within gender categories.
Gender expression	How an individual presents themselves to the world relative to gender (typically as masculine, feminine, or androgynous). This expression may include, clothing, haircut, body language, vocal tone, and behaviors.
Genderfluid	An individual who does not experience their gender identity in a stagnate form. Their identity shifts between 2 or more genders.
Gender nonconforming	An individual whose gender expression and/or gender identity does not match the social expectations of gender (ie, does not adhere to a category of man/masculine or woman/feminine). Shorthand: "GNC."
Genderqueer	An individual whose gender identity and/or expression falls outside societal expectations.
Intersex	An individual who has primary and/or secondary sex characteristics that do not fit the conventional categories of male or female. This may include variations in chromosomes, hormones, and internal and external characteristics.
Lesbian	A woman who experiences sexual/affectional attraction to people of the same gender.
Nonbinary	An individual whose gender does not solely match the binary construction of man or woman. Nonbinary individuals may have a mix of gender experiences, identify with a neutral gender identity (androgynous), or align with a gender identity beyond the man/woman binary. Shorthand: "NB."
Pansexual	An individual who experiences sexual/affectional attraction to another individual regardless of gender identity or sex.
Queer	"Queer" may be used by individuals who identify as anything other than straight and/or cisgender. "Queer" was often used as a derogatory term and is not embraced by everyone, but some have reclaimed the term to identify themselves.
Sex assigned at birth	The assigned category of sex, given at birth based on external genitalia. Historically, these categories have been male and female. Shorthand: "SAAB" for sex assigned at birth, "AMAB" for assigned male at birth, and "AFAB" for assigned female at birth.
Transgender/trans	An individual whose gender identity is not the same as their sex assigned at birth. Some who identify as nonbinary or gender nonconforming may also identify as trans; however, some may not.
Transgender woman/trans woman	A term used by a woman that affirms gender identity and acknowledges lived experience as a transgender individual.
Transgender man/trans man	A term used by a man that affirms gender identity and acknowledges lived experience as a transgender individual.

(Continued)

TABLE 18-1 • Key Terms and Definitions (Continued)	
Term	Definition
Transition	A term used to describe the process where an individual begins to express their true gender identity. Transition may include social changes such as sharing their gender identity with others, changing their name or pronouns, changing their appearance or the clothes they wear, and/or medical interventions such as surgery or hormone therapy.
Two-spirit	A term used in some First Nations/Native American/Indigenous cultures to describe an individual who may experience gender beyond the binary. Two-spirit may have different meanings depending on the specific culture and may be recognized as a separate gender. Additionally, communities may have terms in their own language to describe these identities. Shorthand: "2S."

GENERAL APPROACH TO CULTURAL HUMILITY AND RESPECT FOR LGBTQ+ PATIENTS

A good approach to all patient care, but particularly for LGBTQ+ individuals, is to stay open-minded, affirmative, and humble. Remember that there is no standard language that will work for all patients—give patients space to tell their story and use the patient's own words when asking questions.

When meeting patients for the first time, they should be asked:

- What name they like to be called (also known as their chosen or lived name)
- What pronouns they use

> PEARL: When meeting all patients for the first time, they should be asked what name they would like to be called and the pronouns they use.

Providers and staff should consider introducing themselves with their name and pronouns. When addressing patients, providers and staff should avoid defaulting to "Mr." and "Mrs." based on the patient's listed name or what is likely to be the patient's sex assigned at birth. If pronouns are not yet known and a patient needs to be verified, the patient's last name should be used to identify them.

Common challenges that can occur may be related to deadnaming (referring to someone by their birth name that they have since changed) or misgendering (intentionally or unintentionally referring to a person or using language to describe a person that does not align with their affirmed gender). When people are deadnamed or misgendered, they can feel invalidated and unseen, which can negatively impact their health and well-being.

Deadnaming, misgendering, and using incorrect terminology will occur. What is most important is how it is addressed when it happens. The best way to handle misgendering a patient is to apologize and try to get it right the next time (ie, "I'm sorry; I meant [correct name/pronoun/honorific]"). Your apology should be brief so that it is not about you and your mistake.

CARING FOR LGBTQ+ INDIVIDUALS

An overarching principle of caring for LGBTQ+ individuals is to remember that their care is similar to that of non-LGBTQ+ patients, and that they are at risk for and experience many of the same health issues as all patients (eg, hypertension, hyperlipidemia, diabetes). However, there are medical conditions for which they are at elevated risk due to a multitude of psychosocial, behavioral, and biological factors. As LGBTQ+ patients experience significant disparities in access to healthcare, it is essential to be aware of specific risks that should be discussed and services that should be offered to these individuals.

> **PEARL:** Care of LGBTQ+ patients should be individualized but also informed by data on risks and behaviors associated with each group.

Although LGBTQ+ is a commonly used term, each group described by the abbreviation has its own unique healthcare needs. Special considerations for a few specific groups are described here.

Lesbian and Bisexual Women

- At increased risk for overweight and obesity
- At increased risk for tobacco use, drug and alcohol use disorders (substance use disorders)
- At increased risk for mood disorders
- Lower likelihood to receive appropriate cervical cancer screening

Gay and Bisexual Men

- At least annual screening for HIV, syphilis, chlamydia, and gonorrhea should be offered to those who are sexually active.
- Preexposure prophylaxis for HIV infection may be appropriate for individuals at risk for HIV.
- Mood disorders
- Substance use disorders

Transgender/Nonbinary Individuals

- *Screen the body parts that patients have* is a principle that can help physicians consider which screening tests to utilize.
- Gender-affirming hormone therapy (GAHT) can help individuals affirm their gender.
- HIV/STI risk
- Substance use disorders
- Mood disorders

THE MEDICAL HISTORY

The core elements of history taking are described in Chapter 1, History Taking. Additional elements that apply specifically to LGBTQ+ care are described here.

History of Present Illness

After welcoming the patient and introducing yourself, begin visits with LGBTQ+ patients by asking, "What brings you into the office today?"
- Do not assume that the visit is related to their sexual orientation or gender identity.
- Some patients may experience discomfort related to their gender, also known as gender dysphoria, which can occur in medical environments.
- Asking patients if they experience any particular dysphoria and terms and/or situations to avoid can be helpful in making them feel comfortable.

Medications

- When reviewing a patient's medications, providers should confirm with transgender individuals if they are taking hormones. If yes, identify which type(s), route, and frequency.
- If patients are using injectable hormones, providers should ask if they have appropriate needles, syringes and safe disposal access.

Sexual Health Assessment

Stay sex-positive and open-minded. Remind patients that you ask these questions of all your patients to understand if there are additional risks of which you should be aware. The Centers for Disease Control and Prevention has championed the "5 Ps" of sexual history taking (partners, practices, protection for STIs, past history of STIs, prevention of pregnancy). A more comprehensive sexual history has expanded to include the "8 Ps," which also include preferences, pleasure, and partner violence (**Figure 18-1** and **Table 18-2**).

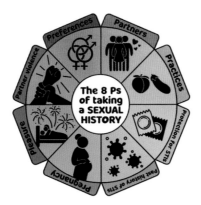

FIGURE 18-1 • The 8 Ps of taking a sexual history, which include preferences, partners, practices, protection from sexually transmitted infections (STIs), past history of STIs, pregnancy, pleasure, and partner violence. (Reproduced with permission from Cathy Cichon, MD.)

	TABLE 18-2 • Clinical Interview Using the 8 Ps	
	"P"	Sample Question
1	Preferences	Do you have language that you use to refer to your body (eg, genitals)?
2	Partners	What are the gender identities of your partners?
3	Practices	What types of sex do you engage in?
4	Protection from sexually transmitted infections (STIs)	Are there some kinds of sex where you do not use barriers? Which kinds?
5	Past history of STIs	Have you ever had an STI? If so, do you remember the site?
6	Pregnancy	Are you interested in getting pregnant?
7	Pleasure	Do you feel you are able to become physically aroused during sex, such as becoming wet or hard?
8	Partner violence	Has anyone ever forced you to do anything sexually that you did not want to do?

Substance Use

Take a complete history of smoking, drugs, and alcohol as you would for all patients, with probing as needed based on patient responses.

Education, Housing, Transportation, and Food Security

It may be important to address certain social issues. Not having basic needs met may significantly impact a person's health and access to medical care. Schools are often unsafe for LGBTQ+ individuals, leading to increased rates of drop out from high school and higher levels of learning, potentially impacting their ability to obtain jobs and health insurance. There are high rates of housing instability and food insecurity among LGBTQ+ individuals, particularly youth and young adults. A lack of reliable transportation may make it difficult to attend in-person appointments or access pharmacies. These same issues also become more prevalent among aging LGBTQ+ patients and may be further compounded by common geriatric issues (eg, social isolation, loneliness—see Chapter 17, Geriatric Exam).

Fertility Intentions

It is important to ask all patients regardless of sexual orientation or gender identity about their fertility goals. Patients should be asked if they or their partner(s) would carry a fetus, if they or their partner(s) would donate eggs, and if they or their partner(s) would donate sperm. Avoid using terms like "mom" and "dad" and instead use parent, unless used specifically by a patient.

THE PHYSICAL EXAM

The technical aspects of the exam can be found in chapters dedicated to each organ system. Those elements that merit adjustment or other special considerations are highlighted below.

> **PEARL:** It is important to ask permission before performing physical exams. Patients should be able to have chaperones present or defer any aspect of their exam.

As with all patients:

- Physical examinations should be conducted in a focused manner based on patients' reported symptoms, concerns and risk factors.
- Unnecessary exams should not be performed, particularly of the chest/breast and/or genitals.
- Unless there is an urgent reason to conduct a sensitive examination, providers should build rapport before performing genital exams.
- When conducting a genital exam, the purpose of the exam should be explained and the patient should be asked about ways to make them feel more comfortable.
- Body parts that are associated with a patient's sex assigned at birth may cause some patients to feel dysphoric; using gender-neutral terms (eg, chest instead of breasts) may be preferable for some patients.
- When discussing genitals, ask patients the words they would prefer you to use (eg, front hole instead of vagina). Providers may also refer to sensitive body parts using "the" instead of "your."
- Physical examinations should never take place simply to satisfy curiosity.

- An anatomic (or organ) inventory allows providers to record in the electronic health record (EHR), as well as update as needed, the organs each patient has at any point in time. Ideally, this inventory then drives any individualized autopopulation of history and physical exam templates. This anatomic inventory should be uncoupled from the patient's recorded gender identity, sex assigned at birth, or pronouns.
  - If no anatomic inventory exists as part of the EHR, specific organs to ask about include penis, testes, prostate, breasts, vagina, cervix, uterus, and ovaries.

TERMINOLOGY COMMONLY USED WITH LGBTQ+ PATIENTS

In the general care of LGBTQ+ individuals, medical language is by and large the same as for non-LGBTQ+ individuals. However, there is some commonly used terminology with which clinicians should be familiar. Furthermore, there are nonmedical aspects of transition that may be important to note. **Table 18-3** provides a list of these words and definitions.

TABLE 18-3 • Commonly Used Terminology

Term	Definition
Gender-affirming hormone therapy (GAHT or hormones)	A form of hormone therapy in which sex hormones and other hormonal medications are administered to TGNB individuals for the purpose of more closely aligning their secondary sexual characteristics with their gender identity.
Binding	This involves the use of tight-fitting sports bras, shirts, bandages, or a specially made binder to provide a flat chest contour. In some people with a chest, multiple garments may be used, and breathing may be restricted.
Tucking	Involves hiding the penis and/or testes, such as moving the penis and scrotum between the buttocks or moving the testes up into the inguinal canals.
Top surgeries	This refers to the group of surgeries that TGNB individuals use to reshape their chests, which includes breast augmentation for transgender women and other transfeminine individuals and chest reconstruction or mastectomy for transgender men and other transmasculine individuals.
Bottom surgeries	Refers to the group of surgeries that TGNB individuals use to reshape their genitalia. Transfeminine surgeries include orchiectomy, vulvoplasty, and vaginoplasty. Transmasculine surgeries include hysterectomy, salpin-go-oophorectomy, vaginectomy, metoidioplasty, and phalloplasty.
Insertive (top) sex	Refers to penetrative sex, with a penis into a vagina and/or anus.
Receptive (bottom) sex	Refers to receiving penetration into a vagina and/or anus.
Versatile sex	Refers to engaging in both or either role of penetration or receiving penetration.

SPECIAL CONSIDERATIONS FOR LGBTQ+ HEALTH

It is important to recognize LGBTQ+ patients as people, not just as their sexual orientation or gender identity. One example of an overemphasis on gender or sex is what is referred to as the transgender broken arm syndrome (ie, their broken arm has nothing to do with their hormones or genitalia). Similarly, a gay man's prehypertension has nothing to do with his sexual preferences or experiences.

There are no symptoms specific to LGBTQ+ individuals that are different than non-LGBTQ+ individuals. While it is important to remember that transgender women and gay and bisexual men and other men who have sex with men are at increased risk for HIV and STIs, clinicians should not promote stereotypes with an overemphasis on HIV and STIs.

LGBTQ+ individuals may have had challenging experiences in the healthcare system that have resulted in medical mistrust. National surveys have shown that LGBTQ+ patients are more likely to have experienced discrimination and been refused healthcare compared to their non-LGBTQ+ counterparts. By creating a welcoming, inclusive environment for all patients, clinicians can help eliminate these healthcare disparities (**Table 18-4** and **Figure 18-2**).

TABLE 18-4 • Considerations for Creating a Welcoming Environment for LGBTQ+ Patients	
What You Should Do	Why You Should Do It
Avoid clinic names and signage that embrace only one gender.	Gender-specific clinic names or centers may not appeal to gender nonbinary people or those in the process of gender affirmation.
Design patient intake forms that collect patient's chosen name, pronouns, gender identity, partner(s), or other family members.	This information will help providers and staff address patients correctly and avoids making assumptions regarding emergency contacts.
Develop EHR templates that allow for the collection of gender identity and sex assigned at birth, including an anatomic inventory.	These data can help providers address specific healthcare needs including prevention services according to their sex assigned at birth and current anatomy.
Create gender-neutral bathrooms and avoid bathroom signs that designate one gender or another.	TGNB individuals should be able to use a restroom that corresponds to their gender identity and expression.
Waiting rooms and clinic spaces should have signage with LGBTQ+ images and people on education materials and brochures, using a variety of ethnic/racial backgrounds.	Seeing LGBTQ+-inclusive and friendly images can increase comfort and make patients feel more at ease during their medical visit.

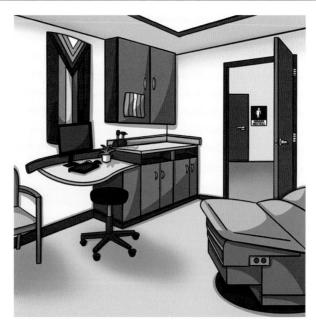

FIGURE 18-2 • **An inclusive environment with LGBTQ+ images, including flags and gender-neutral restrooms, can make patients feel more comfortable in a healthcare setting.** (Reproduced with permission from Cathy Cichon, MD.)

ELECTRONIC HEALTH RECORD TO SUPPORT LGBTQ+ CARE

- An important consideration when using an EHR is the degree to which it supports culturally competent and responsive clinical care.
- Patients should be able to self-report and/or have staff collect appropriate sexual orientation and gender identity data.
- Staff and providers should be easily able to recognize a patient's chosen name and appropriate pronouns.
- EHRs should allow for flexibility in clinical data collection despite the gender marker that is assigned to a chart, which includes, but is not limited to, preventative health screening, lab value ranges, and organ inventories.

TELEHEALTH VISITS

- Telehealth is an excellent way to make patients who are nervous or uncertain about their care feel more comfortable, allowing them to get a sense of their provider before coming into the clinic or hospital.
- For transgender individuals, gender dysphoria can be overwhelming and disabling at times, making in person visits difficult.
- Having the ability to use telehealth on days where a patient's dysphoria/discomfort is unmanageable is preferable to canceling an appointment.
- In addition, LGBTQ+ individuals may not have access to affirming providers locally, and telehealth gives them the option to see someone knowledgeable who works in a geographically distant area.
- Data acquisition and communication should follow the guidance provided in this chapter.
- At the start of the visit, confirm with the patient that they are in a private and comfortable space.
- Telehealth physical exams of sensitive organs may be completed following oral consent of the patient and agreement of the provider that use of the telehealth modality is clinically appropriate. Additionally, a chaperone is recommended for both patient and provider during the exam. Alternatively, it is fine to restrict any physical exam aspects to nonsensitive areas of the body.

BIBLIOGRAPHY

American Psychiatric Association. Gender dysphoria. *Diagnostic and Statistical Manual of Mental Disorders.* 5th ed. Arlington, VA: American Psychiatric Publishing; 2013:451-459.

Centers for Disease Control and Prevention and US Public Health Service. Preexposure prophylaxis for the prevention of HIV infection in the United States—2021 update. A clinical practice guideline. https://www.cdc.gov/hiv/pdf/risk/prep/cdc-hiv-prep-guidelines-2021.pdf.

Coleman E, Radix AE, Bouman WP, et al. Standards of care for the health of transgender and gender diverse people, version 8. *Int J Transgender Health.* 2022;23:(Suppl 1):S1-S259.

Dowshen N, Lett E. Telehealth for gender-affirming care: challenges and opportunities. *Transgender Health.* 2022;7:111-112.

Human Rights Campaign. Glossary of terms. https://www.hrc.org/resources/glossary-of-terms.

Keuroghlian AS. Electronic health records as an equity tool for LGBTQIA+ people. *Nat Med.* 2021;27:2071-2073.

McNamara MC, Ng H. Best practices in LGBT care: a guide for primary care physicians. *Cleve Clin J Med*. 2016;83(7):531-541.

National LGBT Health Education Center, a Program of the Fenway Institute. Creating an inclusive and welcoming health care environment for SGM people. https://www.lgbtqiahealtheducation. org/wp-content/uploads/2020/06/2.-Creating-An-Inclusive-and-Welcoming-Environment.pptx. min_.pdf.

National LGBT Health Education Center, a Program of the Fenway Institute. Sexual health history: talking sex with gender non-conforming and trans patients. https://fenwayhealth.org/wp-content/ uploads/Taking-a-Sexual-Health-History-Cavanaugh-1.pdf.

Payton N. The dangers of trans broken arm syndrome. *PinkNews*. July 9, 2015. http://www.pinknews. co.uk/2015/07/09/feature-the-dangers-of-trans-broken-arm-syndrome/.

Testa RJ, Rider GN, Haug NA, Balsam KF. Gender confirming medical interventions and eating disorder symptoms among transgender individuals. *Health Psychol*. 2017;36(10):927-936.

University of California San Francisco Center of Excellence for Transgender Health. Primary care protocol for transgender patient care. 2016. http://transhealth.ucsf.edu/protocols.

19

Newborn and Infant Exams

Michelle Leff, MD

INTRODUCTION

By definition an infant is a child under one year of age, while a newborn infant is a child 0-28 days of life. The newborn examination is a screening exam that occurs within 24 hours of birth. The goals include the following:

- Identify in utero growth issues.
- Recognize dysmorphic features.
- Note birth trauma.
- Normalize common variations.
- Educate parents about temperament, parent-newborn interaction, and development.
- Model how to hold, interact with, and comfort the baby.
- Provide anticipatory guidance focused on routine newborn care and any concerns that arise from the history.

> **PEARL:** The purpose of the newborn exam is to look for normal growth and development and to identify any deviations.

A similar examination is performed during the first year of life at subsequent well-child checks with some minor variations based on age. A visit for an acute clinical concern would include a focused exam.

HISTORY

General Information

- Newborn: consists mostly of the mom's* pregnancy and delivery history, including:
  - Maternal laboratory results
  - In utero exposures
  - Prenatal ultrasound reports (including placental issues)
  - Birth information
  - Parental observations since the baby's birth
  - You may need to ask visitors, including the partner, to leave the room in order to ask sensitive questions.
  - While speaking with the family, you will get a sense of their dynamics and maternal recovery.
- Infant
  - Feeding
  - Sleep
  - Development
  - Parental concerns and/or any acute issues

Family History

- Newborn
  - Focus on childhood conditions such as:
    - Hip dysplasia
    - Birth defects
    - Sudden infant death syndrome
    - Childhood hearing loss
  - Remember to ask about genetic relatives. The known family history of a donated egg or sperm may be quite limited.
- Infant
  - Ask about any updates.
  - Ask about conditions that are pertinent to the clinical encounter.

Social History

- Newborn
  - Who will be living at home?
  - Are there older siblings?
  - Does anyone smoke?
  - Are there pets that could harm an infant?
  - What are the childcare plans?
  - Does the family have needed supplies such as a safe sleeping space and car seat?

The author recognizes there are many birth stories and uses the terms mom, mother, and maternal for simplicity. The birthing person may not identify as female, may not be biologically related to the newborn, and may not be the intended parent.

- Infant
  - Update the items above.
  - How is parental mental health?
  - Are there any family relationship issues?
  - Is food security a concern?

GENERAL COMMENTS ABOUT THE EXAM

Most newborns in the United States now room-in with their parents rather than going to a separate nursery, so the newborn examination will likely occur in the patient room. As with all patient encounters, the first thing you should do is introduce yourself and your role. Because newborns can get cold quickly, you will want to conduct your exam in a timely fashion in a warm environment. If the room is cold, consider turning up the heat while you interview the parents, and then examine the baby after the room has warmed. Another option is to examine the newborn under a warmer (**Figure 19-1**). Performing an examination on the warmer is especially important if the baby is premature or small for gestational age (weight <10th percentile), as they get cold easily.

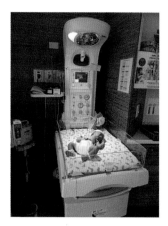

FIGURE 19-1 · **Newborn lying on a radiant warmer. This baby demonstrates the tone of a normal term newborn. Note how elbows, hips, and knees are flexed even while the baby is asleep.** (Photo provided by Michelle Leff, MD.)

You may very well be the first provider examining a newly born infant. Since the average US family has fewer than 2 children, this may be the family's first baby. Approaching the newborn with gentleness will be greatly appreciated. While it is inevitable that many babies will cry during an exam, how you respond to the crying will be noticed by the family.

- Remain calm.
- Speak quietly and reassuringly to the newborn.
- Acknowledge this is a minor stress for the newborn.
- Explain to the family what you are doing and why.
- Discuss your findings as you progress throughout the exam.
- Involve the family if you can. Having a parent offer a finger to suck can be soothing and allows you to evaluate the newborn's suck.

The crying may be anxiety-provoking at first, but as your skill at comforting a baby grows and you are able to teach the family these techniques, they will be amazed and grateful.

While students are often taught a methodical approach to the physical examination, with young children, providers must grab opportunities when they arise. For example, if the baby's eyes are open, go ahead and perform the retinal light reflex; another opportunity may not arise during the encounter. If the newborn is calm and quiet, auscultate the heart; the more the newborn is disturbed, the more likely it is that they will begin to cry. Another technique is to perform some of the examination with the baby in the parent's arms. If the baby is already lying in the crib, unwrap just enough of the chest to listen to the heart and lungs before proceeding with the rest of the exam (**Figure 19-2**). You can also swaddle portions of the newborn while you examine other areas.

> **PEARL:**
> * Keep the baby warm during the examination.
> * Stay calm even if the newborn is crying. The newborn and the family will notice anxiety if present.
> * The provider does not have to follow the head-to-toe examination format; take advantage of opportunities as they arise.

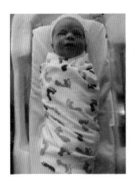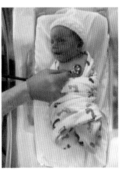

FIGURE 19-2 • Swaddled newborn in a hospital crib (left). Newborn swaddled so heart can be auscultated while they are calm and warm (right). (Photos provided by Michelle Leff, MD.)

VITAL SIGNS

* Typically, you will be assessing vital signs taken by a nurse rather than measuring them yourself, but it is important to know how to measure them accurately if the need arises.
* Vital signs should be done in the order of least invasive to most invasive.
* Growth parameters: Weight, length, and head circumference should be plotted on the appropriate growth chart. Many electronic medical records will auto-plot the data. Make sure the appropriate chart is chosen if the child is premature or has a unique medical condition such as achondroplasia or Down syndrome.
* Weight:
  * Newborns: Birth weight on admission, percent weight loss on subsequent hospital days, weight gain/day for visits in the first month until feeding is well-established

- Infants: Weight for age
- A prefeeding and postfeeding weight may be done to assess transfer of milk anytime during breastfeeding.
● Length:
  - Newborns and infants: Length for age
  - Most accurate using a length board rather than tape measure
● Head circumference:
  - Newborns and infants: Head circumference for age
  - The tape measure should be placed above the ears and brows and the widest diameter obtained (**Figure 19-3**).

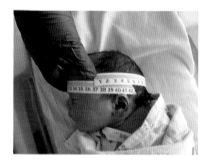

FIGURE 19-3 • **Measuring head circumference. This baby also exhibits typical head molding seen with breech positioning in utero.** (Photo provided by Michelle Leff, MD.)

● Respiratory rate:
  - Rate should be counted over a full minute in the newborn because periodic breathing is normal at this age and can last up to 6 months. This means they may breathe fast, then slow, and then take a pause or deep sigh.
  - In the older infant, you can count over a shorter time frame and multiply like is done with adults.
● Heart rate:
  - In the newborn and infant, auscultate over the apex rather than feeling for a pulse.
  - In the newborn, it is recommended to listen for a full minute as the heart rate can vary greatly in that time.
  - In the older infant, you can listen for a shorter time and multiply.
● Temperature:
  - Temperature may be screened with an axillary measurement.
  - Rectal temperature is the gold standard and should be used to confirm any hypothermic or hyperthermic measurements.
● Oxygen saturation:
  - Critical congenital heart disease screening of the newborn looks for differences in oxygen saturation measurements between the right hand and either foot. This is a mandated screen performed in all 50 states before 48 hours of life. If the screen was not done at birth, such as with a home birth, it can be done at the first outpatient visit.
  - Subsequently, oxygen saturation is only measured during times of concern.

- Blood pressure:
  - Blood pressure is not routinely measured until age 3 but may be done earlier in certain clinical situations, such as concern for coarctation of the aorta.
  - Pediatric blood pressure cuffs come in a variety of sizes including for the smallest premature infants.

> **PEARL:** Normal newborn vitals:
> - Temperature axillary 36.5-37.4°C (97.7-99.3°F) in an open crib
> - Respiratory rate <60 breaths/min
> - Heart rate 100-190 bpm while awake, as low as 70 bpm while asleep

GENERAL OBSERVATION

What you see depends on several factors: how many hours old the baby is, the gestational age of the newborn, what stage of transitioning are they in, and how hungry or satiated the baby is. These factors will affect newborn alertness, lung sounds, the presence of a murmur, vital signs, skin color, and mottling.

- Observe newborn state (asleep, awake, calm, crying).
- Assess intensity and pitch of the cry (if present).
- Hiccups and sneezing are common occurrences in the newborn and do not generally indicate illness.

Findings and Their Meaning: Cry

- An intense cry could indicate pain from birth trauma, withdrawal from an in utero exposure, or an intense temperament.

HEAD AND NECK EXAM

Head

- Remove hat.
- Observe head shape (eg, rounded [**Figure 19-4**], molded [Figure 19-3]).
- Assess the location and number of hair whorls. Whorls are the spiral distribution of hair around an axis. Most individuals have one in the parietal region (Figure 19-4).
  - An abnormal location or number of hair whorls can indicate problems with brain development.

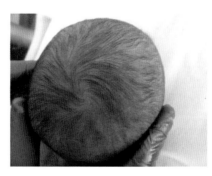

FIGURE 19-4 · Normal hair whorl and rounded head shape. A hair whorl is the spiral distribution of hair around an axis. (Photo provided by Michelle Leff, MD.)

- Look for bruising, abrasions, and other forms of birth trauma.
  - A cephalohematoma and subgaleal hemorrhage (**Figure 19-5**) are typically from birth trauma and increase an infant's risk for jaundice.

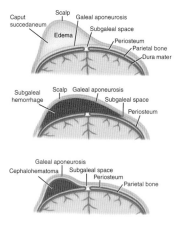

FIGURE 19-5 • **Examples of scalp birth trauma.** (Reproduced with permission from Cunningham FG, Leveno KJ, Dashe JS, et al, eds. *Williams Obstetrics*. 26th ed. New York: McGraw Hill; 2022.)

- For an older baby, assess for abnormal head shape (plagiocephaly) by observing from above while the seated parent holds the child upright (**Figure 19-6**).

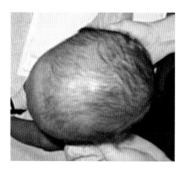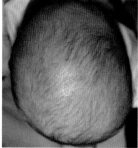

FIGURE 19-6 • **Assessing for plagiocephaly. Baby seated on parent's lap and provider looking down from above. Photo on left is a normally shaped head. Photo on right shows plagiocephaly, with left occiput flatter than the right.** (Left photo provided by Michelle Leff, MD. Right photo reproduced with permission from Schaefer GB, Thompson JN Jr. *Medical Genetics: An Integrated Approach.* New York: McGraw Hill; 2014, Figure 3-23A.)

- Using both hands, rub and gently press the scalp (**Figure 19-7**), feeling for:
  - The sutures (metopic, coronal, sagittal, lambdoid)
  - Fontanelles (anterior, posterior)
  - Swelling

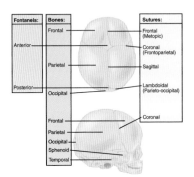
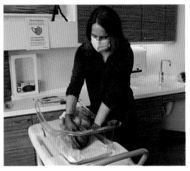

FIGURE 19-7 • **Fontanelles and sutures of the head (left). Palpation of the head (right).** (Left illustration reproduced with permission from Biller J, Gruener G, Brazis PW. *DeMyer's the Neurologic Examination: A Programmed Text.* 7th ed. New York: McGraw Hill; 2016. Right photo provided by Taylor Wrinkle, MD.)

Findings and Their Meaning: Abnormal Head Shape

- An abnormal head shape could indicate positional plagiocephaly associated with too little tummy time, or premature fusion of sutures (craniosynostosis) (**Figure 19-8**).

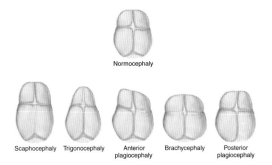

FIGURE 19-8 • **Examples of different skull shapes due to craniosynostosis.** (Reproduced with permission from Brunicardi FC, Andersen DK, Billiar TR, et al, eds. *Schwartz's Principles of Surgery.* 11th ed. New York: McGraw Hill; 2019.)

Ears

- Newborn
  - Look to see if the ears are normal in shape and position.
  - Canals should be patent, but tympanic membranes are not visible due to vernix and small canals, so an otoscopic exam is not typically performed until about 4 months.
- Infant
  - After 4 months, use an otoscope with the smallest speculum to look for the tympanic membranes. See the toddler chapter (Chapter 20) for more details about how to perform this exam.

Findings and Their Meaning: Preauricular Tags or Pits

- These are usually a normal variant but are sometimes associated with a syndrome. If other dysmorphic features are noted, you should consider evaluation for a syndrome.

Eyes

- Visually inspect the eyes looking for symmetry, discharge, and signs of trauma.
- Use a direct ophthalmoscope to assess the retinal reflex in both eyes (**Figure 19-9**).

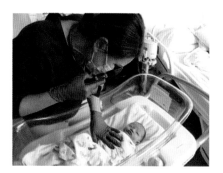

FIGURE 19-9 • **Proper positioning of examiner, baby, and ophthalmoscope for a retinal reflex examination.** (Photo provided by Michelle Leff, MD.)

- Low lighting helps.
- It is ideal to assess both eyes at the same time but often not practical.
- Hold the ophthalmoscope to your eye and look through it while aiming the light below or to the side of the eyes of the infant.
- Swing light onto infant's eye quickly to catch eyes open.
- You can use gentle pressure with your fingers to separate the lids if needed (**Figure 19-10**).

PEARL: Retinal reflex is a more inclusive term than red reflex as darkly pigmented individuals have more pale or even whitish retinal reflexes.

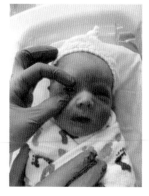

FIGURE 19-10 • **How to open an infant's eyes. Use gentle pressure to spread lids apart.** (Photo provided by Michelle Leff, MD.)

- In the older child, check for strabismus using the corneal light reflex (**Figure 19-11**). The examiner holds the ophthalmoscope like a flashlight and stands far enough away from the child that the light shines on both eyes at the same time (For additional information, see Chapter 20, Toddler exam). Intermittent nonconjugate gaze is normal for the first several months of life.

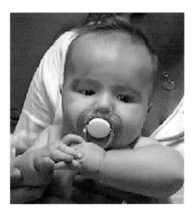

FIGURE 19-11 • **Corneal light reflex. Shine the ophthalmoscope from far enough back that it reflects off both eyes at the same time. Note that the light reflex is symmetric in both eyes for this patient.** (Photo provided by Chris Cannavino, MD.)

Findings and Their Meanings: Common Eye Abnormalities

- Clear or yellow eye discharge usually indicates lacrimal duct stenosis, a common finding in newborns that usually resolves with time.
- Green discharge and scleral injection are signs of infection.
- An abnormal retinal reflex indicates an obstruction of the light beam somewhere along the visual axis. This can include glaucoma, cataract, vitreous hemorrhage, or retinoblastoma.
- An abnormal corneal light reflex in an infant over 6 months can indicate strabismus and necessitates an ophthalmology referral.

Nose

- Look and listen to assess for patency of both nares, congestion, discoloration, and deviation.
- You can hold your stethoscope over the infant's nose, but not touching it, to listen for stertor (the sound you hear when trying to breathe through a stuffy nose). You might want to do this during the lung exam if you cannot tell if noises are coming from the lungs or nose.

Findings and Their Meaning: Bluish Swelling at Nasal Bridge

- A bluish swelling over the nasal bridge can indicate a dacryocystocele.

Mouth

- To visualize the inside of the mouth, use a tongue depressor in your dominant hand and a light (typically the ophthalmoscope, utilized as a flashlight) in your nondominant hand (**Figure 19-12**).

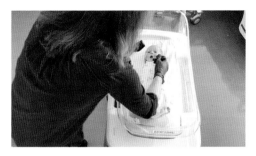

FIGURE 19-12 • **Technique for examining the mouth using the ophthalmoscope as a flashlight. This image also demonstrates how it is easier to do this exam while the baby is swaddled so the arms do not get in the way.** (Photo provided by Taylor Wrinkle, MD.)

- Use the tongue depressor to gently move the lips up and down to visualize the gums.
- Push down gently on the tongue, working your way to the back of the mouth until you can visualize the uvula in order to rule out a cleft palate. It is important to not scrape the palate with the tongue depressor as that can be painful and cause bleeding.
- At some point, the newborn may gag and then provide a thorough view of the uvula. Note, at times, the uvula will flip up into the nasopharynx with gagging.
- Examine for teeth. In most infants, teeth will start emerging by 6 months but may not appear until after a year.

PEARL: Save the eye and mouth exam until the very end. Both maneuvers tend to upset the baby and are easier to do with a baby who is not flailing. Swaddle the newborn with the arms down before performing the exam to keep the hands from interfering with your visualization.

Neck

- Visually inspect and palpate for pits, tags, and masses.
- Examine for congenital torticollis by gently moving each ear to the ipsilateral shoulder (**Figure 19-13**).

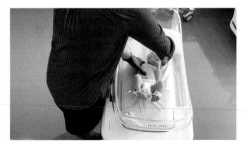

FIGURE 19-13 • **Assessing for congenital torticollis. Hold one shoulder in place while using your other hand to push the ear to the ipsilateral shoulder assessing for tightness and symmetry.** (Photo provided by Taylor Wrinkle, MD.)

- Palpate the clavicles with your fingertips feeling for crepitus and observing for signs of pain, indicative of injury that might occur during birth.

Findings and Their Meaning: Pits, Tags, and Masses of the Neck

- Pits, tags, and masses of the neck could indicate branchial cleft or thyroglossal duct remnants (**Figure 19-14**).

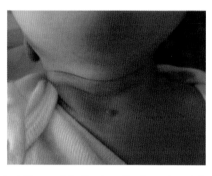

FIGURE 19-14 • **Skin tag of midline neck indicative of a thyroglossal duct remnant.** (Photo provided by Michelle Leff, MD.)

LUNG AND CHEST EXAM

- **Visually inspect:** Assess color and for increased work of breathing.
  - Nasal flaring is when the alae nasi move with respirations.
  - Retractions are when the skin is moving between the ribs.
  - Abdominal breathing is normal in the newborn period.
  - Newborns have periodic breathing where they may breathe fast, then slow, and then take a pause or deep sigh.
  - The xyphoid process is quite noticeable in many newborns due to a thin chest wall with little fat or musculature.
- **Auscultate:** Listen to both sides of the chest.
  - Preferably use an infant stethoscope, but a pediatric one will do. Using the diaphragm is generally adequate.
  - Differentiation of lung segments at this age is not practical given the small size. Listening over the upper chest on the right and left side is adequate.
  - Typically, lung sounds are equal and clear bilaterally. Crackles may be heard if the baby is examined during their first couple hours of life while still transitioning from the in utero environment where the lungs are full of fluid.

Findings and Their Meaning: Breast Buds

- Breast tissue may be enlarged due to stimulation from maternal hormones, and drops of milk might even be present. This resolves over time (**Figure 19-15**).

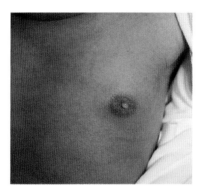

FIGURE 19-15 • **Newborn breast enlargement with a drop of milk.** (From Knoop KJ, Stack LB, Storrow AB, Thurman RJ, eds. *The Atlas of Emergency Medicine.* 5th ed. New York: McGraw-Hill; 2021, Figure 14.7. Reproduced with permission from photo contributor: Michael J. Nowicki, MD.)

HEART EXAM

- **Assess color:**
  - Perfusion in a newborn is quite different than in an older child. Acrocyanosis (**Figure 19-16**) is normal, including perioral cyanosis. The lips and tongue, however, should be pink.
  - Perfusion may be symmetric or asymmetric depending on positioning. A well-known benign phenomenon in newborns called harlequin color change is a dramatic example of asymmetry where one whole side of the newborn will be redder than the other.

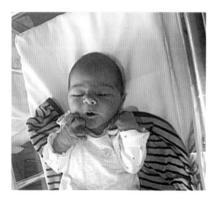

FIGURE 19-16 • **Acrocyanosis of the hands in a 2-day-old newborn. Note the blue tinge to the hands compared to the color of the face. This is a normal finding in newborns and can come and go for a few weeks.** (Photo provided by Emily Golden, MSN, RN, CPNP.)

- **Inspect and palpate the precordium**: You may notice a slight lift, meaning your hand will feel upward pressure as the heart beats.
- **Auscultate:**
  - Use the diaphragm of your stethoscope and listen in several locations. Sinus arrhythmia is common in the newborn. Premature ventricular and atrial contractions are frequent in the first few days and slowly resolve.

- A systolic murmur can be heard as the ductus arteriosus is closing. Sometimes breath sounds can be confused with murmurs.
- Pay attention to chest wall movements while listening. If the sound occurs every time the baby breathes, you are likely hearing breath sounds instead of a murmur. If the sound occurs even when the chest wall is not moving and corresponds to the heart sounds, it is likely a murmur.

ABDOMINAL EXAM

- **Visually inspect:** The newborn belly can be protuberant, especially if the baby recently ate.
- **Palpate:** Using one hand, typically your dominant, feel in all 4 quadrants. You can use your other hand to support the infant's back (**Figure 19-17**), or help the abdomen relax

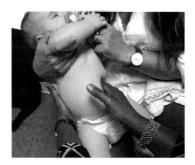

FIGURE 19-17 • Abdominal exam of infant in the parent's lap. (Photo provided by Chris Cannavino, MD.)

by holding the infant's feet and flexing the knees and hips (**Figure 19-18**). Feel for masses and organomegaly. It is not uncommon to be able to feel the liver and spleen in a newborn, but they should be no more than 2 cm below the costal margin. If the belly is especially soft, you might even feel the kidneys.

- The older infant might be more comfortable in a parent's lap (Figure 19-17), allowing for a better exam.

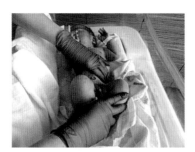

FIGURE 19-18 • Holding the feet with one hand and flexing the knees helps the stomach musculature relax, allowing for better palpation of the abdomen with the opposite hand. (Photo provided by Michelle Leff, MD.)

Findings and Their Meaning: Bulge in the Abdomen

- Diastasis recti and umbilical hernias are common.
- A bulge in the mid-abdomen but cephalad to the umbilicus represents a ventral hernia. These are less likely to close and more likely to strangulate than an umbilical hernia and so should be followed closely for closure (**Figure 19-19**).

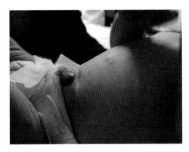

FIGURE 19-19 · **Ventral hernia in a newborn. This may require surgical correction later in life.** (Photo provided by Michelle Leff, MD.)

Umbilicus

- Inspect the skin and cord. Some infants have a long shaft of skin attached to the umbilical cord. This is called umbilicus cutis. In other newborns, the connection to the skin seems deeply buried.
- Look for signs of infection such as redness and discharge. A red rim can be seen at the edge of separation but should not spread further out. A normal dried cord stump can be seen in Figures 19-18 and 19-19.
- An odor as the cord dries and separates is not uncommon.
- The umbilicus usually separates by 2 weeks of life. A granuloma may arise after separation.

Findings and Their Meaning: Delayed Separation of the Umbilical Cord

- Delayed separation of the umbilical cord can indicate a defect in neutrophil function, a disorder called leukocyte adhesion deficiency.
- It can also indicate a lack of drying, as can be seen with certain cultural practices, or seepage of fluid from urachal or omphalomesenteric duct remnants.

Femoral Pulse

- Use 2 fingers (not your thumb, which has its own pulse) to lightly touch the inguinal area (**Figure 19-20**). Too much pressure may occlude the artery completely, making it impossible to feel.
- The goal is to identify a weak or absent femoral pulse, which may indicate coarctation of the aorta or other left-sided obstructive malformation. It takes practice feeling many pulses to be able to distinguish normal from abnormal. The sensitivity of this test is quite low (<20%) but the specificity is high (>99%), so the technique is worth learning.
- This test may be more sensitive at the first outpatient visit when the ductus arteriosus has likely closed.

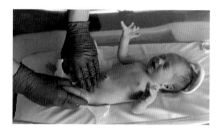

FIGURE 19-20 • Palpation of femoral pulse. Apply gentle pressure or you will fully compress the femoral artery and not be able to feel a pulse. (Photo provided by Taylor Wrinkle, MD.)

GENITAL EXAM

Penis and Scrotum

- Visually inspect for normal development. Look at both the ventral and dorsal sides of the penis to ensure the foreskin is complete.
- The urethra may be visible, allowing you to assess for hypospadias, but not always. The newborn foreskin adheres to the glans, so do not try to retract.
- Feel for descended testicles. Place your nondominant hand at the top of the scrotum to keep testicles from moving up into the inguinal canal while you palpate. Use your dominant hand to milk down the scrotum rather than starting from the bottom of the scrotum.
- Visually inspect for a patent anus (**Figure 19-21**).
- A digital exam of the rectum is not typically performed.

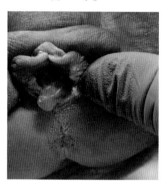

FIGURE 19-21 • Normal anus. Appearance is same for male or female patients (photo is of female). Small pieces of meconium can be seen on the surrounding skin. Note that this patient also has a hymenal tag. The white material in the picture is vernix, the protective material that coats a fetus's skin. (Photo provided by Michelle Leff, MD.)

Findings and Their Meanings in the Scrotal Area

- **Testicle not palpable:** Approximately 1% to 4.6% of term newborns will have an undescended testicle. Usually, the testicle will descend over the first few months, so watchful waiting is fine. A lack of both testicles could indicate a disorder of sex development and requires prompt evaluation.
- **Enlarged scrotum:** This could indicate a hydrocele or inguinal hernia. Hydroceles are collections of fluid around the testicles. They are common findings in newborn boys and can be differentiated from a hernia using transillumination. Touch any light, but usually an ophthalmoscope or otoscope, to the side of the scrotum (**Figure 19-22**). A fluid-filled hydrocele will glow, whereas a hernia-filled sac will not.

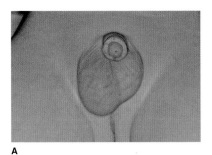 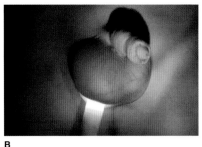

A   **B**

FIGURES 19-22 • **(A and B)** Hydrocele. Part A shows an enlarged scrotum in a circumcised boy. Part B shows how transillumination can reveal an empty sac, which differentiates a hydrocele from a hernia. (From Knoop KJ, Stack LB, Storrow AB, Thurman RJ, eds. *The Atlas of Emergency Medicine.* 5th ed. New York: McGraw-Hill; 2021, Figure 14.123. Reproduced with permission from photo contributor: Kevin J. Knoop, MD, MS.)

Vulvovaginal Area

- Visually inspect for normal development.
- Use your fingers to separate the labia to look for a vaginal opening (**Figure 19-23**).

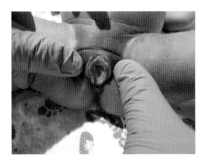

FIGURE 19-23 • Normal vulvovaginal genitalia. The image demonstrates how to separate the labia majora to look for vaginal and hymenal openings. A normal hymenal tag is also demonstrated at the 6 o'clock position. (Photo provided by Michelle Leff, MD.)

- Swollen labia (**Figure 19-24**) and hymenal tags are common (Figure 19-23).
- Vaginal discharge (Figure 19-24) and even bleeding can be seen in the first 2 weeks of life due to the withdrawal of maternal hormones.

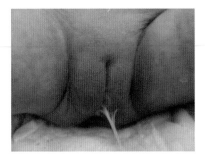

FIGURE 19-24 • Normal vulvovaginal genitalia with normal vaginal discharge. Note swelling and erythema of the labia majora. (Photo provided by Michelle Leff, MD.)

- Visually inspect for a patent anus (Figure 19-21).
- A digital exam of the rectum is not typically performed.

Findings and Their Meaning: Lack of Anal Opening

- Lack of an anal opening or one in an abnormal location is a congenital defect that requires surgical correction (**Figure 19-25**).

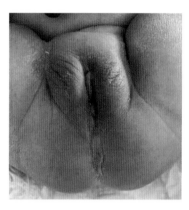

FIGURE 19-25 • **Imperforate anus. No anal opening can be seen.** (Photo provided by Richard Silva, MD.)

MUSCULSKELETAL EXAM

Back and Spine

- The best way to flip a baby over to examine its back is to use one hand to support its chest and the other to help roll. When you first start flipping babies over, do it in the crib, only elevating as much as you need (**Figure 19-26**).
- It is okay for a newborn to lay on its abdomen during the exam while you are present. Repeat the maneuver to return the baby to a supine position.

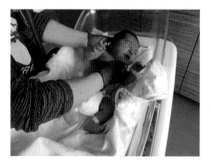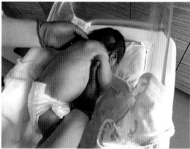

FIGURE 19-26 • **Technique to turn a baby over to examine the back. Place one hand on the chest and use the other hand to roll the baby over.** (Photo provided by Michelle Leff, MD.)

- Visually inspect that the spine is straight and without concerning lesions. Lesions such as dimples above the gluteal cleft, masses, or tufts of hair (**Figure 19-27**) along the midline may indicate occult spinal dysraphism. Dimples in the intergluteal region are less concerning and usually normal, especially if you can feel the coccyx underneath. Certain

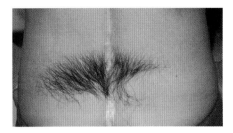

FIGURE 19-27 • **Abnormal tuft of hair. This infant had a tethered cord. Note a scar from surgical repair is visible.** (Reproduced with permission from Kang S, Amagai M, Bruckner AL, Enk AH, Margolis DJ, McMichael AJ, Orringer JS, eds. *Fitzpatrick's Dermatology.* 9th ed. New York: McGraw Hill; 2019, Figure 103-10.)

ethnicities have more hair on the back than others, which should be distinguishable from a concerning tuft that is more localized.

Findings and Their Meaning: Pit, Mass, or Tuft of Hair

- A pit, mass, or tuft of hair along the spine may be an indicator of abnormal spinal column or cord development (Figure 19-27).

Extremities

- Check for normal flexion and extension by passively moving the joints. For instance, straighten the knees and hips and then return to neutral. Positional deformities of the feet are common and need to be differentiated from pathologic problems such as talipes equinovarus, more commonly known as clubfoot. This is a congenital defect where the foot is flexed and inverted in a fixed position. It cannot be brought to a neutral position.
- Ensure the proper number and formation of digits and nails.
- Newborn and infant feet appear flat compared to older children due to differences in adipose tissue distribution.
- Hips:
  - Check for hip stability via Ortolani and Barlow maneuvers (**Figure 19-28**) until 2 months.
    - Proper hand placement is important.
    - Assess one hip at a time, with your second hand used to hold the infant in place as seen in photo on left. Cup the knee between your thumb and first finger, placing the tip of your middle finger over the greater trochanter of the femur.

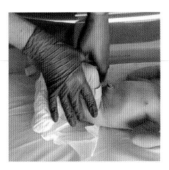
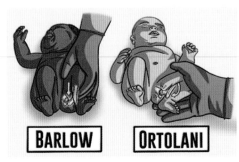

FIGURE 19-28 • **Ortolani and Barlow maneuvers.** (Left photo provided by Taylor Wrinkle, MD. Right drawing Reproduced with permission from Cathy Cichon, MD.)

- For the Barlow, adduct and push back using your middle finger to feel for dislocation.
- For the Ortolani, abduct and pull up slightly on the joint feeling for relocation of a dislocated femur.
* After 2 months, assess for hip abduction of at least 60 degrees and symmetry both in abduction and leg length.
* Thigh skinfold symmetry can also be assessed but is less reliable. Twenty percent of normal infants have asymmetric thigh skinfolds. Current guidelines do not recommend referral based solely on this finding. However, if asymmetry is present along with another subtle finding, referral may be warranted.

Findings and Their Meaning: Abnormal Ortolani or Barlow

* An abnormal Ortolani or Barlow can indicate developmental dysplasia of the hip and requires urgent orthopedic referral.

SKIN EXAM

* Visually inspect and use your hands to palpate any lesions.
* Look for sinus pits, skin tags, birth marks, trauma, and rashes.
* Common newborn skin findings are described in **Table 19-1**.
* Newborn skin is quite variable. The amount of vernix caseosa, lanugo, and peeling varies with gestational age.

TABLE 19-1 • Diagnoses at a Glance: Common Newborn Skin Findings

Finding	Description	Photo
Erythema toxicum (E tox)	Papules surrounded by erythema that come and go over the first 2 weeks; not present at birth but can develop in the first day; few to hundreds of lesions	(Photo provided by Michelle Leff, MD.)
Transient neonatal pustular melanosis	A progression from pustules to collarette of scale to small melanotic macules present at birth that eventually resolves	A B (Reproduced with permission from Kang S, Amagai M, Bruckner AL, Enk AH, Margolis DJ, McMichael AJ, Orringer JS, eds. *Fitzpatrick's Dermatology.* 9th ed. New York: McGraw Hill; 2019, Figure 103-4.)

(Continued)

TABLE 19-1 • Diagnoses at a Glance: Common Newborn Skin Findings (Continued)

Finding	Description	Photo
Nevus simplex/ salmon patch/ stork bite/ angel kiss	Blanching erythematous macules that can be present anywhere but most commonly on the face and nape of the neck; brighter with crying	(Reproduced with permission from Kang S, Amagai M, Bruckner AL, et al, eds. *Fitzpatrick's Dermatology*. 9th ed. New York, McGraw Hill; 2019, Figure147-2A.)
Congenital dermal melanocytosis/ slate gray patches	Bluish patches that can be found anywhere but most commonly on the low back and buttocks of darker pigmented newborns	(Photo provided by Michelle Leff, MD.)
Sebaceous gland hyperplasia	Prominent sebaceous glands usually present on the nose at birth; may be flat or palpable; present at birth; slight yellow tinge	(Photo provided by Michelle Leff, MD.)
Milia	White papules on the face present at birth	(Photo provided by Michelle Leff, MD.)

- Perfusion is discussed under the cardiac exam.
- Jaundice, or yellowing of the skin, should not be visible prior to 24 hours of life. After that time, many newborns have some degree of jaundice secondary to breakdown of red blood cells, immature processing by the liver, and poor excretion in the first few days of life. As jaundice tends to progress from the head to the feet as the serum bilirubin increases, it can be described by the area of the body in which it is observed (eg, jaundiced to the neck or jaundiced to the belly).

LYMPH NODE EXAM

- Approximately one-third of newborns and over half of infants have palpable lymph nodes, usually inguinal or cervical.
- In the newborn, you are not looking specifically for lymph nodes, but you or the parent may notice them while performing the other aspects of your exam.
- They are typically small (<0.5 cm in diameter), rubbery, mobile nodules in the subcutaneous tissue without overlying erythema or tenderness.
- In an older child with an infection, you may note a larger nodule with overlying erythematous skin and tenderness to palpation.

NEUROLOGIC EXAM

- The most important neurologic findings to assess in all newborns are tone, state, suck, and symmetry of movements.
  - Tone refers to how floppy the baby is. Most newborns lie with their elbows, hips, and knees flexed (Figures 19-1 and 19-3), and as you move them around, you feel some resistance. When you pull up on their arms, the elbows stay bent, and their head usually follows (**Figure 19-29**).

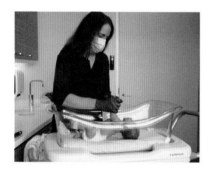

FIGURE 19-29 • Assessing head lag. Pull gently up on both arms and watch how the baby is able to bring the head along. This less than 24-hour-old has mild head lag as expected for age. Do not perform if concern for brachial plexus injury or clavicular fracture. (Photo provided by Taylor Wrinkle, MD.)

  - State refers to how alert or sleepy the baby is as well as how calm or upset. Babies typically alert easily with the exam and can be calmed within a few minutes once upset. The newborn in Figure 19-1 is asleep. The babies in Figures 19-9 and 19-12 are alert and calm. The newborn in Figure 19-20 is alert and crying.
  - To assess newborn suck, use a gloved finger (usually your pinky is a good size).
    - If mouth is not open, tickle the baby's lips with your finger.
    - Once mouth is open, gently rub the anterior hard palate with the dorsal aspect of the gloved finger to elicit the suck.
  - The newborn's right and left sides should move similarly (symmetry). For instance, both elbows should be flexed to an equal extent and move about an equal amount of time. When the baby cries, the right and left sides of the mouth should both descend.
- Many reflexes do not need to be elicited as part of a routine exam, but it is good to know what is normal. For instance, a Babinski (see Chapter 12, Neurological exam) is normal until 2 years. A couple beats of clonus at the ankle is normal. Benign neonatal myoclonus, quick jerky movements, can be seen while the baby is falling asleep.

- The Moro reflex occurs when the baby is startled such as with a loud noise or quick motion. The arms will extend, possibly shake some, and return to a neutral position. The baby's face may have a startled expression and the baby will frequently cry (Figure 19-20).
- Deep tendon reflexes are not part of a typical exam because it is hard to get a relaxed newborn.

Findings and Their Meaning: Asymmetric Arm Movements

- Asymmetric arm movements could indicate an in utero stroke, a brachial plexus injury, or a clavicle fracture.

MATERNAL BREAST

- Given that over 80% of women in the United States initiate breastfeeding, consideration of the maternal breast is an important aspect of the newborn encounter.
- The newborn's feeding success depends on their anatomy and ability, as well as the mom's anatomy and comfort.
- Visually inspect nipples for type (flat, inverted, or everted) as well as for signs of trauma.
- Visually inspect the breast for scars indicating prior surgeries, hypoplasia, and signs of filling.
- You or the mother can hand express to look for milk production (**Figure 19-30**).
- You might want to observe the baby breastfeeding to assess their technique.

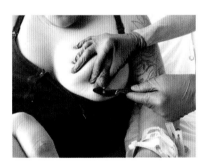

FIGURE 19-30 · **Hand expression into a spoon. Hand expression can be done to assess for milk production or to feed milk to a baby that will not latch.** (Photo provided by Michelle Leff, MD.)

CULTURAL CONSIDERATIONS

- Some cultures wait to name their baby until a specified time.
- Circumcision is a religious practice in some faiths.
- Families may value the placement of religious icons near their newborn.
- Amulets may be placed around the baby's neck or wrist to ward off evil.
- The decision-maker may differ depending on the culture.
- Refusal of care, such as for vaccines or prophylactic medications, may occur with certain religious, cultural, or personal beliefs.
- Women from certain cultures may be more comfortable with a female provider in the room or request time to place a head covering.

🖥️ TELEHEALTH TIPS

- Telehealth in the first year of life can be useful for parenting questions about such things as sleep issues, feeding issues, and stooling concerns.
- Telehealth can sometimes provide information that could not be obtained in a clinic visit as you have the opportunity to visualize the home environment. For instance, you might note an unsafe sleeping situation for which you can provide education.
- Make sure the family knows to have the infant present for a telehealth appointment. Sometimes the family calls from work while the child is at daycare because they mostly want advice, but this does not allow an opportunity for observation.
- Temperature is likely the only vital sign you will be able to have the parent obtain. You may be able to count a respiratory rate if the chest is visible and the camera is aimed from the side. This is also an opportunity to assess the infant's general level of comfort or distress.

✅ SUMMARY OF SKILLS CHECKLIST

- ❏ Wash your hands
- ❏ History
- ❏ Vital signs
- ❏ Observe infant
- ❏ Head and neck
- ❏ If swaddled or clothed, unwrap or undress infant
- ❏ Lungs and chest
- ❏ Heart
- ❏ Abdomen
- ❏ Genitalia
- ❏ Back and spine
- ❏ Extremities, including Ortolani and Barlow
- ❏ During the exam, observe infant tone, movements, and response to the exam; assess suck (all are components of general neurological assessment)
- ❏ During exam, visually inspect for any congenital defects
- ❏ Reswaddle infant
- ❏ Examine retinal reflex and mouth (done last, as they tend to upset)
- ❏ Wash your hands

BIBLIOGRAPHY

Bamji M, Stone RK, Kaul A, Usmani G, Schachter FF, Wasserman E. Palpable lymph nodes in healthy newborns and infants. *Pediatrics*. 1986;78(4):573-575.

Benitz WE; Committee on Fetus and Newborn, American Academy of Pediatrics. Hospital stay for healthy term newborn infants. *Pediatrics*. 2015;135(5):948-953.

Centers for Disease Control and Prevention. Growth charts. Accessed April 1, 2023. https://www.cdc.gov/growthcharts/index.htm.

Jackson JC, Runge MM, Nye NS. Common questions about developmental dysplasia of the hip. *Am Fam Physician*. 2014;90(12):843-850.

Kelly DH, Stellwagen LM, Kaitz E, Shannon DC. Apnea and periodic breathing in normal full-term infants during the first twelve months. *Pediatr Pulmonol*. 1985;1(4):215-219.

Khammari Nystrom F, Petersson G, Stephansson O, Johansson S, Altman M. Diagnostic values of the femoral pulse palpation test. *Arch Dis Child Fetal Neonatal Ed.* 2020;105(4):375-379.

Rozanski TA, Bloom DA. The undescended testis theory and management. *Urol Clin North Am.* 1995;22:107-118.

Shah M, ed. *Transcultural Aspects of Perinatal Health Care: A Resource Guide.* National Perinatal Association. Washington, DC: American Academy of Pediatrics; 2004.

World Health Organization. Growth standards. Accessed April 14, 2023. https://www.who.int/tools/child-growth-standards/standards.

Yang S, Zusman N, Lieberman E, Goldstein RY. Developmental dysplasia of the hip. *Pediatrics.* 2019;143(1):e20181147.

20

Toddler and Early Childhood Exams

Vanessa P. Scott, MD, MS

INTRODUCTION

In this pediatric age group (1-year-old to approximately 10 years, old), cooperation with the history and physical exam may take time, patience, and skill development on behalf of the provider. You will see children from a variety of socioeconomic and cultural backgrounds, developmental levels, and medical histories, and their desires, needs, anxieties, and fears will differ. Your goals will vary based on whether the patient presents for an acute illness, a well-child check, or a behavioral concern. Therefore, be flexible in your approach, with the goal of developing personalized tools that work for you.

Some key tips for approaching a young child's physical exam:

- Let the child play around the room while you talk to their caregivers and give them distance for the first few minutes. This facilitates trust when they see you chatting with people they know.
- Avoid sudden movements. Call out what you plan to do or examine before you move your instrument or hands there and use words which they understand. This also informs the caregivers and allows them to try and help as much as possible.
- Allow the child to sit wherever they want to when starting the exam: in their caregiver's lap or in their own chair. Avoid starting on the exam table until you build trust, unless that is where they want to start.
- Let them touch and play with the instruments as much as safely possible!
- If the child has an acute illness, once you gain trust, focus on the pertinent physical exam maneuvers.
- Be malleable with your exam—you will not always go in the same order (eg, head, eyes, mouth, neck, heart, lungs). You may need to approach the heart first if they take an interest in the stethoscope and then move to other areas.
- Speak to them gently but firmly, using simple commands (eg, "Open your mouth please.")

HISTORY TAKING

The history is obtained in discussion with the caregivers. The initial information presented in this section focuses on the outpatient, primary care setting, where the bulk of pediatric care is delivered. Additional tips related to the inpatient setting are presented at the end of this section. It is also relevant to mention that elements covered in the newborn/infant section around birth and family history can be repeated if those aspects are unknown. Children presenting for an acute concern (eg, sore throat, cough) typically undergo a focused history and examination, capturing core domains of a concern as described in Chapter 1, History Taking.

Wellness Visits

- From infancy into adolescence, children are seen at various time intervals for well-child checks, as recommended by the American Academy of Pediatrics (AAP) Bright Futures Guidelines for Preventive Care Screening and Health Supervision (ie, wellness) Visits.
- These wellness visits are used to assess growth, development, nutrition, mental health, past medical issues, the overall health of the family dynamics, social determinants of health, and adverse childhood experiences (ACEs).
- Primary care offices use validated screening tools (surveys) to help gather this information beforehand in order to have a tailored and effective visit. The AAP recommends the following:
  Developmental and behavioral screening at:
  - 9 months
  - 18 months
  - 30 months
  Autism spectrum disorder (ASD) screening at:
  - 18 months
  - 24 months
- Ask the clinician with whom you are working about which screening tools they use and review them before entering the room.
- If you have any questions about a survey answer, speak with the parents or patient directly for clarification.
- Certain answers or concerns elucidated from these survey questions may help focus your physical exam.

> **PEARL:** Review your patient's chart and medical history, including any screening tools parents may have answered before you begin, in order to help you during the clincal encounter.

Milestones

A major focus for toddlers and children is on the achievement of developmental milestones. These milestones fit into a number of broad categories including motor skills (gross motor [can climb up stairs] and fine motor [can self-feed]), problem solving (object permanence), communication (expressive and receptive language), and emotional/social skills (imaginary play). By observing thousands of children at various ages, pediatricians have been able to develop age-based lists of behaviors and abilities that define typical development. Failure to reach these benchmarks often indicates an important problem that needs to be additionally defined and addressed. Early identification of developmental problems is a significant focus of the pediatric evaluation, as early interventions are more effective in addressing the underlying root cause(s). A link to the AAP

Ages and Stages developmental screening tools (highlighting the different milestones at each age) is provided in the Bibliography.

Key Historical Information to Gather When Working With This Age Group

Some of these elements will be covered in the screening tools mentioned earlier. While these questions may be part of electronic health record templates, it is important to understand the general categories and rationale. Note also that the transition to adolescence does not occur at a specific moment, so knowing when to focus on elements appropriate to that group requires an awareness of each child's developmental stage.

Behavior History

- Sleeping patterns
- Appetite/feeding issues
- Interaction with kids and siblings
- Friends
- School behavior and learning
- Mood
- Temper tantrums
- Any parental concerns

Home Safety and Anticipatory Guidance

- Does anyone smoke at home?
- Bike safety (eg, helmets)
- Exercise
- Screen time
- Car safety (eg, appropriate seats)
- Guns in the home
- Child-proofing the home (eg, lock up medicines, safely store household cleaners, address environmental fall risks)

Social History

- Who is involved in bringing up the child?
- Caregivers' marital status or support system
- Caregivers' work status
- Living arrangements/home stability
- Siblings and their ages
- Methods used to teach and discipline the child

Family History

- Any potentially heritable conditions in family?
- Family allergies

Dental Health

- Regular dental visits
- Dental hygiene: brushing, fluoride, flossing
- Excessive sweets, juice consumption

Immunization History

- Which vaccinations were given and when? See Centers for Disease Control and Prevention (CDC) vaccination schedule for list (Bibliography).
- If there is vaccine hesitancy, questions should explore reasons/concerns and not be accusatory.

Past medical history, including birth history, surgical history, and medication history should also be obtained.

Inpatient Setting Specifics

When a child is hospitalized, both the family and the child are likely to be in an elevated state of anxiety or stress. A few things to consider:

- Ask the nurse taking care of the child if you can perform a physical exam before entering the room. They are the gatekeepers!
- Ask the parents for permission to examine their child, and involve them as much as possible, as this may provide comfort and ease anxiety.
- Take particular care when examining a child with lines, tubes, or monitors.
- If you are concerned about anything, speak to the nurse, the appropriate resident, or the attending physician immediately. Your voice is important!

Initial Approach When Working With A Child

It is important to establish rapport with both the child and their caregiver upon entering the room.

- Introduce yourself, your role, the attending physician you are working with, and the purpose of the interaction (eg, "I understand that Charlie is here because he's had a cough for the past few days").
- Children between the ages of 8 and 24 months may show developmentally appropriate signs of stranger anxiety and/or separation anxiety, so consider initiating the physical exam on the caregiver's lap to gain trust with your patient.
- As you perform the exam, explain to your patient (and their caregiver) what you are about to do so they can anticipate your actions.
- Receptive language in this age group is developing, and if they hear the word "eyes" or "head," they are more likely to understand that is the next area of focus. These verbal cues are important to decrease child anxiety, and they help educate the parents.
- For example, *"Now I'm going to touch the top of your head. I'm checking the soft spot, or anterior fontanelle, to see if it's still open; usually it closes between 12 and 24 months old."* With these few sentences, you alert the child where you will examine next while educating the parents using both layman's terms and medical terminology.

What follows is a suggested order to perform a physical exam on a toddler but remember that it can change. The key is to be adaptable and calm.

VITAL SIGNS

All physical exams start with a review of the vital signs.

- Ensure all vital signs needed for that day's visits are documented by clinical staff, and if not, take the vitals yourself when feasible. Normal ranges for respiratory rate and heart rate for this age group are found in **Table 20-1**.

TABLE 20-1 • Pediatric Respiratory Rate and Heart Rate Normal Ranges (10th-90th Percentiles) by Age		
Age	Respiratory Rate (breaths/min)	Heart Rate (bpm)
1 to <3 years	22-46	98-140
3 to <6 year	20-29	81-123
6 to <12 years	16-24	67-111

- Normal temperature ranges from 96.6°F to 100.3°F.
- Oxygen saturation levels (SpO_2) should be 95% to 100%.
- Normal blood pressure ranges depend on age, height, and sex assigned at birth and may be found in the latest AAP guidelines.
- If you notice the patient's respiratory rate or temperature is high, for example, this will encourage you to investigate and have a more productive physical exam.

GROWTH

This includes head circumference, height, weight, and body mass index percentile (BMI%).

- All children are assessed using standardized growth charts from the World Health Organization (WHO) for 0 to 2 years old and from the CDC for 2 to 19 years old.
- Growth charts are used to compare growth in infants, children, and adolescents with a nationally representative reference based on children of all ages and racial or ethnic groups. They enable healthcare providers to monitor growth and identify potential health- or nutrition-related problems.
- When plotted correctly, a series of accurate weights and measurements of length offer important information about a child's growth pattern, which may be influenced by such factors as gestational age, birth weight, and parental stature. Parental stature, for example, is considered before assuming there is a health or nutrition concern.
- During normal growth, a child consistently follows a percentile curve (5th to 95th).
- It is concerning if one metric is significantly different than the others or if there is a significant change (ie, crossing 2 percentile curves or more) in one metric from previous measurements. This may indicate an underlying medical condition requiring additional investigation.
- Children with specific conditions may have specialty growth charts (eg, genetic conditions such as trisomy 21 or children with BMI% above 95th percentile)
- Head circumference is followed up until 2 years old.
- The WHO and CDC growth charts are excellent reference tools (see Bibliography).

Findings and Their Meaning: Growth Chart Abnormalities

- Crossing 2 percentile lines for weight or BMI may indicate inadequate caloric intake (eg, food insecurity, breastfeeding problem, or eating disorder) or inadequate absorption of nutrients (eg, inflammatory bowel disease or cancer).
- A rapid increase in head circumference percentile may indicate increased fluid in the brain (hydrocephalus).
- A decrease of length (crossing 2 percentile curves) may indicate an endocrine abnormality such as growth hormone deficiency or hypothyroidism.

INSPECTION

Visual inspection can help your assessment significantly, especially with younger children who may become upset (cry, try and hide, push the examiner away) when you start to examine them due to developmentally normal stranger anxiety. Do not be dismayed; there are ways to have a successful physical exam, even with crying!

The 6-Foot Away Exam

- Before you approach, watch the child with their caregiver (**Figure 20-1**).
  - Ask the parent to remove the child's shirt or clothes, especially for a sick visit.
  - Are they retracting their chest muscles at rest? Nasal flaring? If they start screaming or crying, this part of the exam is much harder to assess.
  - Any dysmorphic features, chest wall abnormalities, or skin findings?
  - How do they move around the room? This is helpful for assessing gross and fine motor skills.
  - For a well-child visit, watch for developmental milestones. For example, are they putting 2 words together? Do you understand what they are saying?
  - How do they interact with their caregiver or the environment?

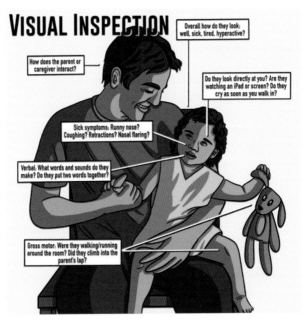

FIGURE 20-1 • **Key initial observations when assessing a child.** (Reproduced with permission from Cathy Cichon, MD.)

Findings and Their Meaning: Things to Note During Initial Observation

- Speech delay (eg, a 2-year-old who can say only 5 words) or fine motor delay (eg, a 6-year-old who does not hold a pencil with a tripod grasp)
- Spasticity with movement (eg, cerebral palsy)
- Abnormal gait (eg, fracture, alignment issues [genu valgum], infectious or rheumatoid [joint pain/preference], neuromuscular [Duchenne muscular dystrophy])
- Hyperactivity (eg, attention deficit hyperactivity disorder)

- Autistic features (eg, limited or no eye contact, does not point to things of interest, speech delay and decreased interest in communication, stereotypies, repetitive behaviors [spinning, rocking, toe-walking])
- Mental state (eg, angry, flat affect, anxious)
- Behavioral considerations including family dynamics. Pay attention to parent-child interactions, signs of inappropriate parental discipline.

CARDIOVASCULAR EXAM

Often parents have introduced the idea of the doctor's visit to their child with books or pictures, which usually show a stethoscope. So beginning the exam by listening to the heart is often a safe and welcomed approach.

Auscultation

- Engage the child, and give verbal cues:
  - For the younger child, have them sit on a caregiver's lap. Listen to the heart of the caregiver or the child's stuffed animal to demonstrate first, and then transition to the child's cardiac exam. *"First, I'm going to listen to Mom's heart; now it's [child's name] turn!"*
  - Older children are often more comfortable and you can listen directly.
  - You may have a child, depending on their comfort level, start in a chair or caregiver's lap, and then move to the physical exam table.
  - For toddlers with developmentally appropriate anxiety, you may do the entire physical exam on the parent's lap.
- Use the diaphragm of the stethoscope to auscultate the main cardiac positions; use the mnemonic **APE To Man** for order of listening (see Chapter 6, Cardiovascular Exam for additional details).
  - Aortic valve
  - Pulmonary valve
  - Erb's point (third intercostal space)
  - Tricuspid valve
  - Mitral valve
- Listen in both sitting and supine positions, the latter of which may occur toward the end of the exam when the child has learned trust.
  - Note any murmurs or irregular rhythms (**Table 20-2**).

TABLE 20-2 • Diagnoses at a Glance: Pediatric Cardiac Murmurs		
Murmur Type	Location Best Heard	Description
Benign		
Still's murmur	Mid-left sternal border in supine position (often disappears or gets softer with sitting)	Most common benign murmur in children; soft (grade I-II) systolic ejection murmur likely due to turbulent flow; "buzzing," "vibratory," "musical"
Pulmonary flow murmur of childhood	Left upper sternal border, sometimes with radiation to the back (often disappears or gets softer with sitting)	Systolic ejection murmur (grade I-III) without harshness or click; often heard when cardiac output increases such as with fever or anemia
Venous hum	Infraclavicular region while sitting (disappears supine)	Low-pitched, soft (grade I-II), continuous murmur due to blood flowing into the superior vena cava

(Continued)

TABLE 20-2 • Diagnoses at a Glance: Pediatric Cardiac Murmurs (Continued)

Murmur Type	Location Best Heard	Description
Pathologic		
Continuous murmurs	Throughout the precordium	Murmur throughout systolic and diastolic phase (that is not a venous hum), such as the patent ductus arteriosus murmur ("machine-like")
Harsh ejection murmurs	Depends on location of obstruction	Harsh and/or loud (grade III or higher), such as aortic stenosis, which has a crescendo-decrescendo quality
Diastolic murmurs	Dependent on location of etiology	Lower-pitched, softer, and often difficult to hear; try to differentiate early (aortic or pulmonic regurgitation) versus mid-to-late (tricuspid or mitral valve stenosis)

Palpation

- Palpate the child's radial pulse for strength and regularity when auscultating in the supine position.
- Examine for normal cap refill (<3 seconds), cyanosis, or clubbing (distal fingers and nails).

Blood Pressure

- Blood pressure (BP) screening begins at 3 years old at well-child visits.
- Some children need a BP measurement at every clinic visit (eg, history of obesity, on certain medications, history of prior hypertension), and some children younger than 3 years old may need a BP if they have a specific risk factor (see current AAP BP guidelines).
- Medical assistants will use an automated BP machine to assess.
- If abnormal, ask them to repeat using a manual BP cuff.
- Ensure measures were taken using appropriate techniques (see Chapter 3, Vital Signs).
  - Patient should be sitting for 5 minutes with feet on the ground prior to the measurement.
  - Use the nondominant arm and measure at the level of heart.
  - Use an appropriately sized cuff.
  - BP parameters are dependent on the child's height and weight and therefore important to note for interpretation.

CHEST AND PULMONARY EXAM

Assess for chest symmetry or deformities of the rib cage such as pectus excavatum (see Chapter 7, Pulmonary Exam, Figure 7-12), or pectus carinatum, normal breast buds (premature thelarche), early signs of puberty, or normal breast development (see Chapter 21, Adolescent Exam, Figure 21-2).

Ensure you know the respiratory rate and SpO_2 (oxygenation) from the vital signs assessed by the medical assistants. Are they normal or abnormal?

Observation

- Are they breathing comfortably?
- Is there any increased work of breathing such as retractions (ie, pulling in of their skin at the supraclavicular, intercostal, or subcostal areas) or nasal flaring?

- Do you hear noisy breathing? Wheezing? Stridor? (See Chapter 7, Pulmonary Exam).
- Respirations per minute:
  - Recheck the respiratory rate yourself for sick visits. Respiratory status can change in minutes.
  - For younger children, count respirations over a full minute to accommodate for any irregular breathing patterns.
  - If you are having trouble seeing the respirations, use your stethoscope to listen.

Auscultation

- Listen directly to all lung fields with your stethoscope by having the child lean forward while in their parent's lap or on the exam table.
- Start at top left, then listen and compare to top right, working your way down to the lower lung fields.
- If the child is upset, have them hug their caregiver and place the stethoscope on their back. They may cry at first, but if you are patient, they will often calm down after a few breaths.
- Differentiate between transmitted upper airways sounds (eg, nasal congestion) and lung pathology:
  - Place the stethoscope in front of the nose or at the superior lateral side of the neck, and memorize that sound.
  - Listen again to the lung fields.
  - If it is the same sound but quieter, it is likely an upper airway sound transmitted to the lungs.
  - If it is a different or louder sound in the lung field, then the lung is likely the origin and there may be underlying pathology.

Findings and Their Meaning: Pulmonary Exam Abnormalities

- Noisy breathing, often with mouth breathing, is usually from nasal congestion or obstruction (eg, mass, foreign body).
- Stridor is a noise heard on inspiration and expiration associated with infections (eg, croup) or anatomic narrowing (eg, laryngomalacia, foreign body) at the level of the trachea/upper airway.
- Focal crackles may indicate a community-acquired pneumonia or atelectasis.
- Crackles throughout the lung fields may be a viral pneumonia or atypical bacterial pneumonia.
- Wheezing is usually associated with an asthma exacerbation or wheeze-associated respiratory infection (WARI, or more recently termed *bronchospasm*).
- Asymmetry of aeration may be heard in children with asthma or focal pathology (eg, pleural effusion).
- Children with severe asthma symptoms may have decreased aeration to the bases of their lungs. This quietness can be a sign of a moderate to severe respiratory situation (ie, limited air movement due to bronchoconstriction) that needs immediate attention.

> PEARL: Close your eyes while listening; this can help increase your hearing sensitivity and focus.

HEAD AND NECK EXAM

Head and Neck Palpation

- By 12 to 24 months, the anterior fontanelle (AF) should close.
  - Announce to the toddler that you will feel their head and palpate softly (**Figure 20-2**).
  - Differentiate between an open AF and closed one.
  - Often there will be the beginning of the cortex formation, and there may still be a depression in the area of the AF, but it is technically closed. If still open, note on your exam and in your medical note to follow up until it closes normally.
- If the head circumference growth chart showed significant deviation, remeasure yourself (largest diameter, see Chapter 19, Newborn and Infant Exam).
- If there has been a significant change in head circumference (ie, crossing 2 lines on the growth charts), it may warrant imaging.
- Next, announce that you will "feel the neck area."
  - Tell the parents you are palpating for lymph nodes to ensure they are normal in size (<1 cm, nontender, mobile).
  - Palpate the pre- and postauricular, posterior, anterior, and supraclavicular lymph nodes. (See Chapter 4, Head and Neck Exam, Figure 4-2)
  - Note any areas of swelling, defects, or asymmetry.

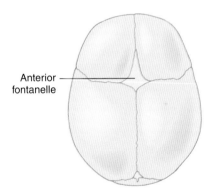

Anterior
fontanelle

FIGURE 20-2 · Location of anterior fontanelle. (Reproduced with permission from Biller J, Gruener G, Brazis PW. *DeMyer's The Neurologic Examination: A Programmed Text.* 7th ed. New York: McGraw Hill; 2017.)

Findings and Their Meaning: Head and Neck Abnormalities

- If the AF remains open after age 2, it can be the result of failure of the bones to fuse, increased intracranial pressure, Down syndrome, or congenital hypothyroidism.
- Early closure of the AF (before 12 months old) may indicate craniosynostosis (premature fusion of the skull bones) or hyperthyroidism.
- An acutely bulging fontanelle is a sign of increased intracranial pressure, whereas a depressed fontanelle can occur with severe dehydration.
- Lymph nodes most commonly enlarge secondary to infections within the areas that drain to those nodes (eg, pharyngitis causes lymphadenopathy at the angle of the jaw to become acutely tender and enlarged). The patient should have other symptoms (eg, sore

throat), and the lymph nodes become smaller after the process resolves. (See Chapter 4, Head and Neck Exam, Figure 4-4)

- Lymph nodes can also be enlarged secondary to cancer (eg, lymphoma) and autoimmune disorders. These are much less common and are associated with additional symptoms (eg, fever, sweats, weight loss) and findings.

EYE EXAM

Visual Acuity

- Beginning around 3 years old, children are tested for visual acuity. Most clinics use the Snellen (literate; ie, letters) and the Allen or Lea (preliterate; ie, shapes) eye charts to assess visual acuity. The average 6-year-old has 20/20 vision; however, before that, there is a range of normal (**Table 20-3**).

TABLE 20-3 • Average Visual Acuity Scores for Children by Age	
Age	Normal Visual Acuity Scores
2.5-3 years	20/60 or better
3-4 years	20/50 or better
4-5 years	20/40 or better
5-6 years	20/30 or better
>6 years	20/20

Assessing for Retinal Light Reflex

- Flashlight fun time! Let the toddlers see the light circle the ophthalmoscope makes on your hand or theirs to show them that these tools do not cause pain.
- Have the child sit comfortably in their parent's lap, facing you (the examiner). If the room is too light, turn down the lights, as a dark room is preferable.
- Looking through the ophthalmoscope, verify the presence of the retinal light reflex in each eye from about 18 to 24 inches away. Then look at both eyes from 2 to 3 feet away. Symmetry in color, clarity, and intensity is key. The reflex color can be a bright reddish-yellow or light gray (especially in patients with darkly pigmented eyes).

Findings and Their Meaning: Absence of the Retinal Light Reflex

- Loss of the retinal light reflex means that something is blocking light from hitting the lens, vitreous, or retina and the light is reflecting back. This is called leukocoria and requires urgent pediatric ophthalmology evaluation.
- The most common reasons for leukocoria in this age group are cataracts and retinoblastoma.

Assessing for Eye Alignment: Corneal Reflex

- To assess for strabismus (eye misalignment), shine the ophthalmoscope light into both of the patient's eyes at the same time while you observe directly for the reflection of the light (called the corneal reflex).
- The normal reflection of light should be centered over the pupil of each eye and appear symmetric.
- If asymmetric, assess for type of strabismus: tropia or phoria.

- Tropias are present even when binocular vision (seeing with both eyes) is intact and can be intermittent or fixed. Phorias are considered latent strabismus, meaning they are only seen when binocular vision is disrupted (ie, one eye covered), and usually an examiner can only elicit them during the cover/uncover test (discussed later in this chapter).
- The prefixes below describe the direction the eye goes:
  - Eso-: The eye deviates inward.
  - Exo-: The eye deviates outward.
  - Hyper-: The eye deviates upward.
  - Hypo-: The eye deviates downward.
- Pseudostrabismus, the most common being pseudoesotropia (the child appears "cross-eyed"), is an optical illusion due to a wide nasal bridge or larger epicanthal folds, which children may have for first few years of life. The corneal reflex will still be symmetric.

Findings and Their Meaning: Esotropia and Exotropia

- If the corneal reflex is asymmetric, there is likely strabismus, which requires a referral to a pediatric ophthalmologist for evaluation and treatment to restore proper vision (**Figure 20-3**).
- The most common reason for strabismus is an imbalance of the extraocular muscles.

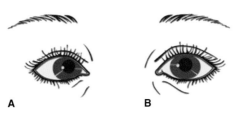

A   B

FIGURE 20-3 • **Corneal reflex in A is temporally displaced, indicating esotropia of right eye. In B, reflex is nasally displaced, indicating exotropia of left eye.** (Reproduced with permission from Bunik M, Hay WW, Levin MJ, Abzug MJ, eds. *Current Diagnosis and Treatment: Pediatrics.* 26th ed. New York: McGraw Hill; 2022.)

Assessing for Misalignment: Cover/Uncover Test

- The cover/uncover test is used to:
  - Confirm a tropia
  - Detect latent strabismus (phoria), which may often present only if the child is tired
- Tropia usually can be seen with corneal reflex exam; however, if subtle, you can use the cover/uncover test to confirm:
  - Cover the eye you are not concerned about for 5 seconds.
  - If the other eye which seems slightly deviated moves toward fixation (straight ahead), then this is a tropia.
- Phoria screening requires the cover/uncover test:
  - Have the child fixate on an object in front of them.
  - Place a cover over one eye for 5 seconds and then rapidly remove.
  - If the eye that was under the cover shifts back to looking straight ahead (orthotropic), this is called a refixation movement and signifies latent strabismus.
- If you do not see an asymmetry on exam but a parent has concerns and reports seeing these types of movements, the child warrants referral to a pediatric ophthalmologist.
- Further references, including a strabismus simulator demonstrating the cover/uncover test, are provided in the Bibliography.

EAR EXAM

Otoscopic Exam

- Ear infections are very common in this age group. The ears should be examined during all sick and well visits.
- First examine the outer ear, including the skin overlying the mastoid bone, for any deformities, trauma, erythema, or swelling.
- Then use the largest speculum possible for the child's ear canal size and have the toddler sit in the parent's lap. There are 2 main approaches for holding a toddler for the ear canal and tympanic membrane exam: the side hold and the hug (**Figure 20-4**).

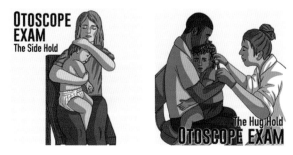

FIGURE 20-4 · **Side hold and hug techniques for holding child during ear exam.** (Reproduced with permission from Cathy Cichon, MD.)

- Once in a hold, gently pull the helix of the ear out, slightly upward and posterior, to create an excellent view of the tympanic membrane. Hold the otoscope like you would a pen, as this will provide better control and optimal viewing of the ear canal and tympanic membrane.
- Remember before you make any movements to tell the child what you are doing. "I'm checking your ears now." Some examiners or kids may enjoy a game-like scenario, such as "Let's see if you can hear the birdies," and the examiner whistles to distract the child while looking in the ear.
- Note your main landmarks (sometimes the canal can deceivingly look like the tympanic membrane!). If there is an abundance of ear wax (cerumen), there are techniques used for removal including plastic curettes, a micro-tipped cotton swab, or warm water lavages if necessary (ask for guidance from your attending physician with all these procedures) (**Figure 20-5**).

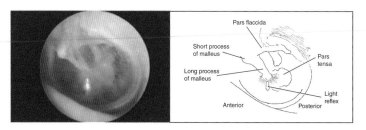

FIGURE 20-5 · **Normal tympanic membrane.** (Reproduced with permission from Knoop KJ, Stack LB, Storrow AB, Thurman RJ, eds. *The Atlas of Emergency Medicine*. 5th ed. New York: McGraw-Hill; 2021, Figure 5.1. Reproduced with permission from photo contributor: Richard A. Chole, MD, PhD.)

Findings and Their Meaning: Common External and Internal Ear Abnormalities

- Otitis externa: Infection in the external canal. There is tenderness upon palpation of the tragus or pinna. There may be discharge, and the ear canal will appear inflamed (**Figure 20-6**).

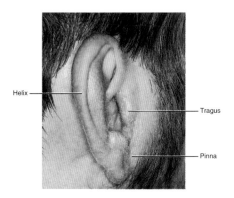

FIGURE 20-6 · **Otitis externa with discharge and swelling of external canal. Photo is of adult, with similar findings in kids.** (From Knoop KJ, Stack LB, Storrow AB, Thurman RJ, eds. *The Atlas of Emergency Medicine*. 5th ed. New York: McGraw-Hill; 2021, Figure 5.14. Reproduced with permission from photo contributor: Frank Birinyi, MD.)

- Acute otitis media: A common problem in this age group, where the child usually complains of ear pain and/or pulls at their ears. They may have fever, upper respiratory symptoms, increased fussiness, or decreased appetite. On otoscope exam, the tympanic membrane (ear drum) is red, bulging, and no longer has a light reflex (**Figure 20-7**).
- Acute otitis media with perforation: Pus and built-up pressure behind the tympanic membrane will sometimes lead to perforation. Signs and symptoms include an event of extreme pain and irritability in the child and white discharge (pus) in the ear canal

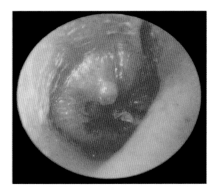

FIGURE 20-7 · **Acute otitis media. Note bulging, red, opaque membrane with loss of light reflex.** (From Tintinalli JE Stapczynski J, Ma OJ, et al. *Tintinalli's Emergency Medicine: A Comprehensive Study Guide*. 7th ed. New York: McGraw Hill; 2009. Reproduced with permission from photo contributor: Dr. Shelagh Cofer, Department of Otolaryngology, Mayo Clinic.)

often occluding the examiner's view of the tympanic membrane. If the tympanic membrane is visible, the perforation may be apparent. (See Chapter 4, Head and Neck Exam, Figure 4-14)

Hearing Tests

- Routine conventional screening audiometry is started at the 3-year-old well-child check and often performed by the medical assistant staff.
- Each ear should be tested at 500, 1000, 2000, and 4000 Hz. Any hearing threshold levels of greater than 20 dB at any of these frequencies should be referred to a pediatric audiologist.
- Often at the 3-year-old well-child visit, patients may not be able to complete the hearing test, as it requires behavioral cooperation.
- If there are no concerns from parents and the patient is developing normally without speech delay, you can repeat in 6 to 12 months.
- If the caregivers have any concerns, there is family history, or there is speech delay, refer to a pediatric audiologist for more formal hearing tests.

NOSE EXAM

- Assess for any nasal discharge.
- Use the otoscope to examine nasal mucosa.

Findings and Their Meaning: Common Nasal Abnormalities

- Upper respiratory infections may cause purulent nasal discharge; however, note that both viral and bacterial infections can cause thick green mucus. A key difference between the two processes is the duration, with viral infections improving in 5-10 days, while bacterial infections will last >10-14 days.
- Assess for a "nose crease," a sign of a child rubbing an itchy nose often, which may indicate allergic rhinitis.
- With the otoscope, assess nasal turbinates for erythema and edema in allergic rhinitis or for foreign bodies or polyps (See Chapter 4, Head and Neck Exam, Figure 4-17, nasal polyp).

MOUTH EXAM

The mouth can be difficult to examine in this age group. Some children can follow the directions of "Please stick out your tongue and say 'Ahh'" to depress the tongue. However, many may not. Some toddlers will cry during the exam, so take advantage and look in the mouth area quickly!

- You may need parents to hold patients in a hug facing forward and gently look with a tongue depressor.
- Note the number of teeth. Children typically have 20 primary teeth, which begin to fall out and are replaced by permanent (adult) teeth starting at age 5 to 7.

Findings and Their Meaning: Common Mouth Abnormalities

- Assess for tooth trauma: a gray-colored tooth signifies nerve trauma and increases risk for an abscess, which requires referral to a pediatric dentist.

- Look for signs of plaque buildup and caries (cavities). Cavities are erosions in the enamel (outer layer) of the tooth. They can extend to variable depth, sometimes causing pain.
- Dental problems can be indicative of excessive intake of foods or drinks that are high in sugar and/or poor dental care. This should prompt a discussion about diet, dental hygiene, and history of visits to a dentist and/or access to dental care.
- Gum bleeding is typically a sign of inflammation, which occurs with poor dental hygiene. It may also be associated with infection and, less commonly, bleeding disorders (eg, thrombocytopenia).
- Note any ulcers, focal swelling or redness, tonsillar enlargement or tonsillar exudates, asymmetry of the pharynx (retropharyngeal abscess), or other abnormalities. Most of these are associated with symptoms (eg, fever, cough, pain, difficulty swallowing).
- See Chapter 4, Head and Neck Exam, for photos of oral pathology.

ABDOMINAL EXAM

- For toddlers, have them lay back on their caregiver's lap with their legs extended onto your lap to ensure they feel comfortable. Older children usually can be evaluated on the exam table.
- Visually assess for distension or protrusions (midline or from umbilicus).
- Palpate the abdomen in all 4 quadrants. Assess for any tenderness or guarding, masses, and enlarged spleen or liver (sweep fingers up from umbilicus).
- Palpate the kidneys for tenderness or masses.
- If there is concern for a urinary tract infection with pyelonephritis, a slightly firm strike to each flank (mid to lower back) may also elicit renal tenderness (see Chapter 8, Abdominal Exam, Figure 8-10).
- If the child is ticklish or nervous, have them bend the knees to relax their abdominal wall, and take deep breaths. Palpate when they exhale.

Findings and Their Meanings: Common Abdominal Exam Abnormalities

- A soft bulge from the umbilicus is usually a hernia. Ensure it can be gently reduced (pushed back into the abdomen) and there are no surrounding skin color changes or tenderness, which can be a sign of incarcerated bowel.
- A soft mass in the lower left quadrant of the abdomen in a child with constipation may be a stool ball.
- A liver palpated more than 2 cm below the right costal margin indicates hepatomegaly and may be a sign of liver or cardiac disease.
- A spleen palpated more than 2 cm from the left costal margin indicates splenomegaly and may be a sign of infection (Epstein-Barr virus, malaria), malignancy (leukemia or lymphoma), hemolytic anemia, liver disease (hepatitis, biliary atresia), or heart failure.

BACK AND SPINE EXAM

- Examine the back for symmetry including shoulder and hip alignment, and look for signs of spinal deformities such as scoliosis or kyphosis. You can identify subtle scoliosis by assessing for shoulder height asymmetry when looking at the child's back while they reach down to touch their toes. A handheld device called a scoliometer (not shown) is used to measure the amount of spinal curvature. Severe scoliosis will be easier to detect (**Figure 20-8**).

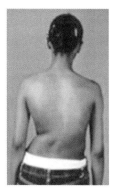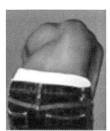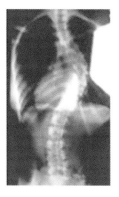

FIGURE 20-8 • **Scoliosis, in this case severe, with obvious curvature and shoulder height asymmetry.** (Reproduced with permission from Mitra R, ed. *Principles of Rehabilitation Medicine.* New York: McGraw Hill; 2019, Figure 65-7.)

- Congenital spinal deformities are rare and often syndromic.
- The most common spinal deformity you may see is idiopathic scoliosis in the older child (often there is a family history).
- The onset is related to when a child starts puberty. Screening should therefore start yearly at the first signs of puberty.

GENITOURINARY EXAM

- Note that this part of the exam is sensitive, and the approach differs depending on the patient's age and the family's preferences.
- Usually, visual inspection of the genitourinary area will suffice and is recommended at yearly well-child visits or acute visits with referable symptoms.
- The main goal is to assess for any abnormalities (eg, undescended testes, labial adhesions) and to monitor for signs of puberty.
- Confirm with your institution at which age you are required to have a chaperone present. Also discuss with your attending whether you should do this part of the exam on your own first or wait until you see the patient together.
- It is recommended to ask for permission to examine the entire body, including more private areas beneath undergarments. Verbally cue the caregiver and the patient that it is permissible for a physician to do this in the presence of the patient's parent or legal guardian. Once there is verbal consent given by caregiver (it is good to see the child nod their assent as well), proceed with the exam. Depending on age and comfort of the patient, you may need to engage the caregiver to either have the child sit on their lap or help reassure the child while they are on the examination table. Use simple, developmentally appropriate statements to explain each part of the exam.

> PEARL: For the toddler and child exam, ask for permission to examine the entire body, including genitalia, and proceed only after consent is given from the caregiver and patient.

Male Genital Exam

- Inspect the appearance of the penis and assess whether the patient is circumcised or uncircumcised. Note the location of the urethral meatus, as well as the testes and scrotum.

- In the uncircumcised penis, the foreskin is usually not retractable until school age; do not attempt to retract.
- If there is a specific issue in that area, have the patient retract their own foreskin for comfort and tolerability.
- Palpate the testes to confirm they are in the scrotal sac to evaluate for undescended testes versus retractile testes.

Findings and Their Meaning: Common Abnormalities to Note During the Male Genitourinary Exam

- Note any rashes or discharge from the urethral opening, edema of the foreskin and head of penis (balanitis), or trauma.
- In the circumcised penis, the foreskin may reattach, causing penile adhesions.
- The meatus is typically in the center of the glans. Congenital abnormalities can occur, where the opening is located along the bottom (hypospadias) or top (epispadias) of the glans or shaft. These would typically have been identified at an earlier age and corrected after 1 year old.
- Referral to pediatric urology is warranted if both testes are not down in the scrotal sac by 1 year old, as this is indicative of an undescended testis.
- Acute testicular pain should prompt consideration for torsion, which is an emergency and needs evaluation and treatment in the emergency department.
- Early signs of puberty (precocious puberty), such as dark, coarse hair around the penis and scrotum in males less than 9 years old, warrant referral to a pediatric endocrinologist. See Chapter 21, Adolescent Exam (Table 21-3, Figure 21-2), for description of normal secondary sex characteristic development.

Female Genital Exam

- A general external exam usually suffices. However, if the parent or patient is complaining of abnormal sensations or discharge, further examination may be necessary.
- Have the patient in the frog position (on the parent's lap or on the examination table) and gently open the labia majora.
- If the child is anxious, consider asking the caregiver for help.
- Inspect the appearance and size of the labia majora and then the labia minora, urethral meatus and clitoris, and hymen (see Chapter 11, Gynecologic and Obstetric Pelvic Exam, for anatomic images).

Findings and Their Meaning: Common Abnormalities to Note During the Female Genitourinary Exam

- Rashes, abnormal discharge, labial adhesions, signs of trauma, or foreign bodies (eg, toilet paper).
- Assessing development of secondary sex characteristics is important to monitor normal growth and puberty, while early signs may reveal underlying endocrine or genetic abnormalities. See Chapter 21, Adolescent Exam (Table 21-3, Figure 21-2), for description of normal secondary sex characteristic development.
- Early signs of puberty (precocious puberty), such as dark, coarse hair on the mons pubis of females less than 8 years old, warrants a referral to a pediatric endocrinologist.

RECTAL EXAM

- Generally, a rectal exam is not performed unless the patient presents with anal pain, anal pruritis, a history of blood on the stool, or constipation.
- Have the child lie on their side with their knees toward their chest.
- With a good light source, gently spread the buttocks and observe the anus, noting any anal fissures, hemorrhoids, erythema, pinworms, or skin tags.
- If assessing with a digital exam (eg, abscess), slowly insert a lubricated, gloved index finger to palpate for masses, asymmetry, or tenderness.
- Throughout the rectal exam, verbally reassure the patient and explain all your movements.

Assessing for Signs of Sexual Abuse

- Signs of sexual abuse on physical exam include blunt or penetrating injuries of the genitalia such as hematomas, lacerations, abrasions, perforations, and excessive bleeding.
- Any signs or evidence of sexual abuse requires careful documentation and a referral to child protection services and a child abuse pediatrician. Discuss any concerns with your attending preceptor for mandatory reporting.

EXTREMITY AND MUSCULOSKELETAL EXAM

- Most of this assessment can be done by watching the patient walk in the room or in the office hallway.
- Gait:
  - Most infant are bow-legged until 18 months to 2 years old and then they slowly transition to have knock-knees, followed by a straightening of the legs by 10 years old.
  - Some toddlers (1-2 years old) will toe-walk in the beginning of their gait, but eventually they should walk on flat feet.
- Examine the patient's symmetry of arms and legs, size and range of motion in all joints, noting any deformities (eg, clinodactyly, webbed toes).
- Examine the hands, feet, and nails.

Findings and Their Meaning: Common Musculoskeletal and Distal Extremity Abnormalities

- If patients have persistent toe-walking, examine calf tightness and consider a physical therapy referral.
- Note any asymmetry in gait and alignment. The most common are tibial torsion (a cause of in-toeing), genu varum (bow-legged), and genu valgum (knock-kneed) (**Figure 20-9**).
- Young children may have mild genu varum, which is normal and will resolve between 2 and 3 years old.

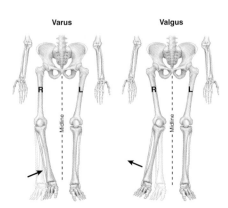

FIGURE 20-9 · **Anatomy of genu varum (bowlegged) and genu valgum (knock-kneed).** (Reproduced with permission from Mitra R, ed. *Principles of Rehabilitation Medicine*. New York: McGraw Hill; 2019.)

- Asymmetric gait could be due to leg-length discrepancy, neuromuscular etiology, or hip disease. Trendelenburg sign, indicative of hip disease, is positive when the pelvis drops on the contralateral side during a single leg stand on the affected side (**Figure 20-10**).
- Acute avoidance of using a limb (eg, limping or only using one hand to do everything) usually indicates an injury (eg, fracture, nursemaid's elbow, or radial head subluxation

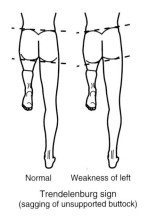

Normal   Weakness of left

Trendelenburg sign
(sagging of unsupported buttock)

FIGURE 20-10 · **Trendelenburg sign.** (Reproduced with permission from Suneja M, Szot JF, LeBlond RF, Brown DD. *DeGowin's Diagnostic Examination*. 11th ed. New York: McGraw Hill; 2020.)

[when a child's elbow partially dislocates after being pulled]), and less likely infection, inflammatory, neurologic, or oncologic etiology.
- Note signs of nail biting or picking or infection such as paronychia or onychomycosis. (See Chapter 16, Dermatologic Exam, Table 16-6, for representative photos.)

> **PEARL:** If a pediatric patient presents complaining of joint pain, always examine the joint above and below where the child complains of pain because the child may be experiencing referred pain (eg, if a child presents with knee pain, ankle or hip pathology may cause referred pain to the knee).

SKIN EXAM

Assess for birthmarks, freckling, moles, hypopigmentation, scars, bruises, rashes, or other abnormalities or areas that are causing symptoms. Common abnormalities are shown in **Table 20-4**.

TABLE 20-4 • Diagnoses at a Glance: Common Skin Disorders in Children

Skin Condition	Image
Eczema/atopic dermatitis: common skin condition in children defined by dry skin, often with erythematous, hyperpigmented, or hypopigmented dry patches, often with lichenification	(Reproduced with permission from Saavedra AP, Roh EK, Mikailov A. *Fitzpatrick's Color Atlas and Synopsis of Clinical Dermatology*. 9th ed. New York: McGraw Hill; 2023, Figure 2-14.)
Acanthosis nigricans: hyperpigmented, velvety-appearing plaques, most often found on the nape of the neck or in the axillary or groin areas; it is an early marker of insulin resistance and suggests risk for diabetes	(Reproduced with permission from Loscalzo J, Fauci AS, Kasper DL, et al, eds. *Harrison's Principles of Internal Medicine*. 21st ed. New York: McGraw Hill; 2022, Figure A5-70.)
Verruca vulgaris: warts caused by human papillomavirus; common in kids; often found on hands and feet	(Reproduced with permission from Soutor C, Hordinsky MK. *Clinical Dermatology: Diagnosis and Management of Common Disorders*. 2nd ed. New York: McGraw Hill; 2022, Figure 13-12.)
Tinea corporis: fungal infection that can occur anywhere on body; well circumscribed, with scaly border and central clearing; often itches	(From Usatine RP, Smith MA, Mayeaux EJ Jr, Chumley HS. *The Color Atlas and Synopsis of Family Medicine*. 3rd ed. New York: McGraw Hill; 2019, Figure 144-7. Reproduced with permission from Richard P. Usatine, MD.)

(Continued)

TABLE 20-4 • Diagnoses at a Glance: Common Skin Disorders in Children (Continued)

Skin Condition	Image	
Impetigo: acute crops of vesicles with a honey-colored crust; caused by *Streptococcus* or *Staphylococcus* infection	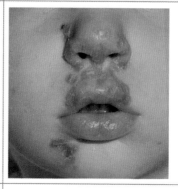	(Reproduced with permission from Wolff K, Johnson RA, Saavedra AP, Roh EK. *Fitzpatrick's Color Atlas and Synopsis of Clinical Dermatology.* 8th ed. New York: McGraw Hill; 2017, Figure 25-8.)
Hives (urticaria): typically acute, raised, red, itchy wheals; usually associated with exposures (eg, cold, food, medications)	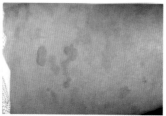	(Reproduced with permission from Bondi EE, Jegasothy BV, Lazarus GS, eds. *Dermatology: Diagnosis & Treatment.* Originally published by Appleton & Lange. Copyright © 1991 by The McGraw-Hill Companies, Inc.)
Molluscum contagiosum: small papules caused by pox virus. Common in kids, and typically asymptomatic and resolve spontaneously	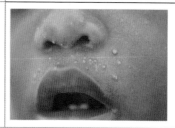	(Reproduced with permission from Soutor C, Hordinsky MK. *Clinical Dermatology: Diagnosis and Management of Common Disorders.* 2nd ed. New York: McGraw Hill; 2022, Figure 13-10.)

- Bruises in this age range can be common, especially on the lower legs and shins, but always ask about any bruising found on examination and confirm etiology. There are specific bruising patterns that may alert the provider to child abuse and would require careful documentation and referral to child protective services and a child abuse pediatrician for a complete evaluation.
- Examples of bruises found on physical exam that would be concerning include hand slap–shaped bruise, ear bruises, or bruises on the face, neck, or torso that are multiple or uniform in shape.

NEUROLOGIC EXAM

- To help tailor your neurologic exam, always review developmental screening tools as children with developmental delays may have abnormal neurologic findings.
- Start with observation of movement. Then perform the cranial nerve exam, assess strength, check sensation, and lastly assess reflexes.

- If a patient is resistant to the neurologic exam, enlist the caregiver to help perform any pertinent tests, but otherwise move on to another part of the exam. Resistance will yield false results, and it is better to perform at another time or after the patient calms.
- Most healthy children do not require an in-depth neurologic examination. However, it is important for learners to attain comfort with these skills so practice any time you have the chance with a cooperative patient.
- Images demonstrating specific neurologic exam techniques can be found in Chapter 12, Neurologic Exam.

Gross and Fine Motor

- Most motor skills can be assessed with the combination of developmental screening tools (surveys answered by the parents) and observing the child interact with their caregiver (eg, walking, climbing, jumping, drawing, eating a snack).

Cranial Nerves

Assessment of cranial nerves II to XII is attainable in a timely manner after practice and more practice! See **Table 20-5** for tips on this exam in the pediatric setting (note that we do not go in numbered order of the cranial nerves), and see Chapter 12, Neurologic Exam, for further details and techniques.

TABLE 20-5 • Cranial Nerve Assessment		
Cranial Nerve Number	Nerve/Function Tested	Methods for Testing
I	Olfactory nerve	Not tested routinely; may assess in older children if any concerns.
II	Visual acuity (optic nerve)	Usually tested with a standardized vision screen for age 3 years or older (see "Eyes" section). Visual field tests can be done as you would for an adult: have the child look at your nose and hold up numbers with your hands in various visual fields. For toddlers, this may be difficult, and if any concerns, refer to ophthalmology for evaluation.
III, IV, VI	Extraocular movements (oculomotor, trochlear, abducens nerves)	Use a fun light or toy to test tracking while the child sits on the caregiver's lap and they hold the child's head still. Alternatively, you can move a toy and hold their head still by placing a finger on their chin.
V	Motor (trigeminal nerve)	Use light touch with your fingers or a cotton ball to test sensation of the face; ask if it feels the same on both sides (forehead, cheeks, mandible). Ask the child to bite down and/or chew a snack to assess strength of the temporalis and masseter muscles of the face via palpation.
VII	Facial	Make silly faces with the child and ask them to copy you: squeeze eyes shut, lift eyebrows up, big smile, puff out cheeks.

(Continued)

Cranial Nerve Number	Nerve/Function Tested	Methods for Testing
TABLE 20-5 • Cranial Nerve Assessment (Continued)		
XII	Hypoglossal	Ask the child to stick out their tongue straight and move side to side or push out their cheek from the inside with their tongue.
IX, X	Swallow and gag reflex (glossopharyngeal and vagus nerves)	During the oral exam (see above), when child protrudes tongue and says "Ahhh," note symmetry of palate and uvula.
XI	Spinal accessory	Ask child to turn their head to one side and then the other (if any concerns and you want to further evaluate strength, place the back of your hand on their cheek and have them push it out of the way). Ask child to shrug their shoulders up ("I don't know!").
VIII	Hearing (vestibulocochlear nerve)	For ~1-2 years old: Watch the child turn to noises or their name. Any concerns by parents or speech delay should be referred to audiology for a formal hearing test. For school-aged children and general screening: Whisper a familiar word in each ear and have them repeat it back to you. Note that children age 3 years and older will have a standardized hearing screen during their well-child check. For older verbal children who have a hearing concern, use a tuning fork to perform the Weber and Rinne tests (see Chapter 12, Neurologic Exam, for details) to assess for conductive versus sensorineural hearing loss.

Strength

- Have the child sit on the exam table. Ask them to put their arms out straight and hold them there for a few seconds, close their eyes, and turn their hands over (if weak, they will not be able to hold this position).
- Have the child grab the examiner's 2 fingers on each hand and squeeze: "Try and break my fingers!"
- Have the child push your hands away, and then pull your hands toward them.
- Have the child relax their arm completely, and as you hold their hand, rotate their wrist and elbow to assess tone.
- Square test for tone: Have the child bend their finger and hands forward toward their elbow. There should be a square shape made by their arm, hand, and fingers if tone is normal.
- Place your hands on the child's knees and have them push their legs out and then in.
- Have the child make their legs straight and tell them to push against you as you gently push down.
- Have the child relax their legs and feet; rotate each foot to assess for tone.

Sensory

- Using a tuning fork and light touch will suffice for a general sensory screening.
- Apply light touch to hand, shoulders, knees, and feet bilaterally and ask if both sides feel the same or different.

- Apply a vibrating tuning fork to the above locations and ask if both sides feel the same or different.
- Apply the end of the cold tuning fork or the examiner's warm hand/finger and ask if they feel "cold or warm." (Make sure your hands are warm!)

Deep Tendon Reflexes

- Show the child the reflex hammer and let them touch it before use for reassurance (you can even hit yourself gently to show them it doesn't hurt).
- The adult techniques are applicable for this age group; see Chapter 12, Neurologic Exam, for details.
- Hold each hand and test for the brachioradialis, bicep, and triceps reflexes. Holding the limb is important because sometimes you feel instead of see the reflex.
- Hold each foot and test for the patellar and ankle reflexes.
- Hold the calf and dorsiflex the foot to test for clonus; there should be none at this age.
- Babinski reflex: At this age down-going toes are normal, while up-going toes are abnormal.

Coordination, Gait, and Posture

- Assess gait, balance, and postural movements by asking the patient to:
  - Touch each finger to their thumb
  - Touch their nose and extend fully to touch the examiner's finger
  - Stand still: look at weight distribution to make sure it is even on both sides
  - Balance on one foot, then the other
  - Jump on one foot, then the other
  - Walk straight ahead with one foot in front of the other "on a balance beam" or "on a straight line"
  - Walk on heels, walk on toes, walk normally

TELEHEALTH TIPS

- Ensure you are in a quiet, private space that is well-lit and that your camera and microphone are working.
- Look directly at the camera as much as possible (instead of your screen) to make eye contact.
- If appropriate, have parents send you high-definition pictures of the child's body (eg, rash) prior to the visit as photographs are often easier to assess and video can make close-up views blurry.
- Ask parents to:
  - Create a calm and quiet atmosphere to decrease interruptions or distractions.
  - Be prepared to do simple games to keep the child's interest during the physical assessment or to help with the assessment (eg, decreased movement of a toddler's limb: have the child sit on a blanket and play with blocks placed around them).
- Walk the parents through a physical exam using a telehealth template note (if available).
- Those with concerning symptoms or findings usually need to be referred for in-person evaluation with appropriate urgency.

✓ SUMMARY OF SKILLS CHECKLIST

- ❏ Clean your hands
- ❏ History: obtained from caregiver, with contributions from child as they get older
  - Ask for any specific concerns to assess during visit
  - Developmental milestones
  - Behavior
  - Home safety and anticipatory guidance
  - Social history
  - Family history
  - Dental history
  - Immunizations
  - Other past medical, surgical history; Medications
- ❏ Engage with child and create trust; Be flexible, gathering exam information as opportunities arise (ie, don't expect to follow an ordered list)
- ❏ Visual inspection using "6-foot away exam"
- ❏ Vital signs
- ❏ Growth
- ❏ Heart
- ❏ Lungs and chest
- ❏ Head and neck
- ❏ Eyes
- ❏ Ears
- ❏ Nose
- ❏ Mouth
- ❏ Abdomen
- ❏ Back, spine and extremities
- ❏ Genitourinary, skin, and neurologic exams if specific concerns
- ❏ Thank patient for their cooperation; ask if they have any questions
- ❏ Discuss findings with caregiver; ask if they have any questions
- ❏ Clean your hands

BIBLIOGRAPHY

ACES Aware. Adverse childhood events. Accessed April 1, 2023. https://www.acesaware.org/.

American Academy of Pediatrics. Ages and stages of development. http://www.healthychildren.org/ENGLISH/AGES-STAGES/BABY/Pages/default.aspx.

American Academy of Pediatrics. Bright Futures Guidelines for preventive care screening and health supervision visits. Accessed April 1, 2023. https://www.aap.org/en/practice-management/bright-futures.

American Academy of Ophthalmology. Strabismus simulator. Accessed April 23, 2023. https://www.aao.org/education/interactive-tool/strabismus-simulator.

Bower C, Reilly B, Richerson J, Hecht J. Committee on practice and ambulatory medicine, section on Otolaryngology-Head and Neck Surgery; Hearing Assessment in Infants, Children, and Adolescents: Recommendations Beyond Neonatal Screening. *Pediatrics* September 2023; 152 (3): e2023063288. 10.1542/peds.2023-063288.

Centers for Disease Control and Prevention. Adverse childhood events (ACEs). Accessed April 1, 2023. https://www.cdc.gov/violenceprevention/aces/index.html.

Centers for Disease Control and Prevention. Childhood vaccinations. Accessed April 14, 2023. https://www.cdc.gov/vaccines/schedules/index.html.

Centers for Disease Control and Prevention. Developmental milestones and screening. Accessed April 1, 2023. https://www.cdc.gov/ncbddd/childdevelopment/screening.html.

Centers for Disease Control and Prevention. Growth charts. Accessed April 1, 2023. https://www.cdc.gov/growthcharts/index.htm.

Felitti VJ, Anda RF, Nordenberg D. Relationship of childhood abuse and household dysfunction to many of the leading causes of death in adults. The Adverse Childhood Experiences (ACE) Study. *Am J Prev Med*. 1998;14:245-258.

Fleming S, Thompson M, Stevens R, et al. Normal ranges of heart rate and respiratory rate in children from birth to 18 years of age: a systematic review of observational studies. *Lancet*. 2011;377:1011.

Flynn J, Kaelber D, Baker-Smith C, et al. Clinical practice guideline for screening and management of high blood pressure in children and adolescents. *Pediatrics*. 2017;140(3):e20171904.

Gold J. Neurology exam in a child. Accessed April 21, 2023. https://canvas.ucsd.edu/courses/37712/modules/items/1352023.

Gonzalez V, Kyle W, Allen H. Cardia examination and evaluation of murmurs. *Pediatr Rev*. 2021;42(7):375-382.

Pan Y, Tarczy-Hornoch K, Cotter SA, et al. Multi-Ethnic Pediatric Eye Disease Study Group. Visual acuity norms in pre-school children: the Multi-Ethnic Pediatric Eye Disease Study. *Optom Vis Sci*. 2009;86(6):607-612.

Scharf R, Scharf G, Stroustrup A. Developmental milestones. *Pediatr Rev*. 2016;37(1):25-38.

Scoliosis Research Society. Position statement: screening for the early detection of idiopathic scoliosis in adolescents. Accessed April 3, 2023. https://www.srs.org/about-srs/news-and-announcements/position-statement—screening-for-the-early-detection-for-idiopathic-scoliosis-in-adolescents.

World Health Organization. Growth standards. Accessed April 14, 2023. https://www.who.int/tools/child-growth-standards/standards.

Adolescent Exam

Maya Michelle Kumar, MD

"Adolescence" is a stage, not an age; however, the World Health Organization defines adolescence as age 10 to 19 years. Our physical, social, and emotional growth during adolescence defines who we will be as adults and our long-term health outcomes. Just as babies achieve important developmental milestones as they grow, so do adolescents (**Figure 21-1**). Failure to progress normally through these adolescent milestones may result in significant functional impairments in adulthood.

Key developmental milestones that adolescents must navigate include the following:

- Separating from their parents and learning to exist independently in a world of their peers
- Coming to terms with physical changes associated with puberty and achieving acceptance of their adult bodies
- Developing a sexual identity
- Developing their moral codes, values, and ideals
- Experiencing stronger emotions while improving their executive functioning (eg, sound judgement, reasoning, and understanding the consequences of their actions)
- Identifying their sense of purpose and desired vocation
- Increasing their capacity for abstract thought

Clinical assessment of adolescent patients uses many of the same history and physical examination techniques described in the chapters about adults, but also requires the provider to give special consideration to the adolescent's stage of development.

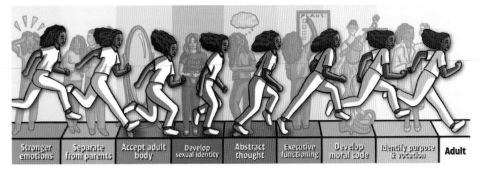

FIGURE 21-1 · Normal developmental milestones of adolescence. (Reproduced with permission from Cathy Cichon, MD.)

SPECIAL CONSIDERATIONS IN ADOLESCENT HISTORY TAKING

Confidentiality

Confidentiality in a healthcare setting means that the practitioner is required to keep the patient's information private. Pediatric patients who can talk to practitioners by themselves have the right to confidential healthcare, even if they are not old enough to consent to their own medical care. There are, however, limits on the right to confidential healthcare. If a practitioner is concerned that the patient (or another minor) is at risk of being seriously harmed or that the patient is at risk of harming someone else, then the practitioner is obligated to break the patient's confidentiality and share whatever information will ensure the safety of the parties involved. The limits of confidentiality should ideally be explained to a patient *before* any sensitive topics are discussed privately. This discussion achieves 2 purposes:

- Assures the patient that they can freely discuss sensitive health topics privately with their practitioner without fear of their caregivers knowing
- Allows the patient to understand the conditions under which the practitioner might need to disclose their health information so they can choose what *not* to share and are prepared for the consequences if they do share information that must be disclosed to others

If a practitioner must break an adolescent's confidentiality, it is preferable to let the adolescent know before making a disclosure and to assure them that the disclosure will be limited to whatever portion of information is relevant for safety. It is helpful to offer the adolescent choices as to how the information will be shared. For example:

- The practitioner can offer to make the disclosure in front of the adolescent, so they know exactly what is being shared.
- The adolescent can be given an opportunity to disclose the information themselves to their caregiver, with the practitioner present to provide support.
- Some adolescents prefer to have the practitioner make disclosures as needed without their presence or involvement, as participating in the disclosure may cause anxiety and/or retraumatization.

Adolescents and Their Caregivers

Unlike clinical interactions with younger children, questions should be directed toward adolescent patients rather than their caregivers as often as possible. As emerging adults, adolescents should be guided toward the driver's seat of their healthcare management with their caregivers shifting toward a more supportive role.

- Adolescents should be offered at least some one-on-one time with their providers at healthcare visits without their caregivers present.
- The American Academy of Pediatrics recommends that this should begin as early as age 11 years, depending on the patient and clinical context.
- Seeing adolescents alone allows them to express their own concerns about their health, ask questions, and provide confidential answers to sensitive health questions without fear of being judged or punished by their caregivers.
- Providers can set the expectation at the start of an appointment that it is routine to speak to the adolescent alone for at least a few minutes during the visit.

- Caregivers can also be offered an opportunity to speak alone with the provider without their child present, as they too may feel more comfortable sharing certain information privately.

> PEARL: If a caregiver expresses hesitancy about leaving the room, explain the rationale for giving adolescents the opportunity to speak confidentially with their providers, and reassure them that if any divulged information suggests that the adolescent (or anyone else) is in danger, it will not be kept secret.

Minor Consent

Practitioners should familiarize themselves with country-specific and state-specific laws about a minor's ability to consent to medical treatment. Many states allow minors to provide their own consent for sensitive medical services, such as:

- Contraception
- Pregnancy-related care including pregnancy termination
- Testing and treatment for sexually transmitted infections and HIV
- Medical care following sexual assault
- Substance abuse treatment
- Mental health treatment

However, there is wide variability as to the ages at which youth can consent, the specific services for which they can consent, and whether parental notification is required even if the minor can consent. See Bibliography for websites that summarize many minor consent laws by state.

Emancipated Minors

An emancipated minor is legally able to consent to their own medical, psychiatric, and dental healthcare services without parental notification or consent. Specific criteria must be met for a minor to be declared legally emancipated. Emancipation laws vary from state to state, but a minor is most commonly emancipated by joining the military or by getting married, both of which require parental consent. Providers cannot assume that a child living apart from their parents is emancipated as it requires a specific legal adjudication.

THE ADOLESCENT SOCIAL HISTORY: THE "HEADS" HISTORY

An adolescent social history can be structured using the mnemonic **"HEADS": Home, Education/Employment, Activities, Drugs/Diet/Depression, and Sex/Safety (Table 21-1).**
The limits of confidentiality should be explained to the adolescent *before* obtaining this history.

> PEARL: Here is an example of how to introduce confidentiality and its limits to an adolescent patient: "You have the right to expect that anything you discuss with me will be kept private, but there are certain exceptions to this. If I am concerned that you or someone else is at risk of serious harm, then I may have to share some of your information to ensure that everyone is safe."

> PEARL: A basic screening HEADS history can be conducted in a few minutes. However, if the adolescent has concerning responses, the provider can explore the topic further. If you are pressed for time, focus on elements of history that might indicate the adolescent is in danger (eg, presence of suicidal ideation, exposure to violence).

TABLE 21-1 • Summary of the HEADS History

	Sample Questions	Other Tips
Home	• Who lives with you? • Who are your primary guardians/caretakers? • Do you have siblings? • How do you get along with everyone at home?	• If parents are no longer together, determine physical and legal custody arrangements. • If parents have romantic partners or if there are step-parents, ask the adolescent about their relationship with them.
Education	• Are you in school? • How much schooling have you completed? • What do you like about school? Are there things that you do not like? • What grades do you typically get? What are your favorite and least favorite subjects?	• If struggling in school, ask what supports are in place to help (eg, individualized education plan, tutoring). • Gauge how much academic stress the adolescent experiences. • Find out whether they have had to change schools and the reason for changing.
Employment	• Do you work? Where do you work? • How many hours a week do you work? • What do you like about your job? Are there things that you do not like? • How would you describe your financial situation?	• Determine whether the adolescent is having a good experience at work or if they are stressed/overwhelmed by work. • Determine whether they are working out of financial necessity or just for experience. • Assess whether work interferes with their ability to participate in school or other important activities.
Activities	• What do you like to do for fun? • What are some activities that help you relax? • Do you have a good group of friends or at least 1 or 2 close friends?	• Disinterest in activities that used to bring enjoyment suggests depression. • The absence of positive connections with peers is a concern that should be further explored.
Diet	• Do you ever worry about your body weight or shape? • What do you like about your body? Is there a part of your body that you do not like? • Have you ever changed the way you eat or exercise because of concerns about your weight or shape?	• If body image concerns are identified, determine whether the adolescent has changed their eating or exercise behaviors due to poor body image. Also inquire about self-induced vomiting and use of laxatives, diet pills, supplements, or teas for losing weight, suppressing appetite, or "detoxing."
Drugs	• Have you ever used any of the following substances? Ask specifically about tobacco, nicotine products including vapes and e-cigarettes, alcohol, marijuana, misuse of prescription and over-the-counter drugs, psychedelic drugs, club or party drugs, and injected or snorted drugs. • Have you ever shared injection equipment with anyone else?	• Use the word "substance" rather than "drug," because many adolescents do not consider alcohol or marijuana a "drug." • Avoid the phrase "illicit drugs" because most drugs used by adolescents are legal (eg, tobacco, nicotine, alcohol, marijuana, prescription and over-the-counter drugs). • If the adolescent currently uses drugs, determine the frequency of use and affect on function. • Ask about driving, sexual activity, or other behaviors while intoxicated with any substance.

(Continued)

TABLE 21-1 • Summary of the HEADS History (Continued)		
	Sample Questions	Other Tips
Depression	• How do you cope with stress? • How would you say your mood has been most of the time in the last couple of weeks? • Have you ever seen a counselor/ therapist or taken medicines for your mental health? Did this help? • Have you ever been so stressed that you had thoughts about wanting to hurt yourself or wanting to die, or seriously hurting someone else? If so, have you ever acted on those thoughts?	• Lack of effective coping skills is often associated with mental health problems. • Even if an adolescent states that their mood is currently good, ask about whether they have ever had thoughts or behaviors of self-harm in the past. • Always assess for any *current active* thoughts of suicidality or harming others. If present, providers are legally required to notify caregivers and immediately refer the adolescent for an urgent mental health assessment. • If the adolescent describes stress or mood concerns, consider further screening using validated questionnaires or DSM criteria.

Sex and gender	• Is there any romance in your life right now? If so, does it make you happy?
	• When you have romance, is it with boys, girls, both, other/neither, or not sure?
	• Have you ever had sex before or any type of sexual contact (including oral sex, sexual touching, etc.)?
	• How would you describe your gender? On the inside, do you feel like you are male, female, both, neither, or unsure?
	• What name and pronouns do you use?
		• "Romance" is a good general word that does not necessarily imply dating or a relationship.
		• Screen for unhealthy relationships in which the adolescent's partner appears controlling, invasive, or jealous. If so, explore whether there is any forced or coerced sexual activity or pressure not to use birth control or condoms.
		• For patients who identify as LGBTQ+, ask whether they feel supported by their family, friends, school, and communities, as lack of support and acceptance is the primary risk factor for poor outcomes.
		• Avoid the terms "preferred name" or "preferred pronouns" in gender diverse patients. They are not "preferred"; they simply are what they are.
		• If the adolescent has had sex before, obtain a more thorough sexual history, including:
		  • Number and types of past and current partners
		  • Types of sexual activity
		  • Previous sexually transmitted infections (STIs)
		  • Last STI/HIV test
		  • History of pregnancy
		  • Use of birth control
		  • Use of barriers (eg, condoms, dental dams) to prevent STI/HIV transmission
		  • Other risk factors including history of incarceration, involvement in commercial sex work, use of injection drugs, living in an endemic area, or a sexual partner with any of these risk factors

(Continued)

TABLE 21-1 • Summary of the HEADS History (Continued)		
	Sample Questions	**Other Tips**
Safety	• Do you feel safe at home? • Do you feel safe at school? • Do you feel safe in your neighborhood? • Do you feel safe online and in your social media activities? • Are there any places that you go where you don't feel safe? • Have you ever experienced or witnessed violence (eg, kicking, hitting, punching, slapping, use of weapons)? • Have you ever experienced bullying or harassment, in person or online? • Have you ever had any unwanted sexual contact, in person or online?	• If they do not feel safe in any environment, explore further. • Even if someone states that they have never had sex, you should still ask about unwanted sexual contact; they may not think of this as sex. • If the patient has experienced any kind of verbal, physical, or sexual abuse, determine whether it has already been reported to child protection services or law enforcement.

Abbreviation: DSM, Diagnostic and Statistical Manual of Mental Disorders.

Additional Tips When Eliciting a HEADS History

• The HEADS history should typically be elicited one-on-one with the adolescent alone, without caregivers present.

• The order of the topics covered by the HEADS history is intended to begin with less sensitive questions (eg, about home and school) and progress to more sensitive questions by the end (eg, about drugs and sexuality). However, the practitioner should assess each individual adolescent patient and ask questions in order of what they feel would be least sensitive to most sensitive for *their particular patient*. For example, for some adolescents, their home life might be the hardest thing for them to discuss and it may be wise to leave this until the end.

• Try to ask open-ended questions.

• Avoid making assumptions or using labels when you phrase your questions; the adolescent may not be operating at the same wavelength as you. Ensure your language is concrete and direct (see examples in **Table 21-2**).

TABLE 21-2 • Examples of Language to Use and Language to Avoid When Obtaining a HEADS History	
Suboptimal	**A Better Option**
"Do you have a boyfriend?"	"Is there any romance in your life? What does that look like for you?"
"You've never had sex, right?"	"Have you ever had sex?"
"Are you gay or straight?"	"When you have romance, is it with boys, girls, both, neither, or are you unsure?"
"Are you a smoker?"	"Do you use cigarettes, e-cigarettes, vapes, or any other nicotine or tobacco products? Do you smoke marijuana or use any other cannabis products?"
"Do you do drugs?"	"Have you ever used [name of substance]?"
"Any chance you could be pregnant?"	"Have you ever had sex before? When was your last period? Have you ever had sex without birth control or a condom?"

Trauma-Informed Care

Trauma-informed care refers to providers being aware of the impact that trauma may have had on a patient and recognizing the patient's individualized response to it. Being mindful of this allows the provider to create an environment for patients in which they feel their needs can be safely met. There are many ways through which a provider can incorporate principles of trauma-informed care.

- Present yourself as open, caring, and professional.
- Respect boundaries of touch. Do not casually touch patients. Ask permission before performing the physical examination.
- Ensure the purpose of the patient's visit is achieved. Do not ask questions that are not relevant to the care they are seeking, as it may be perceived as invasive. For example, a full HEADS history does not need to be elicited if an adolescent is presenting with a sprained ankle, but certain elements related to home environment, school environment, and safety concerns may be clinically relevant.
- Read the patient's nonverbal body language throughout your encounter with them. If they seem angry, afraid, shutdown, or overly eager to please, they may be having a trauma response.
- If you ask a question that seems to elicit a trauma response, clarify the reason why you are asking the question. If they still seem uncomfortable with answering the question, assure them that they do not need to answer it if they feel uncomfortable.
- Remember that you do not need to gather the entire history in one visit. Going slower allows time for building rapport and trust with your patient, which may increase their comfort with sharing information.
- Avoid the temptation to "rescue" patients who have a history of trauma; instead, assume that the goal is to empower them to take charge of their health. In the same vein, it is preferable to refer to patients as *survivors* of trauma rather than *victims*.

PHYSICAL EXAM CONSIDERATIONS

The physical exam for an adolescent is generally the same as for adults. The following special considerations are important to note.

Remain Trauma Informed

Even for general examinations that do not involve the breasts or genitals, principles of trauma-informed care can be consistently incorporated.

- Request adolescent patients to disrobe only when necessary; consider letting them wear light clothing (eg, shorts and T-shirt) rather than a gown.
- Consider placing your stethoscope directly on their skin underneath their clothing so they remain covered.
- "Signpost" your exam: At each step of the exam, inform the adolescent what part of their body you are about to examine before you do so. If an adolescent seems uncomfortable with an aspect of the exam, it can be helpful to first explain its purpose. It may also be helpful to ask the adolescent if they prefer a provider of a certain gender.
- Ultimately, if an adolescent does not want to wear a gown or disrobe, their wishes should be respected.

If the adolescent declines examination due to discomfort, ask whether there are certain parts of the exam they would feel comfortable doing (eg, listening to their lungs on their back, but not on their chest) or if you can offer modifications to make them more comfortable (eg, allow the patient to place the stethoscope on their own body while you listen).

Performing Sensitive Examinations

Be familiar with policies at your institution that may require the presence of a chaperone, but otherwise, it is reasonable to give adolescents a choice as to whether they want a chaperone. Many adolescents feel less comfortable having a chaperone present. If a chaperone is used or if the patient declines a chaperone, this should ideally be documented in the medical record.

Speak to your supervising resident or attending about whether it is preferable for the medical student to perform any sensitive examinations in their presence, so that the adolescent does not need to go through it more than once.

A key component of the adolescent physical exam is the sexual maturity rating, or Tanner staging, of the breasts and genitals. The purpose of assessing the sexual maturity rating is to ensure that the patient is progressing as expected through puberty. See **Table 21-3** and **Figure 21-2** for a description of the sexual maturity ratings and Tanner stages.

TABLE 21-3 • Description of Sexual Maturity Rating (Tanner) Stages		
	Males Testes development	**Penis development**
I	Prepubertal (<4 mL)	Prepubertal
II	Testes enlarge (≥4 mL), scrotum reddens and changes texture	Slight enlargement
III	Larger	Longer
IV	Scrotum darkens	Larger, wider with development of glans
V	Adult size	Adult size
Breast development		
I	Prepubertal	
II	Breast and papilla elevated as small mound with palpable subareolar bud, areolar diameter increased	
III	Enlargement and elevation of whole breast	
IV	Areola and papilla form secondary areolar mound	
V	Mature breast contour, nipple projects	
Pubic hair development		
I	None	
II	Sparse, short, straight, at base of penis or medial border of labia	

(Continued)

TABLE 21-3 • Description of Sexual Maturity Rating (Tanner) Stages (Continued)		
Pubic hair development (cont.)		
III	Darker, longer, coarser, and curlier, sparsely over pubic bones	
IV	Coarse, curly, resembles adult hair; but spares thighs	
V	Adult distribution with inverse triangle pattern and spread to medial thighs	

Source: Reproduced with permission from Shah SS, Zaoutis LB, Catallozzi M, Frank G. eds. The Philadelphia Guide: Inpatient Pediatrics. 2nd ed. New York: McGraw-Hill; 2016.

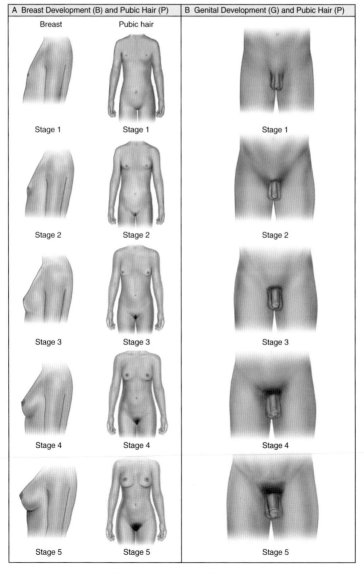

FIGURE 21-2 • **Sexual maturity rating (Tanner) stages.** (Reproduced with permission from Styne DM. *Pediatric Endocrinology: A Clinical Handbook.* Switzerland: Springer International Publishing; 2016.)

Breast Examination

- Breast development is the earliest sign of puberty in biologic females. Routine visual inspection of the chest to determine the patient's sexual maturity rating should begin at no later than 8 years old.
- Assessing the child's breast sexual maturity rating should occur annually until menarche is achieved. After menarche, there is no need for routine breast examination or visual inspection of the breasts for otherwise healthy adolescents.

Findings and Their Meaning: Breast Development Indicating Delayed or Advanced Puberty

- Signs of *delayed* puberty warranting further investigation:
  - No sign of breast buds (Tanner stage 2) by age 13 (Table 21-3, Figure 21-2).
  - No menarche by age 16
  - No menarche >4 years after breast buds appear
  - No menarche >1 year after reaching Tanner stage 5 (fully developed)
- Signs of *advanced* puberty warranting further investigation include any breast development before age 8, although breast development as early as 7 years may be normal in certain ethnic groups.
- While routine breast self-examination is not recommended, it is reasonable to teach adolescents to have breast "awareness" (ie, to be familiar with their normal anatomy and to seek medical attention if they notice any changes).

Assigned Male at Birth: Genital Examination

Inspection

- Penile inspection should be performed as part of the annual exam in adolescent biologic males.
- Visual inspection of pubic hair to determine sexual maturity rating (Tanner stage) can begin at age 9 for biologic males. See Table 21-3 and Figure 21-2 for a description of the Tanner stages.

Testicular Exam

- Testicular enlargement is the earliest sign of puberty in biologic males. Routine palpation of the testicles to determine the patient's sexual maturity rating (Tanner stage) should begin at no later than 9 years old.
- Testicular examination should occur annually throughout adolescence, as the highest prevalence of testicular cancer is between the ages of 15 and 35. This includes palpation of both testicles to ensure normal size, texture, location, and mobility with no associated abnormal lumps, swelling, or overlying skin changes. See Chapter 9, Male Genital Exam, for discussion of technique.
- The adolescent should be standing during the testicular examination. Self-examination can be taught to adolescents in this age group, although guidelines differ in their recommendations as to who should routinely perform testicular self-examination.

Findings and Their Meaning in the Male Genital Area

- Pubic hair present before age 9 in boys suggests early puberty that warrants investigation.
- Signs of *delayed* puberty warranting further investigation include no initial enlargement of the testicles (Tanner stage 2) by age 14 (Table 21-3, Figure 21-2).

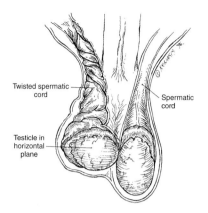 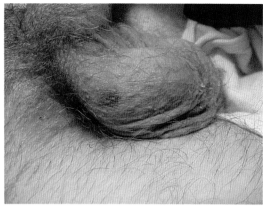

FIGURE 21-3 • Testicular torsion (left) and blue dot sign from torsion of testicular appendage (right). (Reproduced with permission from Knoop KJ, Stack LB, Storrow AB, Thurman RJ, eds. *The Atlas of Emergency Medicine.* 5th ed. New York: McGraw-Hill; 2021. Photo reproduced with permission from photo contributor: Alan B. Storrow, MD.)

- Signs of *advanced* puberty warranting further investigation include any testicular development before age 9.
- Acute testicular pain can result from a number of processes, including: testicular torsion, orchitis, epididymitis, or torsion of a testicular appendage.
- Testicular torsion is an emergency (risk of testicular necrosis), typically requiring prompt evaluation in an Emergency Department. Pain is acute and severe. On exam, the testicle is tender, enlarged, often higher in the scrotum and with a horizontal orientation (**Figure 21-3**). It occurs most commonly <6 months and between ages 12 and 20.
- Torsion of a testicular appendage also causes acute pain and may present with "blue dot" on the scrotal skin (Figure 21-3).
- See Chapter 9, Male Genital Exam, for description of other common genital area pathologies and findings.

> **PEARL:** The cremasteric reflex is seen in healthy males. If you lightly stroke the skin on the medial thigh, the cremasteric muscle contracts and pulls the ipsilateral testicle up toward the inguinal canal (a positive test). In the presence of acute scrotal pain, absence of the cremasteric reflex is one of the most sensitive signs for testicular torsion. Beware of the following, however:
> - Rarely, the cremasteric reflex may be preserved in the presence of a torsion.
> - Even in the absence of disease, the cremasteric reflex may not be seen in young healthy children under age 2 to 3 years old.

Assigned Female at Birth: Genital Exam

- Visual inspection of pubic hair to determine sexual maturity rating (Tanner stage) can begin at age 8 for biologic female (Table 21-3 and Figure 21-2).
- An external vulvovaginal examination does not need to be done routinely but should be performed if there is a clinical concern. For example in the setting of itching, pain, discharge, or the presence of a lesion or sore. The technique and common findings are described in Chapter 11, Gynecologic and Obstetric Pelvic Exam.

- A pelvic exam only needs to be performed when clinically indicated. In these situations, the technique (and common findings) is described in Chapter 11, Gynecologic and Obstetric Pelvic Exam.

Findings and Their Meaning: Early Development of Pubic Hair in Girls

- Pubic hair present before age 8 in girls suggests early puberty that warrants investigation.

CONCLUSIONS

Clinical evaluation of adolescent patients is similar to what is practiced with adults, but special consideration must be given to the adolescent's developmental status as an emerging adult. Offering opportunities for private conversations with their practitioners, protecting patient confidentiality, allowing minors to consent to sensitive health services when legally permitted, and engaging adolescents directly in their healthcare interactions are all important ways that practitioners can encourage youth to start taking charge of their health. The HEADS history is a useful tool to assess an adolescent's psychosocial health and safety. Principles of trauma-informed care are critical to incorporate into both history taking and physical examination.

TELEHEALTH TIPS

- Telehealth is a reasonable modality for performing history and physical examinations for adolescents.
- Before asking the adolescent any sensitive questions, the provider should ask the adolescent whether they are in a confidential space.
- Adolescent patients can be encouraged to use headphones to ensure that their conversation is not overheard.
- Given its sensitive nature, and for comfort of the adolescent, examination of sensitive organs is best conducted in person.

SUMMARY OF SKILLS CHECKLIST

- ❑ Wash your hands
- ❑ Explain confidentiality and its limits
- ❑ In addition to a typical medical history, elicit a HEADS social history using trauma-informed and nonjudgmental language
- ❑ Perform exam using techniques described in the chapters dedicated to adults
- ❑ Perform breast or genital exams when clinically indicated. Wait to perform the exam until your supervising physician is present so the exam only has to be performed once.
- ❑ Respect an adolescent's request to not answer a question or skip elements of the exam
- ❑ Wash your hands

BIBLIOGRAPHY

Caesar RE, Kaplan GW. The incidence of the cremasteric reflex in normal boys. *J Urol.* 1994;152 (2 pt 2):779-780.

Centers for Disease Control and Prevention. State laws that enable a minor to provide informed consent to receive HIV and STD services. Accessed March 19, 2023. https://www.cdc.gov/hiv/policies/law/states/minors.html.

Diaz A, Laufer MR, Breech LL. American Academy of Pediatrics Committee on Adolescence, American College of Obstetricians and Gynecologists Committee on Adolescent Health Care. Menstruation in girls and adolescents: using the menstrual cycle as a vital sign. *Pediatrics.* 2006;118:2245-2250.

Ford C, English A, Sigman G. Confidential health care for adolescents: position paper for the Society for Adolescent Health and Medicine. *J Adolesc Health.* 2004;35:160-167.

Guttmacher Institute. An overview of consent to reproductive health services by young people. Accessed January 15, 2024. https://www.guttmacher.org/state-policy/explore/overview-minors-consent-law.

Hagan JF, Shaw JS, Duncan PM, eds. *Bright Futures: Guidelines for Health Supervision of Infants, Children, and Adolescents.* 4th ed. Elk Grove Village, IL: American Academy of Pediatrics; 2022.

Herman-Giddens ME, Steffes J, Harris D, et al. Secondary sexual characteristics in boys: data from the Pediatric Research in Office Settings Network. *Pediatrics.* 2012;130(5):e1058.

Mellick LB, Mowery ML, Al-Dhahir MA. Cremasteric reflex. June 27, 2022. In: StatPearls [Internet]. Treasure Island, FL: StatPearls Publishing; 2022.

Neinstein LS. *Adolescent and Young Adult Health Care: A Practical Guide.* 6th ed. Philadelphia, PA: Wolters Kluwer; 2016.

Substance Abuse and Mental Health Services Administration. SAMHSA's Concept of Trauma and Guidance for a Trauma-Informed Approach. HHS Publication No. (SMA) 14-4884. Rockville, MD: Substance Abuse and Mental Health Services Administration; 2014.

22

Medical Documentation

Emily Sladek, MD

Medical documentation can edify and enhance patient care, but note writing intimidates many clinicians, both learners and seasoned practitioners alike. Our aim here is to help clarify the rationale for note writing and underscore some best practices to help master the art of effective, efficient documentation.

BRIEF HISTORICAL PERSPECTIVE

The written medical record in Western medicine dates to the time of Hippocrates and initially consisted of anecdotal case histories recorded largely for didactic use. In the 4000 years since its inception, written clinical documentation has evolved significantly, shifting from an occasionally used educational tool to a broadly adapted instrument informing real-time care of individual patients.

While widespread propagation of written medical records improved patient outcomes, clinical notes remained handwritten for most of the 20th century, which left the challenge of deciphering illegible handwriting and difficulty sharing information among providers in different healthcare settings. While doctors, as a group, do not actually have worse handwriting than the population at large, up to 15% of handwritten notes have been found to be illegible, which can have outsized consequences on patient care.

Starting in the 1990s, with the rise of personal computers, electronic medical records (EMRs) began to propagate. Fueled in part by funding from the 2010 Affordable Care Act, EMRs had a meteoric rise, with documented use in 9% of hospitals in 2008, increasing to 96% by 2015. The EMR eliminated the perils of handwritten notes but opened the door to a new set of challenges.

CHALLENGES OF THE EMR

While patient care has benefitted from the development of standardized clinical documentation, negativity surrounds electronic note writing, stemming largely from the volume of time it absorbs. As Thoreau said, "Men have become the tools of their tools." Some challenges are as follows:

Clinical Time Is a Zero-Sum Game

- More time writing notes equals less time spent with patients.
- More than 65% of medicine residents reported spending >4 hours/day working on documentation, whereas <30% reported spending >4 hours/day on direct patient care.

- Clinicians are demoralized to find note writing time supplanting meaningful bedside time, a phenomenon Verghese describes as the "iPatient."

Attempts to Improve Electronic Note Writing Efficiency Can Backfire

- Copy-and-paste is a method of expediting note production, but leads to:
  - Note bloat
    - A snowballing effect wherein notes become haphazardly bloated with disorganized, internally inconsistent, pasted information.
    - Median note length increased by 60% from 2009 to 2018 with a significant increase in note redundancy.
  - Chart lore
    - Inaccurate data carried forward from note-to-note without verification.
- Consequences of electronic copy-and-paste Frankensteinian notes:
  - Worsened patient outcomes
  - Provider burnout and disengagement

Our goal in the remainder of this chapter is to outline a practical approach to electronic note writing that will improve the experience for both reader and writer.

WHAT'S THE WHY?

Let's start with the "why." Note writing developed to serve a vital clinical role. Remembering the rationale behind documentation can help the process feel more productive and result in the creation of better notes.

Note Writing Serves 3 Main Purposes

- Capturing the narrative by:
  - Telling the story that brings data to life
  - Humanizing the patient as someone with a life and connections outside of their medical problems
  - Making the patient "stickier," or more memorable, by relating unique aspects of their story, which also breeds empathy and improves outcomes
- Communicating with others, including:
  - Physicians and other healthcare workers, allowing them to understand a patient's issues in a succinct and reliable way
  - Evaluators, giving them insight into how trainees think and what they know
  - Patients, who have access to the EMR and can read their own notes
- Funding healthcare:
  - Insurers use documentation to help determine reimbursement for services rendered

FUNDAMENTAL FIRST CONCEPTS

- Always review primary data firsthand.
  - Prior notes may inform your initial understanding of a patient, but take the time to verify this understanding by talking with the patient, examining them, and reviewing primary objective data.

- Helps correct cognitive biases, such as anchoring
- Prevents magnification of misinformation
- Allows for identification of missed information
- Fundamentally: **Trust. But verify.**
- Do not write anything in the chart that you would not want your patient to read.
  - Be accurate and use words that are appropriately descriptive and not pejorative.
  - The Health Insurance Portability and Accountability Act (HIPAA) of 1996 gave patients the legal right to access their medical records.
  - As of April 2021, all US healthcare systems are required to electronically share clinical notes with patients at no charge as a part of the 21st Century Cures Act.
- Recognize that the note is a legal document.
  - Document everything that occurs in an accurate fashion.
  - Negligence is often inferred from undocumented events and can form the basis of litigation; as the adage goes, "If it's not documented, it didn't happen."
  - The least credible records are those that are internally inconsistent or incomplete.

THE NITTY GRITTY

There are 2 main types of notes:
- History and physical (H&P)
  - A comprehensive note written when a patient is seen for the first time in a new setting such as a hospitalization or a new clinic
- Progress note (hospital) or follow-up note (clinic)
  - A more targeted follow-up note on an established patient

The format for each of these note types is detailed below. It is worth recognizing that most EMRs use templates that prepopulate the note field with many of the categories described below. This can serve as a helpful reminder system, although it may also create sections that are not needed or omit important areas. EMRs can also auto-import data (eg, medication lists), which may be useful (if accurate) or may perpetuate note bloat if this data is extraneous or incorrect.

As with many other elements of medical education, it is useful to ask for guidance when you are working in a new environment. Inquire about expectations around note-writing. If novel approaches are used and/or you do not grasp the reasoning behind a particular format, ask why. Understanding the rationale for any approach is a critical part of learning and developing your own style. Throughout this chapter, *Examples* are provided for the most common types of notes.

HISTORY AND PHYSICAL (H&P)

Chief Concern (CC)

- A few words that capture the primary reason for a clinical encounter.
- Traditionally referred to as the "chief complaint," "chief concern" is now preferred as a less pejorative and confrontational alternative.
- The Centers for Medicare and Medicaid Services recommends that the CC be "in the patient's own words," but this is not a strict requirement.
- A CC should seldom be more than 10 words.

Examples

CC: Worsening chest pain

CC: "I'm here because my chest hurts."

History of Present Illness (HPI)

- The story of how and why a patient ended up in a clinical setting, described in detail in Chapter 1.
- Should include details about the core elements of the CC, which can be captured by the following:
  - Onset, duration, location and radiation, intensity, what makes it better or worse, characteristics, changes over time, associated symptoms, what worries them and why today.
  - For those favoring mnemonics, **OLD CARTS** can be a useful tool: **O**nset, **L**ocation and radiation, **D**uration, **C**haracter, **A**ggravating and **A**lleviating factors, **R**elated symptoms, **T**iming, and **S**everity.
- The HPI is a **cultivated selection** of content.
  - Should only include **relevant information** that supports the assessment and plan that follow.
  - SHOULD NOT INCLUDE a patient's entire past medical history in the first line!
    By the time a reader learns that a "76-year-old man with a history of hypertension, hyperlipidemia, benign prostatic hypertrophy, bilateral cataracts, eczema, male-pattern baldness, dry mouth, chronic low back pain, tinea pedis, hypersomnia, and chronic fatigue" is presenting with "acute substernal crushing chest pain," the intended audience is adrift in a sea of irrelevant information.
- Should be written in **chronological order**, rather than jumping straight to the highest acuity piece of the story.
  - Identifying when a patient last felt "100%" can help distinguish between acute, subacute and chronic, which can significantly inform the differential diagnosis.
    - Cough, fever, and dyspnea in someone who felt perfectly well a week ago suggest acute pneumonia.
    - Cough, fever, and dyspnea in someone who has not felt well for months, with a recent 20-lb weight loss and weeks of fatigue, are more suggestive of an underlying malignancy or a subacute infection such as subacute bacterial endocarditis.
- Should include pertinent aspects of the rest of the H&P, including relevant Review of Systems (See Chapter 2 for details):
  - Pertinent ROS positives: Factors related to the most likely diagnoses
  - Pertinent ROS negatives: Factors that are not present, making alternate diagnoses less likely

Examples

If a case is relatively straightforward, the HPI can consist of a paragraph of prose.

HPI: Mr. Jones is a 40-year-old man with no significant medical history whose wife was diagnosed with COVID-19 one week prior to hospital presentation. Three days after his wife's diagnosis, Mr. Jones developed progressively worsening cough, fever, and dyspnea. Checking his oxygen saturation on his smart watch, he noted it was down to 90%, which is what prompted him to seek medical care on the day of admission. Prior to 3 days ago, he felt completely healthy. He denies anosmia, dysphagia, rhinorrhea, chest pain, and diarrhea.

If the relevant history is more complex, it is worth reformatting data relevant to the CC into a more digestible format. An example of an HPI for more complex case is provided here.

HPI: Mr. Smith is a 70-year-old man presenting with chest pain and worsening lower extremity edema with the following cardiomyopathy and coronary artery disease-related history:

- Status post 3-vessel CABG 11/2008
- Recurrent chest pain at rest 12/2015 → left heart catheterization and mid-LAD stent placement
- Recurrent chest pain at rest 1/2017 → left heart catheterization with no significant change; medical therapy continued with ASA, beta-blocker, and statin
- TTE 11/2018: EF of 40% with inferior and lateral akinesis
- Exercise Tolerance Test 11/2018 with no ischemia at 8 METS of activity

At baseline, he can walk vigorously for 8 to 9 blocks, sleep flat in his bed, and notes no swelling in his legs. He was in this usual state of health until two weeks prior to admission, when he began experiencing chest pain after walking only one block. He described the pain as a "pressure-like" sensation unlike his prior anginal pain. The pain does not radiate but does worsen when he lies down. He has also noted increased swelling in his legs over the same period and has had to use 3 pillows to sleep at night for the 5 nights prior to admission. One day prior to admission, he was so short of breath, he had to stop four times on his way to the bathroom from his bedroom. He reports having had three meals at Red Lobster in the last two weeks to celebrate a series of family events. He denies fevers, chills, cough, wheezing, nausea vomiting, recent travel, or sick contacts.

Past Medical History (PMH)

- A list of all prior illnesses a patient is known to have had.
- Includes important childhood illnesses and hospitalizations.
- The level of detail included in this section may vary by setting.
    - In a setting with a longitudinal provider–patient relationship, a more detailed PMH can help streamline subsequent care.
- Avoid perpetuating chart lore by verifying previously recorded diagnoses rather than blindly cutting and pasting an old PMH from another note.

Examples

PMH (Hospital Setting)
- Congestive heart failure with reduced EF (EF 40%); Admitted for CHF exacerbation 1/2019
- Diabetes mellitus
- Chronic Kidney Disease, Stage 3b
- Hypertension
- Hyperlipidemia
- Peptic ulcer disease
- Glaucoma
- Benign prostatic hyperplasia
- Peripheral arterial disease
- Anxiety

PMH (Primary Care Setting)

- Congestive heart failure with reduced EF (EF 40%): Secondary to ischemic cardiomyopathy. Presented with dyspnea, weight gain 2008, found to have 3-vessel disease, s/p CABG 11/2008 (LIMA → LAD, SVG → RCA, SVG → CX). Recurrent chest pain at rest 12/2015 → PCI: mid-LAD stent placement. Recurrent chest pain at rest 1/2017 → LHC with no targets. TTE 11/2018: EF of 40% with inferior and lateral akinesis, mild mitral regurgitation. Exercise Tolerance Test 11/2018 with no ischemia at 8 METS of activity. GDMT includes carvedilol, lisinopril, empagliflozin, torsemide, and atorvastatin, with some ongoing adherence challenges given distaste for urinary frequency associated with diuretics.
- Diabetes mellitus: Diagnosed 1996. Complicated by neuropathy, which is controlled with gabapentin. Well-controlled on metformin and empagliflozin. Highest A1C from 2001-2021: 7.4 on 4/5/17. Most recent A1c: 6.8.
- Chronic Kidney Disease, Stage 3b: Secondary to diabetes and hypertension. Baseline CR 1.2-1.4, EGFR 35-40. On lisinopril 40 mg po daily.
- Hypertension. First diagnosed in 2000. Well-controlled on carvedilol and lisinopril.
- Hyperlipidemia: 10/14/21 LDL 75, HDL 50, TG 78 on atorvastatin 80 mg po daily.
- Peptic ulcer disease: Status post upper GI bleed, 2020.
- Glaucoma: Followed by Dr. Green in UCSD Ophthalmology, on latanoprost since 2018.
- Benign prostatic hyperplasia: Started on tamsulosin 0.4 mg 6/2017 with improvement in symptoms.
- Peripheral arterial disease: s/p LLE angioplasty on 9/18/19, on daily aspirin. On statin as above.
- Anxiety: For which he takes Anxie-T OTC 1 tab PO daily with reportedly good effect.

Past Surgical History (PSH)

- A list of all past surgeries, along with their rough date
- Include any major traumas

Example
PSH
- S/P appendectomy 5/2017
- S/P MVA 4/1999 with left shoulder fracture treated nonoperatively
- S/P lap chole 12/1995 complicated by SBO requiring lysis of adhesions 1/2021

Medications (Meds)

- A list of **all** prescribed medications, over-the-counter medications, and integrative medicine therapies.
- Includes dosage, frequency, and adherence.
- Be wary of cutting and pasting medication lists or auto-importing them through an EMR template unless you **reconcile the source data firsthand.**
  - Discontinued medications commonly linger on lists (eg, a short course of azithromycin appearing as "active" for months afterward).
  - Medications prescribed outside of a given healthcare system may be missing.
- It can be useful to group medications by indication, in particular for students who are still early in process of learning about which meds are used for each situation. For advanced note writers, meds are simply listed, with a notation about indication for each sometimes added for clarity.

Example

Current Medications (by indication)

Heart Failure with Reduced Ejection Fraction (HFrEF)

- Carvedilol 25 mg PO BID
- Lisinopril 40 mg po daily
- Atorvastatin 80 mg po daily
- Empagliflozin 10 mg po daily
- Torsemide 80 mg PO daily; reports missing 2-3 doses per week
- Potassium chloride 20 mEq PO BID

Pain Control (neuropathy)

- Gabapentin 300 mg PO tid
- Acetaminophen 650 mg PO q6h PRN; takes 2-3 tabs daily

Coronary Artery Disease (CAD) and Peripheral Vascular Disease

- Aspirin 81 mg PO daily
- Atorvastatin 80 mg PO qhs

Peptic Ulcer Disease

- Pantoprazole 40 mg po daily

Glaucoma

- Latanoprost 0.005% 1 drop ou qhs

Benign Prostatic Hyperplasia

- Tamsulosin 0.4 mg po qhs

Anxiety

- Anxie-T OTC 1 tab PO daily (20 mg magnesium, 200 mg L-theanine, 100 mg *Theobroma cacao*, 100 mg Withania somnifera, 100 mg gamma-aminobutyric acid, 100 mg kavalactones, 100 mg theobromine)

Allergies/Reactions (All/RXNs)

- Many adverse reactions are NOT true allergies, but rather intolerances; all offending agents are recorded, along with specifics of the allergy or intolerance.

Example

All/RXNs

Sulfa → anaphylaxis

Ibuprofen → dry eyes

Social History (SHx)

- A broad category, including information that informs both the differential diagnosis of the acute problem and proactive planning for ongoing care.
- A complete social history can include:
  - Alcohol intake: Specify the type, quantity, frequency, and duration.
  - Tobacco use: Include type, "pack-year" history (number of packs × years smoked), and quit date if relevant.
  - Other substance use: Specify type, frequency, and duration.
  - Marital/relationship status; intimate partner violence (IPV) screen.

- Sexual history: Include details about types of activity, protection, and history of sexually transmitted infections (STIs).
- Work history: Type, duration, and exposures.
- Home environment: Specify location, cohabitors, and community support.
- Functional level: Ability to perform activities of daily living (ADLs) and instrumental activities of daily living (IADLs).
- Other: Travel, pets, and hobbies.
- Healthcare maintenance: Age- and sex-appropriate screening and vaccinations.
- Military history: Service branch, type of work, and deployments.
- Religion and spirituality: Identified faith and any associated implications for care.

Example

SHx

- Alcohol intake: 4 12-oz beers weekly; no history of heavy use.
- Tobacco use: 30 pack year cigarette history starting at age 20, quit in 1996.
- Other substance use: Edible THC use 2-3 times per month.
- Marital/relationship status: Married, negative partner violence screen.
- Sexual history: Monogamous with wife of 20 years, uses condoms, no reported history of STIs.
- Work history: Electrician with the City of Vista × 30 years.
- Home environment: Lives with wife in a single-level house with no steps to enter in El Cajon; 2 daughters live nearby.
- Functional level: Independent with ADLs and IADLs.
- Other: No recent travel, has had a beagle for 10 years, no other pets, enjoys woodworking.
- Healthcare maintenance: Colonoscopy 10/2020 with recommendation for repeat in 10 years, influenza vaccine 10/2021, pneumovax 10/2019, COVID-19 Moderna 12/2020, 1/2021, 10/2021.
- Military history: In the Marine Corps from 1966-1973, electrician/utilities chief. Combat deployments to Okinawa and Chulai, Vietnam. + exposure to Agent Orange.
- Religion: Jehovah's Witness; does not accept transfusion of any blood products.

Family History (FHx)

- A focused recording of illnesses within the patient's immediate family.
- Focuses particularly on identifying cancer, vascular disease, and other potentially heritable diseases among first-degree relatives.
- Patients may not always know the exact diagnoses, but these can be described as best as can be recalled.
- Only information relevant to a particular patient's presentation needs to be included.
  - For instance, in a centenarian presenting with cellulitis, it would be appropriate to report: "No relevant family history given patient age and current presentation."

Example

FHx

- Mother – died age 67 of GI (stomach?) cancer
- Father – died in his early 70s with alcohol use disorder and diabetes
- Denies family history of heart disease

Obstetrical History

- Where appropriate, an enumeration of number of pregnancies, live births, duration of pregnancies, complications, spontaneous and/or therapeutic abortions, and birth control.

Example

Obstetrical History

- G2, P1, A1 [2 pregnancies, 1 live birth, 1 abortion]; currently using NuvaRing for birth control

Review of Systems (ROS)

- Often written as a list reflecting the system-based questions asked of the patient.
- The most pertinent positives and negatives should be included in the HPI, as they help to inform the possible diagnoses. See Chapter 2, ROS, for additional details.
- Early in training, it can be useful to record a full ROS in the H&P so that evaluators are aware that a comprehensive assessment was truly completed and to gain familiarity with the questions.

Example of a Comprehensive ROS

ROS

Constitutional: Weight stable, no fatigue

Eyes: No changes in vision, no pain in eyes

Ear, nose, mouth, throat: Denies sore throat, dysphagia, ear pain, nasal discharge

Cardiovascular: Chest pain and peripheral edema as noted in HPI

Respiratory: Dyspnea on exertion as noted in HPI

Gastrointestinal: Good appetite, no heartburn, no diarrhea, no abdominal pain, regular bowel movements

Genitourinary: No incontinence, frequency, urgency, nocturia, flank pain

Endo: Denies heat/cold intolerance, weight changes, polyuria, polydipsia

Heme/Onc: Denies unusual bleeding, bruising, clotting

MSK: Denies joint pain, swelling, muscle aches

Skin: No new rashes or sores, no hair loss

Neurologic: Denies numbness, tingling, tremors

Psychiatric: Denies memory loss, low mood, anxiety

Physical Exam (PEx)

- Generally formatted as a list of observed findings, beginning with vital signs.
- While not all the elements below are included in every PEx, the **order** listed is generally fixed.
- Only include the elements that you actually performed.

Example

PEx

Vitals: Temp 97.2 F, BP 116/78, HR 92, RR 16, O_2 96% RA

Height: 74 inches; weight: 191 pounds; BMI: 25

General: Pleasant older man lying back on gurney in no acute distress, breathing comfortably, conversant

HEENT: NCAT, EOMI, PERRLA, oropharynx clear with no lesions, moist mucous membranes, nonpalpable thyroid, no cervical lymphadenopathy

Pulmonary: + dullness to percussion at the right base, + crackles halfway up the chest bilaterally, no wheezing, no cough noted

Cardiac: RRR, 2/6 holosystolic murmur at apex radiating to axilla, +S3, no S4; PMI displaced laterally toward axilla; carotid pulses 2+ bilaterally, no bruits; JVP 12 cm

Gastrointestinal: Abdomen soft, nondistended, nontender with active bowel sounds, no hepatosplenomegaly

Genitourinary: Penile pouch in place; clear urine in bag, no suprapubic fullness, no CVA tenderness

Musculoskeletal: No joint swelling or erythema

Extremities: 3+ edema to sacrum, warm, no cyanosis or clubbing noted

Pulses: 2+ femoral pulses bilaterally, 1+ PT/DP bilaterally

Skin: Multiple tattoos, no rashes or lesions noted, peripheral IV in right arm, dressing clean/dry/intact

Neuro:

Motor: 5/5 strength in major flexors/extensors in all extremities

Sensory: Distal sensation in legs intact to light touch, pin prick; proprioception toes normal bilaterally; vibration intact at IP joint bilateral great toes

Reflexes: 2+ and symmetric bilaterally: biceps, triceps, brachioradialis, patellar, Achilles

Coordination: Finger to nose testing intact bilateral

Gait: Normal narrow-based gait using FWW, slow with frequent pauses to catch breath

Psych: Alert and appropriate, oriented to self, place, calendar date, purpose

Labs and Data

- A list of relevant labs, imaging, and procedures.
- Be wary of auto-importing data, an option in many EMRs. If using a data-importing shortcut, we recommend:
  - Choosing a format with as little extraneous clutter as possible (eg, most clinicians know the normal values for basic labs, and these ranges can be left out).
  - Altering the data in some way from its imported format to ensure that you have deliberately considered all of the information included in the note.
- An alternative to importing data through the EMR is to manually enter relevant data, as in the example below.
  - In this case, it is also possible to indicate that specific named labs were reviewed and include only the data points of greatest interest.

Example

Labs and Data

Na 128, Cl 96, Bun 59, Glucose 92, K 4.4, CO_2 40.8, CR 1.4 (EGFR 35), WBC 7.9, PLT 349, Hgb 14.7, MCV 96, Alk phos 72, Total Protein 5.6, Alb 3.5, T Bili 0.5, Alt 17, Ast 52, troponin <0.01, BNP 1610.

ECG: NSR at 74, q-waves v1-v5, no acute ST-T wave changes. No change compared with 6/2021 ECG.

CXR: Prominent pulmonary vessels with moderate interstitial edema and moderate right pleural effusion. Cardiomegaly. No parenchymal infiltrates.

Assessment and Plan (A&P)

- The summative analysis and plan stemming from all previously presented subjective and objective data.

- There are 2 main ways to structure the A&P:
  - By named problem; For example: # CHF exacerbation, # diabetes mellitus, etc.
  - By organ system; For example: # neuro, # cardiac, # pulmonary, # renal, etc.
- Every problem or system should have an assessment *and* a plan.
  - Too often, the assessment portion of notes is lacking, which can lead to inappropriate treatments. For example, an A&P that reads, "CHF exacerbation – daily weights, Lasix 20, fluid restriction," leaves out the critical questions of WHY the decompensation occurred, which is critical both for correcting the current pathology and preventing future exacerbations. In the examples that follow, diagnostic and therapeutic plans are presented separately for the sake of clarity. In practice, they are usually contained within a single plan.
- The end of this section should also include notation of diet, deep vein thrombosis (DVT) prophylaxis (ppx), code status, medical decision-making capacity, and disposition.

Example (System Based – ordered primarily head to toe)

Mr. Smith is 70-year-old man with ischemic cardiomyopathy presenting with subacute dyspnea and edema consistent with acute-on-chronic HFrEF exacerbation.

Neuro: Alert and oriented, without evidence of delirium at this time, but given age and multiple comorbidities, is at higher risk for delirium. Neurologic exam nonfocal. Pain well-controlled on acetaminophen as needed. Denies significant anxiety at this time, but will continue to monitor, as we are unable to given his OTC anti-anxiety supplement inpatient. Diabetic neuropathic pain is controlled on gabapentin.

- Continue delirium precautions.
- Continue acetaminophen 650 mg PO q6h PRN and gabapentin 300 mg po BID, monitoring daily renal function as noted below.

Cardiac: Progressive dyspnea and edema over several weeks are most consistent with heart failure in the context of his increased weight, pulmonary congestion, JVP of 12, and elevated BNP. His renal disease is a less likely explanation for his extensive edema as his BUN/Cr remain at their baseline. Similarly, he has nothing to suggest significant liver disease in his history, on exam, or in his initial workup.

The question is what has led to this decompensation in his cardiac function. The most likely possibilities include: (1) worsening LV function, (2) another MI, (3) worsening valvular disease, (4) poor compliance with medications, and/or (5) excess salt and water intake. There is no evidence by history, ECG, or enzymes for current ACS, and his valvular disease does not appear severe enough to be causing symptoms. Given this, the most likely precipitant of his failure is a combination of dietary indiscretion in a patient with depressed EF.

Diagnostic Plan:
- Repeat echo to evaluate for possible drop in LV function.

Therapeutic Plan:
- Strict I/Os; daily weights
- Fluid restriction to 2 L/day
- Low-salt diet
- Lasix 80 mg IV with goal diuresis of 2-3 L/day
- Continue lisinopril 40 mg PO daily and Coreg 25 mg PO BID
- Continue aspirin 81 mg po daily
- Check BMP daily while diuresing
- Education about appropriate diet via nutrition consult

Pulmonary: Dyspnea, crackles on exam, and noted O_2 requirement are likely due to pulmonary congestion from LV dysfunction (above). He has no fever, cough, wheezing, pleurisy, or chest x-ray findings to suggest another primary pulmonary process (eg, infection, COPD exacerbation, PE, pneumothorax).
- Diuresis as above; O_2 to maintain sat greater than 95%

Renal: CKD stage 3 from DM (on basis of prior elevated protein/creat ratio) and hypertension. Currently at baseline, with no evidence of AKI, cardiogenic or otherwise. BPH well controlled on tamsulosin.
- Continue to monitor BID chem 7 w/diuresis
- Continue tamsulosin 0.4 mg po QHS.
- Strict I/Os, as above

Endo: History of diabetes controlled on oral medications. Most recent A1C 6.8.
- Hold metformin and empagliflozin tonight while monitoring renal response to aggressive diuresis. Anticipate restarting in short order however, if renal function remains stable.
- Low-intensity sliding scale insulin coverage + FSBG qAC/HS.
- Carb Consistent 2100 calorie diet, salt restricted, as above.

Infectious Disease: No evidence of infection at this time. Pulmonary symptoms appear to be secondary to CHF exacerbation. No fevers/chills, no new urinary symptoms, no diarrhea or rashes. No antibiotics indicated. Will continue to monitor.

Heme: Anemia is correlated with worsened outcomes in CHF, but hemoglobin within normal limits at present. At increased risk for anemia given CKD, but no indication for further work-up at this time.

GI: History of PUD, but no evidence of active bleeding at this time. Continue pantoprazole 40 mg po daily per home regimen.

HEENT: History of glaucoma. No new visual concerns on admission. Continue outpatient latanaprost.

FEN/GI: Low salt, carb consistent diet as above. Regular texture, thin liquids. Daily lytes while diuresing as noted above.

DVT ppx: Given relative immobility and deconditioning, will start enoxaparin 40 mg sq daily and order PT consult to encourage early, regular mobilization.

Capacity: Patient does have medical decision-making capacity at the time of this note.

Disposition: Anticipate discharge home in 3 days, with close follow-up from heart failure service to assist with maintaining clinical stability, preventing readmissions.

Code Status: FULL CODE/FULL CARE.

PROGRESS NOTE

SOAP Note Formulation
- The standardized format for day-to-day progress notes (PNs) uses the **S**ubjective-**O**bjective-**A**ssessment-**P**lan (or **SOAP**) framework, first codified by Larry Weed in the 1960s.
- Be wary of copy-and-pasting the H&P as a template for daily PNs, as this can lead to note bloat and chart lore.

The sections of the PN are composed as follows.

Subjective: Information a Patient Self-Reports

- No need to recapitulate the entire HPI, PMH, FHx, etc., enumerated in the H&P.
- Can be brief, usually starting with an identifying sentence (the "one liner"), recent/overnight events, and the patient's subjective report from interview.

Example

Mr. Smith is 70-year-old man with ischemic cardiomyopathy presenting with acute-on-chronic HFrEF exacerbation secondary to medication and dietary nonadherence, slowly improving with IV diuresis.

Overnight events: Night float called for 6-beat run of asymptomatic VT on telemetry.

Mr. Smith reports feeling better this morning. Reports that he is breathing somewhat better than yesterday and thinks his swelling is improved. Is having a hard time adjusting to the bland diet, however. No chest pain, no dizziness/lightheadedness. No cough, fevers/chills.

Objective: Information Obtained on Exam or by Laboratory or Radiographic Analysis

- Consists primarily of the physical exam, including a review of recent vitals, as well as any new laboratory or radiographic data.
- Vitals are often paired with input/output (I/O) counts and blood sugar logs.
- **USE CAUTION** in copying forward any physical exam findings, as these should change as a patient's condition evolves.

Example

PEx:

Vitals (reviewed over prior 24 h): Afebrile $\times$ 24 h, Tmax 97.9, BP 100s-110s/70s-80s, HR 80s-97, O_2 98%

Weight 191 pounds 6/11/21 $\rightarrow$ 187 pounds 6/12/21

I/Os 2.4 L/3.9 L, net −1.5 L

Finger Stick Blood Glucose (FSBG): AM 160, noon 187, PM 145, HS 148

General: Pleasant older man sitting up on the side of the bed eating breakfast, in no acute distress, conversant

HEENT: NCAT, oropharynx clear with no lesions, moist mucous membranes

Pulmonary: + dullness to percussion at the right base, + crackles about one-third of the way up the chest bilaterally, no wheezing, no cough noted

Cardiac: RRR, 2/6 holosystolic murmur at apex radiating to axilla, +S3, no S4; JVP 10 cm

Gastrointestinal: Abdomen soft, nondistended, nontender with active bowel sounds, no hepatosplenomegaly

Genitourinary: Penile pouch in place; clear urine in bag, no suprapubic fullness, no CVA tenderness

Extremities: 3+ edema to the midthigh bilaterally

Labs and Data:

BMP and CBC from 6/11/21 reviewed revealing Na 130, K 3.2, bicarb 26, Cl 96, BUN 60, Cre 1.4, glucose 137, Mg 1.7

TTE 6/11/21 with stable EF of 40%, mild mitral regurgitation, no new focal wall motion abnormalities

Assessment and Plan

- Should **change as needed for each day** as you evaluate a patient's response to various therapeutic interventions and incorporate data from new diagnostic interventions.
- The orders of problems can change depending on the acuity of a given problem on a given day.

Example (Problem-based, ordered by relative importance)

Mr. Smith is 70-year-old man with ischemic cardiomyopathy presenting with acute-on-chronic HFrEF exacerbation secondary to medication nonadherence and dietary indiscretion, overall doing well with aggressive diuresis.

Acute exacerbation of chronic ischemic HFrEF: Symptoms improving as expected with IV diuresis, suggesting that the initial diagnosis of medication/diet-related exacerbation was likely correct. Did not quite meet 2-3 L diuresis goal yesterday, however, so will increase Lasix dosing to BID. Mr. Smith dislikes the low-salt diet, so will ask dietary to meet with him again to discuss way to infuse more flavor into his meals without adding salt, as this will be a crucial part of his management on discharge. No evidence of worsening valvular disease or new focal wall motion abnormalities on TTE. Was noted to have low potassium and magnesium this morning with a few beats of VT overnight, so will increase lab check to BID, particularly given increase in diuretic regimen.

- Continue strict I/Os, daily weights
- Continue fluid restriction to 2 L/day
- Continue low-salt diet
- Lasix 80 mg IV, increasing from daily to BID 6/11/21 with goal diuresis of 2-3 L/day
- GDMT: Continue lisinopril 40 mg PO daily, Coreg 25 mg PO BID and atorvastatin 80 mg po daily; continue holding empagliflozin for now given increasing diuresis
- Increase renal function check to BID while aggressively diuresing; replete PRN with goal K 4, Mg 2
- Will ask Nutrition to discuss further way to increase flavor in a low-salt diet

CKD stage 3 b: secondary to DM (on basis of prior elevated protein/creatinine ratio) and hypertension. Remains at baseline even with diuresis. Will continue to monitor.

- Continue to monitor BID chem 7 w/diuresis; increasing to BID checks 6/11/22
- Strict I/Os, as above

Diabetes mellitus, type 2: controlled on oral medications at home. Most recent A1C 6.8. FSBG at goal of 120-180 inpatient. Renal function remains stable with diuresis.

- Held metformin and empagliflozin on admission given increase in diuresis; if renal function remains stable, anticipate restarting soon
- Continue low-intensity sliding scale insulin coverage + FSBG qAC/HS
- Carb consistent 2100-calorie diet, salt restricted, as above

Coronary artery disease and peripheral vascular disease: No evidence of acute occlusion in either vascular system. Continue aspirin 81 mg po daily and atorvastatin 80 mg po daily.

Benign prostatic hyperplasia: No evidence of retention at this time. Using external catheter given increased frequency related to IV diuresis. Continue tamsulosin 0.4 mg po qhs.

Peptic ulcer disease: No evidence of active bleeding at this time. Continue pantoprazole 40 mg po daily per home regimen.

\# Neuropathic pain: Secondary to diabetes. Well-controlled on gabapentin 300 mg po TID, which we will cautiously continued, continuing to monitor renal function, as noted above.

\# Glaucoma: No new visual symptoms at this time. Continue home latanaprost.

\# FEN/GI: Low-salt, carb consistent diet as above. Regular texture, thin liquids. BID lytes while diuresing as noted above.

\# DVT ppx: Given relatively immobility and deconditioning, continue enoxaparin 40 mg sq daily and daily PT to encourage regular mobilization.

\# Capacity: Patient does have medical decision-making capacity at the time of this note.

\# Disposition: Anticipate discharge home in 1-2 days, with close follow-up from heart failure service to assist with maintaining clinical stability, preventing readmissions.

\# Code Status: FULL CODE/FULL CARE

SPECIALTY/CONSULT AND FOLLOW-UP NOTES

- Different specialties can have unique note documentation. Some examples include the following:
  - Surgical notes tend to be much more succinct than those of internists.
  - Ophthalmology notes use diagrams to capture specialized eye exams.
  - In a renal clinic, the assessment and plan often include a standardized set of elements that reflect the multiple systems affected by kidney dysfunction. This includes: chronic kidney disease (CKD) stage, dialysis access, anemia, acid/base, bone mineral density, and hypertension.
- When acting as a consulting service, there are a few customary practices:
  - Word the plan in terms of recommendations rather than orders (eg, "Would recommend starting lisinopril 10 mg PO daily").
  - Thank the service requesting the consult for involving you in the care of a patient.
  - Indicate your intention to continue following a patient (and at what interval) or whether you are signing off.
- Progress notes for a patient seen in clinic are used to document ongoing care. They follow the SOAP format described earlier under Daily PNs. A few additional elements to highlight include the following:
  - The breadth of information presented and focus of this note depend on the type of clinic and the areas of care for which they have responsibility.
  - The note often begins by highlighting important interval events (eg, studies completed, visits to specialty clinicians, ED visits, hospitalizations) that might have occurred since the last visit. New symptoms or any changes in those previously described are then noted.
  - Any elements of the physical exam that were performed should be documented.
  - Medications and adherence should be reviewed during each visit.
  - Important labs or imaging results should be noted.
  - It is not necessary to restate the PMH, PSH, etc., as those elements can be found in the initial H&P and are not typically relevant to a follow-up visit.
  - The assessment and plan should be appropriate to the number of issues being followed in that clinic.
- In any setting, defer to the guidance of the senior provider as to the best way to document.
  - Different specialties will often have special templates for specific clinics or consult recommendations.

PARTING PEARLS

1. **Bigger is not better.** Pay attention to the "signal-to-noise" ratio and deliberately cultivate the story to include only what is needed to make a case for the leading diagnoses and treatment plans.

2. **Trust but verify.** Avoid perpetuating chart lore by verifying that there is objective data to support prior claims in the chart.

3. **Think "copy and EDIT," not "copy and paste."** Avoid including unexamined or erroneous information in your notes.

4. **Don't pick a fight in the chart.** Documentation is no place to air grievances with colleagues, patients, or staff. Conflict mitigation should be done verbally outside the written medical record.

5. **Use calendar dates.** Avoid using words and phrases such as "today," "yesterday," or "a week ago," as these terms lose their meaning in a note that can be accessed an hour, year, or decade after it is written.

6. **Avoid including ethnicity in the HPI.** Think carefully about whether any demographic information is critical to refining your differential diagnosis or treatment before including it, as this can perpetuate bias without meaningfully improving clinical reasoning.

7. **Don't invent acronyms.** It is appropriate to use abbreviations you have seen repeatedly used in other documentation (eg, SBO, small bowel obstruction; NCAT, normocephalic, atraumatic; EOMI, extraocular movements intact; PERRLA, pupils equal and reactive to light and accommodation). But avoid fabricating new acronyms, as it can be very confusing (eg, using ADH in place of "anticipate discharge home").

8. **Solicit feedback.** Be active in getting feedback on your notes from residents and attendings. This is the best way of assuring that what you're providing aligns with what's expected and needed.

9. **Artificial Intelligence (AI) has arrived.** Be prepared for further revolutions in note-writing in the era of AI, remaining mindful of the pitfalls that accompanied the last digital transformation of documentation.

BIBLIOGRAPHY

Aronson M. The purpose of the medical record: why Lawrence Weed still matters. *Am J Med.* 2019;132(11):1256-1257.

Berwick D, Winickoff D. The truth about doctor's handwriting: a prospective study. *BMJ.* 1996;313:1657-1658.

Centers for Medicare and Medicaid Services. Evaluation and management services guide book. Accessed April 20, 2023. https://www.cms.gov/outreach-and-education/medicare-learning-network-mln/mlnproducts/downloads/eval-mgmt-serv-guide-icn006764.pdf.

Collier R. Electronic health records contributing to physician burnout. *CMAJ.* 2017;189(45): E1405-E1406.

Decety J. Why empathy has a beneficial impact on others in medicine: unifying theories. *Front Behav Neurosci.* 2015;8:457.

Gillum RF. From papyrus to the electronic tablet: a brief history of clinical med record. *Am J Med.* 2013;126:853-857.

Goldberg C. Practical guide to clinical medicine: outpatient clinics. Accessed April 20, 2023. https://meded.ucsd.edu/clinicalmed/write.html.

Goldberg C. Practical guide to clinical medicine: write-ups. Accessed April 20, 2023. https://meded.ucsd.edu/clinicalmed/write.html.

Heath C, Heath D. *Made to Stick 2008*. London: Arrow Books.

Henry J, Pylypchuk Y, Searcy T, Patel V. *Adoption of Electronic Health Record Systems among U.S. Non-Federal Acute Care Hospitals: 2008–2015*. ONC Data Brief, no.35. Washington, DC: Office of the National Coordinator for Health Information Technology; May 2016.

Hirschtick RE. A piece of my mind: copy and paste. *JAMA*. 2006;295(20):2335-2336.

Oxentenko A, West CP, Popkave C, Weinberger SE, Kolars JC. Time spent on clinical documentation: a survey of internal medicine residents and program directors. *Arch Intern Med*. 2010;170(4):377-380.

Podder V, et al. SOAP Notes. 2022 Aug 29. In: StatPearls [Internet]. Treasure Island, FL: StatPearls Publishing; 2023.

Public Health Law. Medical records as a plaintiff's weapon. Accessed April 20, 2023. https://biotech.law.lsu.edu/map/MedicalRecordsasaPlaintiffsWeapon.html.

Rule A, Bedrick S, Chiang M, et al. Length and redundancy of outpatient progress notes across a decade at an academic medical center. *JAMA Netw Open*. 2021;4(7):e2115334.

Siegler EL, Adelman R. Copy and paste: a remediable hazard of electronic health records. *J Am Med Inform Assoc*. 2004;11(4):300-309.

Sinek S. Start with why, but know how. In: Sinek S. *Start With Why: How Great Leaders Inspire Everyone to Take Action*. London: Penguin Books; 2009.

Sokol D, Hettige S. Poor handwriting remains a significant problem in medicine. *J R Soc Med*. 2006;99(12):645-646.

Thielke S, Hammond K, Helbig S. Copying and pasting of examinations within the electronic medical record. *Int J Med Inform*. 2007;76(suppl 1):S122-S128.

Thoreau H. *Walden, or Life in the Woods*. 1854.

US Food and Drug Administration. Twenty-first century cures act. Accessed April 20, 2023. https://www.fda.gov/regulatory-information/selected-amendments-fdc-act/21st-century-cures-act.

Verghese A. Culture shock: patient as icon, icon as patient. *N Engl J Med*. 2008;359:2748-2751.

23

Oral Case Presentations

Meghan Sebasky, MD and Brian Kwan, MD

The oral case presentation is a skill central to physician-physician communication and provides a natural venue for the teaching and evaluation of the clinical competency of learners. A well-done presentation:

- Advances patient care
- Provides an efficient vehicle for collaboration and idea sharing
- Highlights areas of uncertainty to further individual or team-directed learning
- Promotes self-reflection on gaps in knowledge
- Provides space for iterative feedback toward skill refinement

Within this chapter, we review the core elements of an oral case presentation and provide examples about how to adapt the content to different settings (ie, the context). The structure of presentations varies from service to service (eg, medicine vs surgery), among subspecialties (eg, cardiology vs gynecologic oncology), and between environments (eg, inpatient vs outpatient). Content delivery changes with different audiences (eg, ward attending vs specialty consultant) or with recipients' familiarity with the patient case (eg, new patient evaluation vs daily update on rounds).

Before getting into the "how," it is important to recognize some of the reasons why mastering an oral case presentation can be challenging.

BLENDING MULTIPLE SKILLS

The oral case presentation requires that a presenter demonstrate aptitude across a range of clinical skills. At the most basic level, a presenter must accurately gather data, perform an appropriate physical exam, and organize the obtained information into a formed clinical impression.

These clinical skills span multiple core competencies (**Figure 23-1**), including the following:

- Patient care (history, physical exam, clinical reasoning, management)
- Medical knowledge (applied foundational sciences, therapeutic knowledge, knowledge of diagnostic testing)
- Practice-based learning and improvement (evidence-based and informed practice)
- Interpersonal and communication skills (patient- and family-centered communication, interprofessional and team communication)
- Professionalism (accountability/conscientiousness)

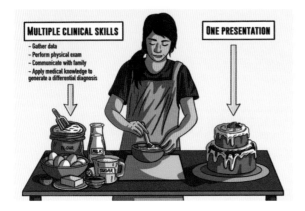

FIGURE 23-1 • A trainee, much like a baker, must combine each ingredient, or skill, to create the final masterpiece. (Reproduced with permission from Cathy Cichon, MD.)

A single shortcoming in any domain has the potential to alter the end product. An effective oral presentation requires fluid synthesis of building blocks coupled with deliberate practice to produce expert delivery. As learners gain mastery over different clinical skills, the oral case presentation tends to evolve in parallel.

NEGOTIATING PROFESSIONAL RELATIONSHIPS

It is important to recognize that while the content and structure of oral case presentations are often explicitly taught, the actual refinement typically occurs via trial and error. Inherent in the mastery of the oral presentation is actively navigating different professional relationships in the practice environment with each recipient possessing their own (sometimes quirky!) presentation preferences (**Figure 23-2**).

Because the oral case presentation is an important way by which teachers gauge a student's clinical performance, students naturally look for ways to adapt their presentation to a preceptor's liking. As a novice who is looking for rules to organize the often-overwhelming mass of data, a teacher's comment to the student can dramatically shape how a student's

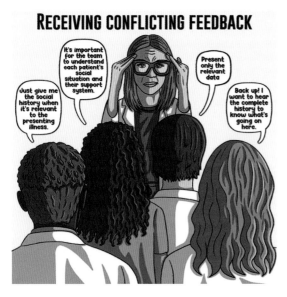

FIGURE 23-2 • It can be extremely difficult navigating contradictory feedback received from different sources. (Reproduced with permission from Cathy Cichon, MD.)

TABLE 23-1 • Challenges for Students Interpreting and Incorporating Feedback About Presentations	
Attending Comment	Maladaptive Student Rule Creation
"Shorten your presentation."	Presents in incomplete sentences or disjointed phrases; speaks in rapid fashion 2 times normal speed
"Present without your notes."	Prioritizes rote memorization over other components of the presentation, such as clinical reasoning
"Skip the review of systems."	Interprets that the review of systems is "never relevant" in a presentation and may omit in other contexts (eg, data gathering or documentation)

rulebook on oral presentations is formed and can create unintended consequences. Let's go through some examples in **Table 23-1**.

Finally, let's consider the commonly given feedback of "Just present what is relevant." "Relevant data" go beyond relaying factually accurate information and require the presenter to actively process and adjust information based on the needs of the receiver. Further complicating this dynamic is the fact that different receivers may have varying interpretations of what actually is relevant.

CHANNELING YOUR PUBLIC SPEAKING

At the end of the day, an oral case presentation is a form of public speaking. Turning a good presentation into a great one may be dependent on other unique communication strategies that are less often taught in medical education. During a presentation, it is natural for the presenter to feel the stress of being on the hot seat, which may uncover underlying speaking tendencies.

Let's consider the auditory cues one might send during a presentation.

- Tone of voice: A voice that is too soft-spoken can be construed as mumbling, whereas an overly booming tone might be interpreted as obnoxious or disruptive.
- Variation in volume: A lack of variation in voice volume could be seen as monotone. Instead, consider how you might dial up or down the volume at points in the presentation you believe are important and should be highlighted.
- Cadence: This refers to the tempo or rhythm of the presentation. If we liken it to music or dance, changes in pace can be utilized to emphasize important moments and to reengage your audience.
- Filler words: One of the most challenging habits to undo is the practice of using filler words (eg, "um," "uh," "like"). These fillers commonly exist in our everyday speech, although they are not normally noticeable. However, in a presentation, these words are often apparent to the listener and can derail the message being sent.

> PEARL: Record yourself doing a presentation and take a listen! What auditory cues did you find out you were sending, consciously or unconsciously?

Presenters also send many nonverbal cues through their posture, facial expressions, body movement, and gestures. Like auditory cues, these nonverbal signals can engage your listener and reinforce points that you want to get across. You might also unintentionally send nonverbal cues that detract from the presentation. For example, some people naturally speak with their hands, and when nervous, they may begin flailing their arms! Your audience will also frequently send you nonverbal cues. Expert presenters will watch for that feedback to gauge the reaction of their audience and use it to adjust their message on the fly.

PEARL: Feeling anxious? Consider the following 2 strategies to calm and focus your energy!

- One of the most powerful auditory cues is "the pause." A masterful speaker carefully utilizes silence or deliberate pauses to accentuate content and maintain audience engagement. Additionally, a pause lets you catch your breath and calm any nervousness or anxiety. Use these moments to focus on your next words.
- A powerful nonverbal tool is the use of eye contact as it can help create connection with the listener and hone your focus.

TIME: A PRECIOUS COMMODITY

One of the greatest threats to learners attempting to refine their oral case presentation is the modern medical environment. Consider an outpatient clinic encounter where a half-hour visit is allotted for a new patient (at some sites, even this amount of time might be considered a luxury!). Incorporating a student into this process (interviewing, examining, and then presenting the patient) creates logistical challenges for the faculty, as they are also trying to keep their clinic running on time.

We will provide some guidelines on general expectations for the duration of each type of presentation, based on both anecdotal experience and the literature. However, it is important to note that time is just one measured component of an effective presentation. How you shorten a presentation to make it concise without leaving out important information is much more critical.

THE POWER OF WORDS

Recent studies have shown that the language we use when caring for patients can influence healthcare quality. For example, compare the phrase "37-year-old alcoholic" to "37-year-old person with alcohol use disorder." The former contains stigmatizing language that may engender negative attitudes toward a patient and can influence care delivery, as compared to the latter's neutral language. Furthermore, the use of words like "insists," "denies," or "claims" risks casting doubt on a patient's credibility and may propagate implicit biases. Similarly, using the phrase "quote unquote" may imply doubt or disbelief about the veracity of a patient's history.

When presenting patients, it is important to use patient-centered and neutral language that avoids imparting judgement. One way to reflect on whether a presentation might require alteration is to consider whether you would feel comfortable delivering it at the bedside in front of your patient.

GENERAL TIPS TO SUCCEED IN DELIVERING A STELLAR ORAL PRESENTATION

- Ask for guidance: At the start of any new rotation, ask your preceptor(s) what is expected in terms of presentations. Many clerkships provide guidance (eg, via documents, videos, orientation PowerPoints) to students about how they want presentations to be given, what to include, and time frames, among other parameters.
- Develop a standardized approach: In learning and repeating any skill, it is important to stick to a given format. Using a similar order and style for each patient every day makes it easier for a listener to follow, such that they can anticipate what is coming next and when they can expect to hear information. It also helps the presenter stay organized, develop a rhythm, and lessen the chance of omitting elements. When you rotate onto

a new service, recalibrate your presentation in the first few days and use feedback to further refine it.

- Tell a story: Perhaps another way to frame this is to present your argument. Presentations are the way we tell medical narratives to one another. When presenting, ask yourself if you have described the story accurately. Will the listener be able to "see" the patient the same way you do? Will they come to similar conclusions? Does the story flow and make sense?

- Complete versus concise: As outlined earlier, it takes time for an early learner to recognize what elements are important to include. Preceptors can also have different expectations that will require adjustment in real-time. When in doubt, prioritize relaying accurate and complete information, understanding that you will be trimming and adjusting your presentation in subsequent encounters.

- Prepare your content: Effective presentations require that you have thought through the case beforehand and understand the rationale for your conclusions and plan. Especially when starting out, give yourself extra time to process new data (eg, overnight events or consultant recommendations), bounce ideas off other team members, or seek additional information to clarify or refine your presentation (eg, online resources, literature search).

- Tap into the power of priming: For those who might be anxious about presentations, consider using the technique of priming, which is a way to get your mindset into a positive place before any presentation. Here is a sample routine that you can try: Before rounds, find a quiet place to ground yourself. Take a few deep breaths and notice your heartbeat. Think of something you are grateful for. Recall a time when you felt confident and accomplished. Visualize how terrific your presentation will be and how you will feel afterward.

- Consider your audience: Think about the clinical situation in which you are presenting so that you can tailor your presentation to the expectations of the recipients. For example, work rounds are clearly different from presenting a case at a conference and mandate a different style of presentation.

- Reflect and seek feedback: Don't just pay attention to your own presentations, but listen to others present as well. When done well, ask yourself, "Why was it good?" and try to incorporate those elements into your own presentation. When a presentation goes poorly, identify the specific things that made it ineffective and avoid those pitfalls. Seek feedback after you present from your listeners (eg, students, residents, faculty), and use that information to guide improvements for the next time.

- Practice, practice, practice: Do this on your own, with colleagues, and/or with anyone who will listen (and offer helpful commentary) before you present in front of other clinicians. Speaking "on the fly" is difficult, as rapidly organizing and delivering information in a clear and concise fashion is not a naturally occurring skill.

CONTENT AND CONTEXT OF ORAL PRESENTATIONS

When preparing an oral presentation, the first aspect to consider is the context in which you will be delivering it. The context will inform the length, format, and level of detail of your presentation as well as the relevant clinical information that should be included.

We will focus on oral presentations given in the following settings and situations:

- In the hospital
  - New admission: A patient admitted by you who is not yet known to your team
  - Holdover admission: A patient admitted by another team, usually the overnight crew, for whom you are assuming care and who is not yet known to your team
  - Daily rounds: A patient known to you and your team

- In the outpatient clinic
  - Initial primary care visit: An unknown patient who presents to establish care
  - Follow-up primary care visit: A known patient coming for a scheduled appointment
  - Acute primary care visit: A known or unknown patient presenting for a specific concern
  - Specialty clinic visit: A new or returning patient

The time parameters listed are general guidelines and will vary based on the complexity of the patient case, the experience of the presenter, and the preferences of the clinical preceptor. With practice, you will be able to present more concisely. Consider timing yourself to get a feel for how you are progressing, noting that time can really fly while giving a presentation!

With clinical experience, it will become more obvious which elements of the history, physical exam, labs, and imaging are relevant to a patient's chief concern. As your clinical reasoning skills grow, you will learn to discern which information should be presented (and which information omitted) to best "make a case" for the diagnosis or diagnoses you consider most likely.

Note that while the written history and physical directly informs the presentation (see Chapter 22, Medical Documentation), the oral presentation is not simply a reading of that document. Rather, the verbal presentation provides a more succinct summary of the key elements. The same applies to oral presentations for all components of healthcare that have written formats (eg, daily progress notes, clinic visits). The key components to include are highlighted below. Examples of presentations are provided at the end of this chapter.

IN THE HOSPITAL

While rotating in the inpatient setting, you will encounter new patients who you will follow longitudinally during their hospitalization. The oral presentation for new versus known patients has several important differences, which will be highlighted in the descriptions that follow.

The New Admission

After taking a comprehensive history and performing an exam for a new patient, thoroughly reviewing the medical record, and formulating an assessment and plan of care, you will need to introduce the patient to your team. Note that the alternating colors for the boxes (blue and pink) are to highlight different sections and time allotted for each.

Duration: 8-10 minutes		
30 seconds	Chief concern (CC) + problem representation (PR)	• One sentence, often referred to as the opening "one liner." • Highlights the reason patient presented to the hospital. This can include a direct quote from them. • The PR contains relevant patient demographics and background (*the who*), length and tempo of illness (*the when*), and clinical syndrome (*the what*).

(Continued)

Duration: 8-10 minutes (Continued)		
3 minutes	History of present illness (HPI)	• If the patient is not able to provide their own history, state the reason why and from whom/where the history was obtained. • Detail symptoms and events leading up to the patient's presentation in chronological order. • Give a thorough description of the characteristics of the patient's chief concern. See Chapter 1, History Taking, for more details. • Include positives and negatives from review of systems that are pertinent to chief concern. • Include a brief discussion of any directly related past medical history/recent hospitalizations that are necessary to better understand the chief concern. If, for example, the patient presents with symptoms suggestive of pneumonia and has untreated HIV infection, this should be made known early in the presentation as this information will critically inform the interpretation of data and formulation of the differential, as well as the diagnostic and therapeutic plans. • Include a brief synopsis of what occurred in the emergency department on the day of admission (eg, medications administered, imaging obtained).
	Review of systems (ROS)	• Do not repeat the portion of ROS discussed in HPI. • Report any other positive responses to an appropriate ROS. See Chapter 2, Review of Systems, for additional information about what questions to consider. • Report any pertinent negative responses.
2 minutes	Past medical history/ past surgical history (PMH/PSH)	• Omit conditions mentioned previously in HPI. • Mention all conditions that may affect patient's current hospitalization and management. • Note if any care is delivered via other health systems, highlighting overlapping and/or potentially redundant aspects. • Omit unrelated and/or minor conditions that will not affect current management (eg, toe surgery 20 years ago).
	Medications and allergies	• List all medications the patient is actively taking, including doses. Include over-the-counter medications, supplements, and herbals, if any. • Comment on adherence to regimen. • If unable to obtain accurate medication history, state why. • List specific allergies and reactions, if known.
	Social history (SH)	• Include alcohol and other substance use history and smoking. • As pertinent to the situation, can mention: past/current work, travel, hobbies, environmental exposures, relationship status, home environment, sexual history, military history, or functional level.
	Family history (FH)	• As pertinent to the CC, can mention conditions among first-degree relatives that are genetically based. • If no conditions fit the above criteria, it is acceptable to say "noncontributory."
1 minute	Physical exam (PE)	• Always list vitals first. • At a minimum, mention pertinent positive and negative findings (as related to chief concern). • If preferred by your supervisor, mention all findings, positive and negative, in each organ system examined.

(Continued)

Duration: 8-10 minutes (Continued)		
1 minute	Labs and imaging	• Report abnormal findings as well as changes from patient's baseline. • If preferred by your supervisor, report values of all labs obtained.
30 seconds	Refined problem representation (PR)	• The initial PR is in the "one liner" that started the presentation. • When restated here toward the end of the presentation, it has been refined based on the data gathered and presented. • Here, it provides a 1-sentence summary that highlights the defining features of the case and is a jumping off point for discussing assessment and plan. • Consists of patient demographics and risk factors (*the who*), length and tempo of illness (*the when*), and clinical syndrome with key signs and symptoms (*the what*).
3 minutes	Assessment and plan *Option A:* Problem based	• Generally preferred for inpatient wards. • List each problem (can be a symptom or a diagnosis) you have identified, starting with patient's chief concern and including patient's other health conditions that will require management during hospitalization. • For each problem, explain your clinical reasoning based on the information you have presented. • For each problem, list the plan, including additional tests, imaging, consults, medications, etc.
	Option B: Organ system based	• Most often used for patients in the intensive care unit. • Present organ systems from "head to toe" and include all systems that have relevant findings or concerns for the patient. • For each organ system (eg, neurologic, psychiatric, cardiovascular, pulmonary, gastrointestinal, renal/genitourinary, hematologic/oncologic, endocrine/metabolic, musculoskeletal, infectious), report associated symptoms and diagnoses as indicated, clinical reasoning, and plan, including additional tests, imaging, consults, medications, etc.

> **PEARL:** You may recall from Chapter 22, Medical Documentation, that the review of systems (ROS) was placed between the family history and the physical exam. When presenting a patient, it generally flows better to mention the pertinent ROS directly after the history of present illness (rather than waiting to present it later to mirror the format of a written history and physical).

The Holdover Admission

A holdover is a patient admitted by another team, most often the overnight admitting crew. The accepting team, most often the day rounding team, assumes care of the patient who already has a history and physical in the chart from the admitting team. As part of the accepting team, you may be assigned to assess the patient and then present the information gathered by the night team to introduce the patient to your team.

The format for presenting a holdover is very similar to the format for presenting a new admission, but there are some nuanced differences. The accepting team will need to review the key components of the patient's history, exam, imaging, and labs and carefully consider the working diagnosis, diagnostics, and treatment proposed by the admitting team. As new data become available, the leading diagnosis or plan of care may change.

The unique elements of a holdover presentation are highlighted below in green.

Duration: 9-11 minutes		
30 seconds	Chief concern (CC) + problem representation (PR)	• One sentence, often referred to as the opening "one liner." • Highlights the reason patient presented to the hospital. This can include a direct quote from them. • The PR contains relevant patient demographics and background (*the who*), length and tempo of illness (*the when*), and clinical syndrome (*the what*).
2 minutes	History of present illness (HPI)	• Details of symptoms and events leading up to the patient's presentation, provided in chronological order. • Give a thorough description of the characteristics of the patient's chief concern; see Chapter 1, History Taking, for additional details. • Include pertinent positives and negatives from review of systems. • Include brief discussion of any directly related past medical history/recent hospitalizations that are necessary to better understand the CC.
	Review of systems (ROS)	• Do not repeat the portion of ROS discussed in HPI. • Report any other positive responses to a full ROS that covers the other organ systems; see Chapter 2, Review of Systems, for additional details. • Report any pertinent negative responses.
30 seconds	Overnight events	• Review events since hospital admission. • Based on your assessment, report how the patient feels currently.
2 minutes	Past medical history/ past surgical history (PMH/PSH)	• Omit conditions mentioned previously in HPI. • Mention all conditions that may affect patient's current hospitalization and management. • Omit unrelated, minor conditions that will not affect current management.
	Medications and allergies	• List all medications the patient is actively taking, including doses. Include over-the-counter medications, supplements, and herbals, if any. • Comment on adherence to regimen. • List specific allergies and reactions, if known.
	Social history (SH)	• Focus on information that informs the current presentation.
	Family history (FH)	• Focus on information that informs the current presentation.
30 seconds	Physical exam (PE)	• Vitals and exam obtained at time of admission.
30 seconds	Updated physical exam (PE)	• Summarize vital sign trends since admission. • Include your own physical exam findings if they differ from the admitting team's.
30 seconds	Labs and imaging	• Key labs and imaging obtained at time of admission.
30 seconds	Updated labs and imaging	• Report labs and imaging that have resulted since the admitting team's initial evaluation of the patient.
30 seconds	Refined problem representation (PR)	• The initial PR is in the "one liner" that started the presentation. • When restated here toward the end of the presentation, it has been refined based on the data gathered and presented previously. • Here, it provides a 1-sentence summary that highlights the defining features of the case and is a jumping off point for discussing assessment and plan. • Consists of patient demographics and risk factors (*the who*), length and tempo of illness (*the when*), and clinical syndrome with key signs and symptoms (*the what*).

(Continued)

Duration: 9-11 minutes (Continued)		
2 minutes	Assessment and plan (usually problem based)	• Review working diagnosis or differential diagnosis at time of admission. • Review key portions of the plan for the working diagnosis as well as for other active problems.
1 minute	Revisit assessment and plan	• Are there any changes to the working diagnosis or treatment plan? • Have any new problems or symptoms been identified? If so, what is the plan for evaluation and treatment?

Daily Rounds

After admitting a patient or accepting a holdover to your team, you will typically follow them each day during their hospitalization. During daily rounds, you will be responsible for presenting an update of events over the past 24 hours and the plan moving forward. Because the patient is already known to the team, your presentation is expected to be a focused and concise discussion of the key facts.

The daily rounds presentation conveniently follows the structure of a daily SOAP note: subjective data (S), objective data (O), and assessment and plan (AP) (**Figure 23-3**).

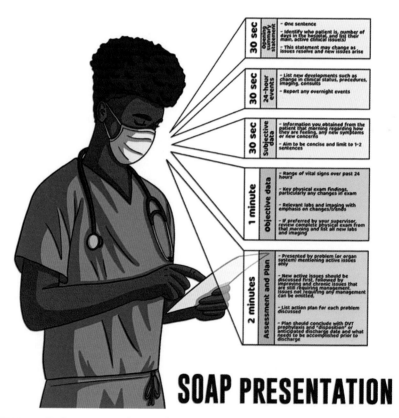

FIGURE 23-3 • **Patient presentations on daily rounds conveniently follow the same format as the daily progress note: Subjective, Objective, Assessment, and Plan.** (Reproduced with permission from Cathy Cichon, MD.)

You will notice that most of this framework is different than the presentations previously discussed, as highlighted below in yellow.

Duration: 5 minutes		
30 seconds	Refined problem representation	• One sentence. • Identifies who patient is and number of days in the hospital, and lists their main, active clinical issue(s). • This statement should change daily as issues resolve and new problems arise.
30 seconds	24-hour events	• Briefly list new developments such as change in clinical status, procedures, imaging, and consults. • Report any overnight events.
30 seconds	Subjective data	• Information you obtained from the patient that morning regarding how they are feeling and any new symptoms or concerns. • Should be concise and limited to 1-2 sentences.
1 minute	Objective data	• Range of vital signs over the past 24 hours. • Key physical exam findings, particularly any changes. • Relevant interval labs and imaging with emphasis on changes/trends. • If preferred by your supervisor, review complete physical exam from that morning and list all new labs and imaging.
2-3 minutes	Assessment and plan	• Presented by problem (or organ system) mentioning active issues only. • New, active problems should be discussed first, followed by improving and chronic issues that still require management. Issues not requiring any management can be omitted. • List action plan for each problem discussed. • Overall plan should conclude with deep venous thrombosis (DVT) prophylaxis and "disposition" or anticipated discharge date and what needs to be accomplished prior to discharge.

IN THE OUTPATIENT CLINIC

During medical school, you will spend time in a variety of clinic settings and work with both primary care physicians as well as specialists. You may have the opportunity to see the same patient multiple times and follow them longitudinally as well as the chance to see new patients for acute concerns.

The Initial Primary Care Visit

When working with a clinical preceptor in a primary care clinic, you may be assigned to see a new patient who is presenting to the clinic to establish care. After you interview and examine the patient, you will need to synthesize a presentation for your preceptor.

Many of the components of this type of presentation differ slightly when compared to presenting a new patient in the inpatient setting. These components are highlighted in orange. The pink and blue boxes will be familiar to you from the prior section.

Duration: 8-10 minutes		
30 seconds	Reason for visit	• 1 or 2 sentences. • Why patient is presenting to clinic (in this case, to establish care). • Mention any other specific goals such as medication refills or referrals. • There may or may not be a "chief concern" for this type of visit.
2 minutes	Relevant acute/ subacute history	• Highlight main issues that are bothering the patient (if any). • Mention any symptoms related to chronic diseases (eg, peripheral neuropathy in patient with diabetes). • Include any "data" related to chronic diseases (eg, blood glucose values for patient with diabetes, home blood pressure readings for patient with hypertension). • For some patients, there may not be anything to mention in this category.
1 minute	Review of systems (ROS)	• This should be appropriate to the clinical situation. See Chapter 2, Review of Systems, for additional information. • May include questions that are epidemiologically appropriate (eg, based on age and sex).
1 minute	Past medical history/ past surgical history (PMH/PSH)	• List all known medical issues, prioritizing those that require ongoing management. • Include time of onset and if followed by a specialist who might co-manage the condition. • Note if any care is being delivered via other healthcare systems, highlighting any overlapping and/or potentially redundant aspects. • If one of these diagnoses was described in detail in the "acute history" section, do not mention again. • List all surgeries, including year performed.
30 seconds	Medications and allergies	• List all medications the patient is actively taking, including doses. Include over-the-counter medication, supplements, and herbals, if any. • Comment on adherence to regimen. • List specific allergies and reactions, if known.
1 minute	Social history (SH)	• May include work, hobbies, and travel exposures. • May include if married or in a relationship and ages of any children. • Sexual activity, which may include type of activity, number and sex of partner(s), and health of partner(s). • Smoking, alcohol, and other substance use, including quantification of use and duration. • Extent of the information presented can be determined in discussion with your preceptor.
30 seconds	Family history (FH)	• Mention conditions among first-degree relatives that are genetically based. • If nothing relevant, can state "noncontributory."
1 minute	Physical exam (PE)	• Always list vitals first. • Report relevant findings (as informed by patient's past medical history or their reported concerns).
1 minute	Labs and imaging	• Report if available and relevant. Include when and where they were obtained.

(Continued)

Duration: 8-10 minutes (Continued)		
2 minutes	Assessment and plan Problem based Or Organ system based	- Include as many organ systems or problems as necessary to cover all active and chronic health issues. - Conclude with "healthcare maintenance" section, which covers age-, sex-, and risk factor–appropriate vaccinations and screening.

The Follow-Up Primary Care Clinic Visit

You will likely see many patients who are already known to your clinic preceptor and are returning for a new concern or for a follow-up visit as requested by their physician. An oral presentation in this situation should provide context regarding the patient's last appointment and interval events as well as the reason for the current appointment. As you might suspect, this presentation is typically shorter and more succinct in comparison with the presentation for a new patient establishing care.

The unique parts of this presentation are highlighted in gray. Note that, in general, past medical and surgical history (PMH/PSH), social history (SH), and family history (FH) are all *omitted* because this information is already known to your preceptor. You may elect to restate some of this information if a new symptom or interval issue has arisen and needs to be addressed.

Duration: 5-7 minutes		
30 seconds	Reason for visit	- 1 or 2 sentences. - State when last clinic visit occurred. - Mention what issues patient is following up on. - There may not be a "chief concern" as patient may simply be returning as requested by their physician.
1 minute	Events since last clinic visit	- Any interval visits to emergency room, specialty clinics, hospitalizations, or surgeries/procedures. - Note if any care was delivered via other healthcare systems, highlighting any overlapping and/or potentially redundant aspects. - Any changes in medications. - Any new symptoms. - Any interval data related to chronic health issues (eg, blood glucose trends, home blood pressure log).
30 seconds	Review of systems (ROS)	- Focused on patient's chronic health issues (eg, if patient has diabetes, include vascular ROS). - If patient lacks chronic health conditions or risk factors, the ROS can generally be omitted. See Chapter 2, Review of Systems, for additional details.
30 seconds	Medications and allergies	- Brief review of medications, including any interval changes if not mentioned previously. - Comment on adherence to regimen.
30 seconds	Physical exam (PE)	- Always list vitals first. - Pertinent positive and negative findings of a general physical exam with focus on organ systems affected by chronic health conditions or new symptoms.

Duration: 5-7 minutes (Continued)		
30 seconds	Labs and imaging	• State reasons why any interval labs or imaging were obtained, as well as results. • Highlight changes from patient's baseline.
2 minutes	Assessment and plan	• State all conditions that are being addressed at the visit followed by a specific plan for that condition. • May include new issue(s) if identified. • Review healthcare maintenance issues.

The Acute Visit to Primary Care Clinic

Another common type of patient you will encounter in the primary care clinic are those who made an appointment to address a particular concern or symptom. Often these are patients who are already known to your preceptor, although this category may also include patients who have another primary care provider but are seeing your preceptor for their acute concern due to appointment availability. Even if the patient is not known to your preceptor, a presentation for an acute visit should be very focused.

The presentation for this type of visit is similar to a follow-up primary care visit with a few nuances. We will use the template above as a starting point with differences highlighted in yellow.

Duration: 5 minutes		
30 seconds	Reason for visit (chief concern)	• One sentence that reports the symptom(s)/concern that prompted patient to make an appointment.
1 minute	History of present illness (HPI)	• Describe the sequence of events and symptoms leading to patient's current condition.
30 seconds	Review of systems (ROS)	• Include systems that are related to chief concern. • Can be abbreviated, but discuss to an appropriate depth that focuses the listener on the main differential diagnoses that must be considered.
30 seconds	Past medical history, past surgical history (PMH/PSH), and medications	• Mention only those elements that might be related to the presenting symptom(s)/concern. • May briefly list all medications if preferred by preceptor.
30 seconds	Physical exam (PE)	• Always list vitals first. • Pertinent positive and negative findings of physical exam that are focused on areas related to presenting symptom(s)/concern.
30 seconds	Labs and imaging	• Report if any were done along with date obtained, and highlight any changes from patient's baseline.
1 minute	Assessment and plan	• In general, will be very focused and relate directly to the main presenting symptom(s)/concern. • May contain only one "problem."

The Specialty Clinic Visit

Specialty clinic visits generally focus on the healthcare domains covered by those physicians. For example, pulmonary clinic visits review events, labs, imaging, and procedures related to the lungs, whereas orthopedic clinic visits focus on musculoskeletal events, imaging, and procedures. Information about other organ systems is typically omitted, although it is good practice to ask your specialty clinic preceptors what information they expect to be included in your presentations. Sometimes disorders may have a dominant effect in one organ (eg, the kidneys) which reflect conditions that are also impacting other areas of the body (eg, diabetes can lead to nephropathy, neuropathy, retinopathy and cardiovascular disease). This often requires a more holistic approach to care.

The presentation structure provided here can be applied to both new and returning clinic patients. Nearly every portion of presentations for a specialty clinic is different from the presentation types discussed previously for the same reason: it is appropriate to focus on the information that is directly related to the organ system the clinic specializes in. To make this distinction, the framework below is highlighted in green to indicate that there are nuances to every portion of the presentation in this setting.

You may be wondering if the framework below can be used in the inpatient setting if you are rotating with a consulting service that specializes in a certain area, and the answer is yes. Apply the guidelines below to the "new admission" patient to present the "new consult" patient and to the "daily rounds" patient to present consult patients that the team follows for more than 1 day.

Duration: 5-7 minutes		
30 seconds	Reason for visit (chief concern)	• If the patient was referred for a consult, state the consult question or reason as well as the referring provider. • If it is a return visit, state the reason the patient is followed in the clinic and the date of the last visit. • If the visit is for an acute issue, then report the chief concern.
1 minute	Relevant acute/subacute history	• For a new patient, describe the reason for referral and related historical information. • For a returning patient, report any interval events related to the reason they are followed in the specialty clinic. You can also include major events (eg, procedures, hospitalizations) related to other areas that would be important to know about. • For an acute visit, outline the history of present illness for the concern. • The key is that the information for any of the above presentations is typically limited to that which is directly related to the specialty clinic's area of care.
30 seconds	Review of systems (ROS)	• Focused on those symptoms relevant to the specialty clinic's organ system. • Many specialties use an expanded ROS that assesses for symptoms in their organ system. Ask your preceptor and/or check specialty-specific resources to see if this applies.

(Continued)

Duration: 5-7 minutes (Continued)		
1 minute	Past medical history, past surgical history, social history, family history (PMH/PSH, SH, FH)	• Review anything that is directly related to the specialty (eg, date and details of coronary artery bypass surgery for cardiology clinic, date of fistula placement for nephrology clinic, tobacco use history for pulmonary clinic). • Note relevant healthcare delivered via other specialty clinics or health systems.
30 seconds	Medications and allergies	• Brief review of medications with emphasis on those related to specialty clinic's focus. • Comment on adherence to regimen. • May mention allergies if pertinent to medications prescribed by specialty clinic.
30 seconds	Physical exam (PE)	• Always list vitals first. • Pertinent positive and negative findings of a general physical exam with focus on organ system(s) related to specialty clinic.
30 seconds	Labs and imaging	• Report recent labs, imaging, and procedures related to organ system(s) relevant to specialty clinic.
2 minutes	Assessment and plan Problem based	• Since the specialty clinic typically deals with one organ system, it makes the most sense to approach the assessment and plan in a problem-based manner. • State all conditions that are being addressed at the visit followed by a specific plan for each condition.

While the scenarios detailed above are not an exhaustive list of every type of presentation you will encounter during your clinical training, if you have a grasp of the basic components of each and an understanding of how the context informs the main differences in the presentations, you will be off to an excellent start. Each clinical preceptor you encounter may have a slightly different set of preferences, which you will need to incorporate into the guidance provided here (**Figure 23-4**).

CONTEXT MATTERS:

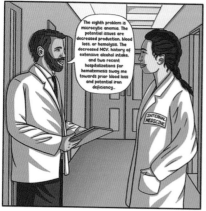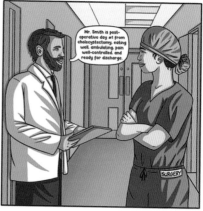

FIGURE 23-4 • **Different contexts call for different types of presentations. Your internal medicine attending will have different expectations than your general surgery attending.** (Reproduced with permission from Cathy Cichon, MD.)

PEARL: It is a good practice to ask each of your clinical preceptors about their preferred presentation style so you can adjust accordingly. Flexibility is one of the keys to success!

SAMPLE PRESENTATIONS

To bring life to the oral presentation guidelines discussed in this chapter, transcripts of 2 of the most common oral presentations—the new admission and daily rounds—are included. The same patient is used for both examples to allow for comparison of the 2 different presentation types. Try reading these out loud to get a feel for the format and flow.

The New Admission

Chief Concern and Initial Problem Representation Frank Johnson is a 55-year-old man with well-controlled type 2 diabetes, hypertension, and chronic lower back pain who presented after an episode of vomiting up what he described as "a cup of blood."

History of Present Illness Mr. J was in his usual state of health until 3 weeks prior to presentation when he developed upper abdominal pain. The pain came on gradually over a few days and is present intermittently. He describes it as "twisting" with general severity of 5 out of 10. Pain improves with eating, and he cannot identify anything that makes it worse. He tried taking an over-the-counter antacid, which made the pain subside for a few hours. He has never had this type of pain in the past. He is anxious about the cause as he had a maternal uncle who recently passed away from stomach cancer.

Earlier today, the pain increased to 9 out of 10 and was accompanied by nausea and lightheadedness. Mr. J had an initial episode of vomiting that was "greenish" in color and then another episode 30 minutes later that contained red blood. He vomited into the toilet, and it seemed to him that the bowl was filled with about a cup of blood. This prompted Mr. J to present to the emergency department. He drove himself here.

Mr. J denies any recent fevers or night sweats. He has had no recent weight loss. His appetite and oral intake have been normal aside from today. He has no shortness of breath or chest pain. He has no diarrhea or black or bloody bowel movements. He usually has 2 to 3 drinks per week (12 ounce bottles of beer), and last alcohol use was about 2 weeks ago. He has no known history of liver disease or prior gastrointestinal bleeding. He takes ibuprofen several times a week for chronic lower back pain with max use of 600 mg × 4 doses in a 24-hour period. He took 2 tablets yesterday.

Review of Systems Review of systems as above. It is also notable for occasional pain radiating from low back to behind right knee. There is no associated numbness, tingling, or weakness. He also reports chronic nocturia 3 times per night and occasional dry eyes.

Past Medical History/Past Surgical History Medical history is notable for well-controlled type 2 diabetes managed with oral medications and patient doesn't check sugars at home. Also, history is notable for hypertension, hyperlipidemia, benign prostatic hyperplasia, and chronic low back pain. Patient has had no prior surgeries. No healthcare delivered outside of our system.

Medications and Allergies Medications include metformin 500 mg twice daily, amlodipine 10 mg daily, hydrochlorothiazide 25 mg daily, atorvastatin 20 mg daily, tamsulosin 0.4 mg daily, lidocaine patch as needed for lower back pain, artificial tears as needed, and an over-the-counter multivitamin. Ibuprofen use as noted previously. He has no medication allergies. He takes all his medications exactly as prescribed.

Social History He has never used tobacco products. He smoked marijuana in the past, but has not smoked for over 5 years. Alcohol use as noted previously. Patient indicates no other substance use, lives with a roommate, and is a high school history teacher.

Family History Father has coronary artery disease and had a stent placed at age 70. Mother has hypertension. Maternal uncle had gastric cancer, diagnosed at age 75.

Physical Exam Afebrile, blood pressure 120/75, heart rate 110, respiratory rate 16, saturating 97% on room air. On exam, he is alert, appears anxious, but can answer questions appropriately and cooperate with physical exam. No icterus or conjunctival pallor. No bleeding from nose or in mouth. Heart rate is tachycardic and regular, no murmurs. Lungs are clear bilaterally. Abdomen is not distended. Tender to palpation in epigastric region, without rebound or guarding. Brown stool on rectal exam. Tender to palpation over lower thoracic paraspinal muscles bilaterally. Lower extremity strength is 5/5 bilaterally. Skin without jaundice or spider angiomas.

Labs and Imaging Labs are notable for a hemoglobin of 11.5 compared to 14 when last checked 1 year ago. MCV 90, platelets 220, coags normal. Electrolytes and liver function tests are also within normal limits. Lactate is normal. Troponin x1 is within normal range. Hemoglobin A1C was 6.5% 1 month ago.

Chest x-ray was normal. Electrocardiogram showed sinus tachycardia with no evidence of ischemia.

Refined Problem Representation Mr. J is a 55-year-old man with well-controlled type 2 diabetes, chronic back pain necessitating frequent ibuprofen consumption and alcohol use who presents with subacute epigastric pain alleviated by oral intake and antacid use, one episode of hematemesis, and anemia.

> PEARL: The refined problem representation should reflect the information you gathered during the history and physical. Compare this updated problem representation to the initial one at the beginning of the presentation.

Assessment and Plan: Problem Based Problem number 1 is epigastric pain with hematemesis, which is concerning for an upper gastrointestinal bleed. Based on the location of the pain and the consistency of ibuprofen use, my highest suspicion is for peptic ulcer disease. Because pain improves with eating, I am most concerned about a duodenal ulcer that is now complicated by bleeding. I think it could be caused by NSAIDs or *Helicobacter pylori*. My differential diagnosis also includes gastritis, esophagitis, and a Dieulafoy lesion. Bleeding esophageal varices is much less likely considering there is nothing on exam or labs to support cirrhosis. Gastric cancer is also possible although less likely given acute presentation and no definite risk factors.

My plan is to make sure the patient has 2 large-bore IVs for adequate access as there is the potential for him to become unstable if blood loss is ongoing. We will follow his hemoglobin every 6 hours and transfuse blood if his hemoglobin drops below 7. I would like to perform an ultrasound to look for any evidence of cirrhosis. I also plan to consult gastroenterology for consideration of an upper endoscopy. We will avoid NSAIDs and keep him NPO for a possible endoscopy. We will start an IV pantoprazole infusion while awaiting endoscopy. Overnight, he will stay in the intermediate care unit for close monitoring.

Problem number 2 is anemia. I suspect this is most likely due to acute blood loss, but I am also considering decreased production due to lack of iron. Folate or vitamin B$_{12}$

deficiency is possible, although the anemia is normocytic rather than macrocytic. I would like to order an iron panel, ferritin, folate, and vitamin B_{12}.

Problem number 3 is diabetes. I plan to hold the metformin he takes at home. Since he will not be eating for now, we can start him on a lispro insulin correctional scale. He has an A1C from last month, so it is not necessary to get another one during this admission.

Problem number 4 is hypertension. I would like to hold his home medications of amlodipine and hydrochlorothiazide as there is the potential for hypotension due to bleeding. We can restart these if his blood pressure is getting high.

Problem number 5 is chronic low back pain. My plan is to avoid NSAIDs due to concern for peptic ulcer disease. He can continue using a lidocaine patch as he does at home. We can add acetaminophen as needed if pain control becomes an issue.

Problem number 6 is hyperlipidemia. We can hold his home atorvastatin until medically stable.

Problem number 7 is benign prostate hyperplasia. We will continue home dose of tamsulosin to help avoid urinary retention during hospitalization.

For deep vein thrombosis prophylaxis, we ordered sequential compression devices instead of pharmacologic prophylaxis due to active bleeding.

Disposition will be pending stabilization of hemoglobin and gastroenterology consult and recommendations, and I expect he will be able to return to his home independently at that time.

Daily Rounds

Opening Summary Statement/Problem Representation This is hospital day 2 for Frank Johnson, a 55-year-old man with chronic low back pain and frequent ibuprofen use who was admitted with anemia due to an acute upper gastrointestinal (GI) bleed from a duodenal ulcer.

> PEARL: Note how the problem representation is refined (compared with day 1) based on newly available clinical information.

24-Hour Events GI performed an upper endoscopy, which showed a nonbleeding duodenal ulcer that was biopsied.

Hypertensive overnight without symptoms. Home dose amlodipine was started.

Subjective Data Mr. J has mild epigastric pain this morning but has not had any episodes of hematemesis since prior to admission. He was able to eat a liquid diet last night and today is without any nausea or vomiting. He is relieved that the endoscopy did not show overt evidence of gastric cancer.

Objective Data Afebrile over past 24 hours. Systolic blood pressure ranged from 130 to 168 with diastolic from 80 to 100. Heart rate has been 80 to 100. Respiratory rate 16 to 20. Saturating 96-100% on room air.

Intake was 1500 mL (1 L IV normal saline, the rest PO) with urine output of 1200 mL. No bowel movements since admission.

On exam, he is sitting up in bed, alert, and appears comfortable. Heart with regular rate and rhythm. Lungs are clear. Abdomen is nondistended. There is mild tenderness to palpation of epigastric region and less pain compared to yesterday. No edema of lower extremities.

Labs today show a hemoglobin of 9.6 compared to 11.5 yesterday. BUN is elevated to 25 compared to normal value of 10 yesterday. Folate and B_{12} levels are normal. Stool antigen test is negative for H pylori. Iron panel and ferritin are pending. Creatinine remains normal. Glucoses have been 220 yesterday (fasting) and 240 prior to eating last night. This morning's glucose was 250 prior to eating.

Upper endoscopy showed a duodenal ulcer with no active bleeding, visible vessel or other high-risk features. GI performed biopsies and the pathology is pending.

Further Refined Problem Representation   This is hospital day 2 for Frank Johnson, a 55-year-old man with chronic low back pain and frequent ibuprofen use who was admitted with anemia due to an acute upper GI bleed from a duodenal ulcer now with hyperglycemia and elevated blood pressure.

Assessment and Plan: Problem Based   Problem number 1 is acute upper GI bleed secondary to a duodenal ulcer. The ulcer appears to be secondary to NSAID use, given endoscopic findings, history and stool antigen test negative for H pylori. We have counseled Mr. J on the need to avoid NSAIDs in the future. Today, we will stop the pantoprazole infusion and start oral pantoprazole 40 mg twice daily. He is doing well with a liquid diet so we will advance to a carb-limited regular consistency diet. I think we can discontinue the abdominal ultrasound, as there is no evidence of any contribution from occult liver disease.

Problem number 2 is anemia due to blood loss. Hemoglobin was 11.5 at admission and is down to 9.6 today. Folate and B_{12} levels were normal, and workup for iron deficiency anemia is pending. I think it is most likely that the anemia is due to the GI bleeding, and I suspect the iron studies will confirm iron deficiency anemia from GI blood loss or be normal if the bleeding was all acute. I will follow up those results. I recommend spacing out hemoglobin checks to every 12 hours today. And we can consider providing supplemental iron at discharge.

Problem number 3 is diabetes. Since we are starting a carb-limited diet and his glucose levels are elevated, we will start insulin. Based on his weight, I calculated a starting dose of glargine 10 units once daily and lispro 3 units 3 times daily with meals. We will continue the lispro correctional scale.

Problem number 4 is hypertension. He has not had any episodes of hypotension, and blood pressures today are above goal. Amlodipine was started last night, and I think we should add back his hydrochlorothiazide this morning and follow his blood pressures.

Problem number 5 is chronic low back pain. We will avoid NSAIDs now and in future. I would like to continue the lidocaine patch, and I talked to Mr. J about trying a scheduled dose of Tylenol and he was in favor. I also discussed that more adjustments may be necessary as an outpatient.

For DVT prophylaxis, he has been out of bed walking in his room and in the hallway, so he is at low risk for a DVT and I don't think pharmacologic prophylaxis or sequential compression devices are needed at this time.

For disposition, I think he will be okay to go home tomorrow if he tolerates a regular diet and does not have further decline in his hemoglobin level. GI was also okay with discharge home tomorrow, and they will follow up on his biopsy results and schedule repeat endoscopy if needed.

PEARL: It is appropriate to omit nonactive issues in a daily rounds presentation. Here, hyperlipidemia and benign prostatic hyperplasia were omitted as no management was necessary.

BIBLIOGRAPHY

Beach MC, Saha S, Park J, et al. Testimonial injustice: linguistic bias in the medical records of black patients and women. *J Gen Intern Med.* 2021;36(6):1708-1714.

Berger G, Lessing J, Connor D. Exercises in Clinical Reasoning Web Series. Accessed November 24, 2023. https://clinicalreasoning.org/

Goddu AP, O'Conor KJ, Lanzkron S, et al. Do words matter? Stigmatizing language and the transmission of bias in the medical record. *J Gen Intern Med.* 2018;33(5):685-691.

Goldberg C. *Practical Guide to Clinical Medicine: Oral Presentations.* UC San Diego School of Medicine. March 2020. Accessed June 21, 2023. https://meded.ucsd.edu/clinicalmed/oral.html.

Green EH, DeCherrie L, Fagan MJ, Sharpe BA, Hershman W. The oral case presentation: what internal medicine clinician-teachers expect from clinical clerks. *Teach Learn Med.* 2011;23(1):58-61.

Haber RJ, Lingard LA. Learning oral presentation skills. *J Gen Intern Med.* 2001;16:308-314.

Olenik J, Kohlwes J, Manesh S, et al. Problem representation overview. *J Gen Intern Med.* 2010. Accessed June 27, 2023. https://www.sgim.org/web-only/clinical-reasoning-exercises/problem-representation-overview.

24

Telehealth and Digital Health

Leonie Heyworth, MD, MPH

INTRODUCTION

The use of telehealth in healthcare has grown exponentially since the onset of the COVID-19 pandemic. From 2019 to 2021, the use of telehealth technology increased for office-based physicians from 15.4% to 85.9%. In 2021, approximately one-third of all Americans had completed a telehealth visit. The landscape shifted dramatically during the pandemic as healthcare systems pivoted to care solutions not requiring in-person interactions. This accelerated the understanding of patients, providers, and health systems about what could be accomplished with telehealth. Today, patients expect to be able to choose telehealth as a part of their healthcare. The evidence to support telehealth as a replacement versus an adjunct to in-person care is beginning to be established for clinical specialties outside of mental health, where its role is firmly established.

This chapter covers core approaches for successfully engaging in telehealth. As in any area of medicine, clinical judgement for when telehealth is an appropriate modality is necessary. Many medical issues can be addressed by telehealth without additional equipment. More sophisticated tools for remote physical exams by telehealth (eg, using a digital stethoscope or otoscope) can be helpful for certain specialties or where a comprehensive remote exam is needed. The wide array of issues that can be readily addressed without tele-specific equipment will be discussed here. Organ-based telehealth tips for equipment-free examinations have been embedded into the end of most chapters of this book. Any urgent or emergent clinical issues identified during a telehealth visit should be rapidly transitioned to a plan for in-person assessment.

WHAT IS TELEHEALTH?

Telehealth involves the use of technology and telecommunication for the purposes of delivering healthcare by a clinician located remotely from a patient. The American Telehealth Association defines telehealth as "a mode of delivering healthcare services through the use of telecommunications technologies, including but not limited to asynchronous and synchronous technology, and remote patient monitoring technology, by a healthcare practitioner to a patient or a practitioner at a different physical location than the healthcare practitioner." However, definitions vary according to the source and no

Reproduced with permission from ATA's Standardized Telehealth Terminology and Policy Language for States on Medical Practice. The American Telemedicine Association. 2020.

single authority exists. Perhaps the broadest definition is 25 USC § 1603, which defines telehealth as "the use of electronic information and telecommunications technologies to support long distance clinical health care, patient and professional health-related education, public health, and health administration."

The simplest and likely oldest example of telehealth is that of telephone-based care, but 2-way audiovisual care has existed since the advent of television in the early 1960s. With modern technology, a wide array of care can be delivered. For example, a clinician may complete an assessment for joint pain by video when their patient is at home, while a dermatologist can offer gap coverage to a distant facility, reviewing images taken of a suspicious mole and imparting a likely diagnosis. Of note, remote communications between healthcare providers where the consultant does not engage in direct patient care or management is referred to as "teleconsultation," rather than telehealth.

Telehealth is an important solution in facilitating access to care for patients in rural or remote locations, for homebound patients, or for those who cannot easily travel. In areas where workforce shortages exist, remote providers can offer services from anywhere. For subspecialized areas of medicine often concentrated in urban centers, telehealth can improve quality of care as well as enable teaching and education of generalist physicians in resource-poor settings.

TELEHEALTH SERVICES IN HEALTHCARE

Types of Telehealth

Synchronous, or video, telehealth is real-time video teleconferencing for healthcare on an app-based and/or web-based video platform where the patient may be at home (**Figure 24-1**) or a non-healthcare location using a personal Internet-connected device with a camera. Alternatively, patients may be located in a clinic setting using video equipment and a camera housed there, a set up seen typically in more rural locations and/or broadband-poor areas.

Video telehealth may be supported by additional monitoring devices (eg, blood pressure cuffs, weight scales, pulse oximeters). These can be plugged into the video-capable device

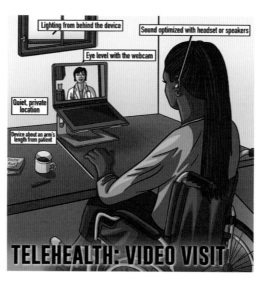

FIGURE 24-1 • **Patient engaged with a synchronous telehealth visit from home with a remote provider.** (Reproduced with permission from Cathy Cichon, MD.)

or connected by Bluetooth with some arrangements enabling the remote provider to visualize patient biometrics within the video session.

Asynchronous, or store-and-forward telehealth, is capture of patient health information (eg, images, data, video/audio clips) that may be stored securely prior to being transmitted to a clinician for interpretation at a later time (**Figure 24-2**). This type of telehealth is used across a wide variety of specialties, including radiology, dermatology, ophthalmology, plastic surgery, and many others. Images or data may be captured with the assistance of a technician in the clinic setting, or self-captured through secure applications by patients at home and stored securely for transmission and interpretation at a later time.

Another commonly used asynchronous feature is communication between patients and their care teams through secure electronic health portals. In addition, patients may be able

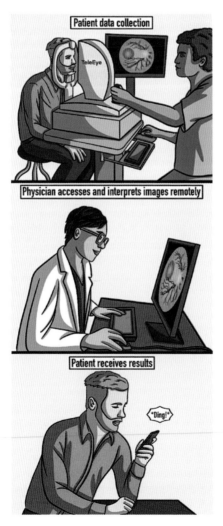

FIGURE 24-2 • A patient's retinal images are captured with the assistance of a technician and securely stored for a provider to interpret asynchronously—typically, remotely and at a later time. (Reproduced with permission from Cathy Cichon, MD.)

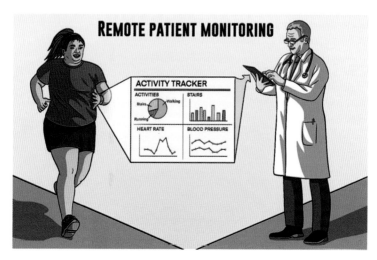

FIGURE 24-3 • A patient runs with her wearable device that is capturing real-time biometric data and transmitting this data in real time to her healthcare team, who can review it synchronously or asynchronously. (Reproduced with permission from Cathy Cichon, MD.)

to directly access their medical records, providing an opportunity to review test results, read notes, and even schedule appointments.

Remote patient monitoring (RPM) uses wearable devices, mobile applications, and other equipment to collect, transmit, report, and interpret patient health data for the purposes of disease management and care coordination. Data collected may be intermittent (eg, blood pressure) or continuous (eg, heart rate and rhythm) in nature (**Figure 24-3**). Following interpretation, patients are notified of results and actions by the clinician. The ability to monitor patients outside the clinical setting has great promise to facilitate access to care, improve outcomes (eg, via early detection and intervention), and reduce costs, particularly for patients with multiple chronic conditions, after hospitalization, or at risk for (re)hospitalization.

Considerations Prior to Embarking on Telehealth With Your Patients

Ultimately, both patient and provider must be interested in utilizing telehealth. It is a powerful tool that requires engagement from both parties. Patients less familiar with technology may be initially apprehensive. Yet with the right support and resources, they can become highly satisfied with telehealth. Everyone involved needs to understand what can be accomplished and then make intentional decisions about putting this approach to use.

The Digital Divide

In some areas of the United States, the digital divide—those who have access to a device and/or connectivity versus those who do not—continues to be a challenge as the option of telehealth does not exist for everyone. Efforts to narrow this divide are underway, including federal and nonprofit programs creating subsidized access to devices and technology in order to promote digital equity.

In broadband-poor areas, healthcare facility–based telehealth offers a potential solution for patients who cannot complete a high-quality home-based telehealth visit or for patients needing a more comprehensive exam facilitated by an on-site technician. Increasingly, non-healthcare locations are also serving as a resource for technology and/or connectivity (eg, community centers, pharmacies, public libraries).

Digital Skills

Participation in any form of telehealth requires that the patient have basic knowledge of the use and function of their internet-connected device and often more advanced digital literacy to effectively navigate platforms and applications. It is therefore critical for healthcare systems and clinicians to support patients by providing the necessary resources to acquire digital skills, including hands-on teaching developed at an appropriate level and language. These are important steps along the road to digital equity.

Digital literacy is quite variable and highest among digital natives who were brought up with technology from an early age. As a general strategy, it is best to not assume that your patient is comfortable or interested in using technology based on their age or other markers that may reflect our biases. A better approach is to ask everyone about their level of comfort and then offer support and teaching from staff as needed, particularly prior to the first telehealth visit. Engaging with family/caregivers on the patient's end can sometimes be helpful. As with most things, skills will improve with time and practice.

THE REMOTE EXAM IN DETAIL

Settings

Telehealth visits can take place in a variety of locations, with the most common being the patient's home or a medical clinic.

Who's Involved?

Most commonly, patients will be in their homes using their own technology and leading their own exam, sometimes with the assistance of a caregiver or family member if available and needed.

Exams via telehealth can also be assisted by a trained healthcare professional, usually a nurse or technician, who is co-located with the patient at one site, communicating with a remote provider and using examination tools such as an exam camera. At this type of visit, the patient will generally be located within a medical clinic.

Requirements

Devices and Connectivity To be recipients of any form of telehealth, patients must have access to a device and connectivity. As computers, smartphones, and other connected devices have become increasingly ubiquitous, the ease with which patients have been able to engage in their healthcare virtually has rapidly increased. This was spurred in particular by the COVID-19 pandemic. Patients who may otherwise have been apprehensive about trying home-based telehealth saw it as a safer option for receiving care.

Patient's Equipment
- Computer (desktop, laptop), tablet, and smartphones will all generally support a video telehealth visit (Figure 24-1).
- A larger screen is preferable to enable the patient to better see you, and any instructions or results shared on the screen.

Provider's Equipment
- Dual monitor: Ideal set up enabling browser window with video on one monitor and electronic medical record (EMR) on the other.

- Single monitor: If limited for space, a single monitor can accommodate a smaller video window size and smaller EMR on the same screen.
- Smartphone: This is the least ideal option given limited screen size and difficulty with positioning and stability.

A landline or smartphone should be available as backup in case of video failure. Sound is optimized by using a headset or speakers.

Connectivity

- Landline: Connection via hardwiring to the internet for clinicians working in an office is highly reliable.
- Wi-Fi: Work-station positioning beside the Wi-Fi router will optimize connection.
- Cellular signal: Cellular signal is best picked up by being close to a window.

Test Call

- This will enable the patient to test their device and connectivity. If doing a video telehealth visit, it is recommended that all new patients be offered a test video call prior to their first visit.

Choice of Video Teleconferencing Platforms

- The clinical interaction via video can take place on a variety of video teleconferencing platforms (eg, Zoom, Skype, Teams). In general, the license to use a particular video platform is purchased by the healthcare organization on behalf of the clinicians. Particular requirements may factor into this decision, including:
  - Ease of use for patient and clinician
  - Built-in features (eg, chat box, picture-in-picture, virtual background, closed captioning, group visits)
  - Privacy, security, and encryption features of the platform
  - System capacity: Ability to accommodate concurrent video volume—more critical to consider for larger healthcare organizations
  - Compatibility with the electronic health record
- Scheduling: The video visit can be scheduled ahead of time, and the link to the visit accessed via email, text, or through a healthcare organization's secure patient portal. Alternatively, visits may also be on demand, particularly if a rapid visual assessment is needed.

During the Telehealth Visit

Patient's Environment

- Identify the best location for the visit. Most important is a quiet, private place. For some patients, this may be their car—in which case, request that it is parked safely (eg, on a street or in a lot, not on the side of a freeway), and make sure that the patient is not actively driving.
- Lighting: If an exam is needed, and patient lighting conditions need to be improved, ask the patient to sit facing a window or next to a light source, such as a lamp (Figure 24-1).
- The background should not be distracting.

Clinician's Environment

- Lighting: Ideally, sit facing a window or next to a light source, such as a lamp, to illuminate your face.

- Sit in a quiet, private place.
- Have a nondistracting background or apply an appropriate simple therapeutic virtual background.
- Avoid shared offices and public settings, where people walking in the background interfere with creating a private or therapeutic environment. If such settings cannot be avoided, clinicians should optimize patient privacy by using headphones during the video visit.

Patient's Position

- If the patient is using a tablet or smartphone, encourage the patient to keep their device still for the best experience—even if this means resting their device.
- Placing the device on a table or stand frees the patient to use their hands and sit a distance from the camera, which makes for a better provider-side experience.

Clinician's Position

- Eyes should be level with webcam.
- Sit an arms-length distance from seated position to webcam.
- Wear professional clothing.

Additional Considerations

- Be on time. A patient waiting online may worry that they have been forgotten. If you are running behind, ask a clinical team member to join the session and share a time update with the patient.
- Review your preparation steps. Make sure that the environment is optimized.
- Center yourself. As you enter the video session, ensure that your head and shoulders are in the center of the screen with some space above your head. Sit upright with good posture.
- Welcome the patient to the video session. Do the following:
  - Confirm that they can see and hear you clearly. Let them know if you can see and hear them clearly.
  - Confirm their identity, if you are unsure.
  - Troubleshooting any audio or visual issues early on in the visit (as needed) will help to set you up for an enjoyable session.
- Make eye contact. For the patient to perceive that you are looking at them, you will want to look at the webcam, or ensure sufficient distance (about an arm's length) between your seated position and the screen (in which case, looking at the patient's face will be perceived as eye contact).
- Acknowledge the presence of individuals attending the video visit with your patient and ensure that your patient approves of their participation.
- Be expressive, relax your facial expression, and smile! Body language cues may be less obvious over video, so talk more slowly. Try to avoid sudden movements or shifting your position outside of the frame.
- Document. Making note of the patient's location, to be used in the event of an emergency, is good practice. Completing documentation during the encounter can be time efficient, and the 2-screen setup will facilitate your ability to document and enter orders in the EMR on one screen and visualize the patient on the other screen.
- Consent for the visit. There may be limitations to the care that you can provide in a single telehealth visit, so explain this to the patient and address any privacy or security

questions they may have. Typically, consent requirements and whether they are documented in the medical record are determined by the healthcare organization.

- Explain your actions. If you are entering orders or looking up information in the EMR, communicate this to the patient. Without seeing you, they may not understand why your focus has shifted.
- Emulate the in-person visit. As you would share a screen to show lab trends or an educational video, do the same virtually as features permit.
- Organ-specific telehealth exam tips are provided at the end of each organ-focused chapter.
- No food or drink. As with an office visit, a professional provider–patient encounter does not occur over a meal or snack.
- Work with your healthcare team (eg, nurses, licensed vocational nurses, pharmacists, appointment schedulers) so that everyone understands their role when engaging with patients in the telehealth environment.
- Try to ensure secure connections. Despite your best efforts to ensure a private and secure session, there may be times when this is comprised for reasons relating to technology security (eg, hacking via "Zoombombing"), a systems issue at the level of the healthcare organization (eg, with scheduling), or patient error (eg, sharing the secure link with another party). If in doubt, terminate the visit and generate a new link for another video session.
- Recording the video visit. Laws differ by state regarding consent requirements for third-party recording. Additionally, secure storage of the recording will need to be considered.

Closing the Visit

- Any clinically urgent or emergent symptoms should be immediately addressed by making plans for the patient to be seen in person, including going to the emergency department or calling 911.
- Document any limitations to your assessment by video, including screenings and health maintenance (eg, "Vaccination due was discussed, with a follow-up plan to receive it in person").
- Without physical cues that the visit is nearing completion, it can be helpful to alert patients verbally (eg, "I wanted to see if you had any other questions before we finish up today").
- Follow-up plans should be discussed, including time and location for the next visit, reminders about scheduling tests, need for labs, process for any planned consults, and methods for communicating between visits. Note that the typical paths for making some of these arrangements (eg, dropping by the lab or radiology space when the visit occurs on site) have been disrupted.

TELEHEALTH CHALLENGES AND OPPORTUNITIES

Emerging patterns of telehealth use during the COVID-19 pandemic suggest that patients living in rural or highly rural areas experience more difficulty with accessing telehealth as an option for care. This digital divide will be critical to address in the postpandemic period as a mixture of telehealth and in-person care becomes more common and healthcare organizations continue to consider equity in healthcare delivery. Evidence for the effectiveness of telehealth, particularly in clinical areas outside of mental health, is limited but rapidly evolving, particularly in the domain of chronic disease management. This means that providers must continue to use their clinical judgement regarding the appropriacy of telehealth visits and its impact on care and the clinician-patient relationship.

Telehealth Licensure and Reimbursement

During the COVID-19 pandemic, licensing compacts between states increased in number, offering providers a faster solution to interstate telehealth practice. Compacts are created when states agree upon a uniform standard of care and both the home and compact states maintain oversight. In addition to compacts, this topic may be addressed in the future by legislation.

Legislation introduced during the COVID-19 pandemic removed barriers to reimbursement of telehealth services that resulted in permanent changes in federal laws. In the majority of states, requirements now exist for reimbursement based on coverage and payment parity (ie, the requirement that telehealth services are reimbursed at the same payment rate as an in-person service).

Telehealth, Artificial Intelligence, and the Future of Healthcare

Patient–clinician–health system interactions with telehealth will continue to increase, as all parties gain comfort with this modality and the technology evolves to make the interactions easier and more productive.

The growing landscape of wearable devices is also set to have a significant impact. For example, a patient may interact with a chatbot to manage their diabetes through a protocol using predetermined algorithms or track sleep patterns through a wearable device that collects data within a mobile application that can be shared with clinical teams. Still in its infancy as far as integration into routine clinical care, patient-generated health data is a rapidly growing field with far-reaching potential to transform healthcare interactions.

Moving forward, artificial intelligence (AI) will further shape patient interactions with healthcare. The expectation is that with the use of these next generation management tools, exchanges will occur in a way that improves care by enhancing precision via early disease detection for patients, while streamlining and securely feeding forward the most relevant clinical data to providers, thereby increasing overall accuracy and efficiency of care (and in the process, reducing clinical burnout). Training in the optimal use of telehealth and other technologies that improve healthcare delivery from the beginning of medical education will presumably enhance clinicians' abilities to efficiently integrate these potentially powerful tools. To ensure digital inclusion for all, availability of digital skills training to patients and clinical teams, access to technology and affordable, high quality connectivity for patients will be essential to mitigating the existing digital divide and enabling all patients, when preferred, to engage in digitally-delivered care.

BIBLIOGRAPHY

Ayers JW, Poliak A, Dredze M, et al. Comparing physician and artificial intelligence chatbot responses to patient questions posted to a public social medium forum. *JAMA Internal Medicine.* 2023;183(6):589-596.

Crowley ST, Belcher J, Choudhury D, et al. Targeting access to kidney care via telehealth: the VA experience. *Adv Chron Kidney Dis.* 2017;24(1):22-30.

Frank JW, Carey EP, Fagan KM, et al. Evaluation of a telementoring intervention for pain management in the Veterans Health Administration. *Pain Med.* 2015;16(6):1090-1100.

National Center for Health Statistics. National Health Interview Survey, 2021. Accessed January 15, 2024. https://www.cdc.gov/nchs/nhis.htm.

Rodriguez JA, Shachar C, Bates DW. Digital Inclusion as Health Care- Supporting Health Care Equity with Digital-Infrastructure Initiatives. *N Engl J Med.* 2022;386:1101-1103.

Tapper EB, Asrani SK. The COVID-19 pandemic will have a long-lasting impact on the quality of cirrhosis care. *J Hepatol.* 2020;73(2):441-445.

US Department of Health and Human Resources. Telehealth information for patients. Accessed June 10, 2023. https://telehealth.hhs.gov/.

US Department of Health and Human Resources. Telehealth licensing. Accessed June 10, 2023. https://telehealth.hhs.gov/licensure/licensure-compacts.

Vogels E. Some digital divides persist between rural, urban and suburban America. Pew Research Center 2021. Accessed June 16, 2023. https://www.pewresearch.org/topic/internet-technology/technology-policy-issues/digital-divide/.

Watts SA, Roush L, Julius M, Sood A. Improved glycemic control in veterans with poorly controlled diabetes mellitus using a specialty care access network-extension for community healthcare outcomes model at primary care clinics. *J Telemed Telecare.* 2016;22(4):221-224.

Wray CM, Sridhar A, Young A, et al. Assessing the impact of a pre-visit readiness telephone call on video visit success rates. *J Gen Intern Med.* 2023;38:252-253.

25

Putting It All Together

Charlie Goldberg, MD

How do you perform the examination in a way that is complete, makes sense, and yet is not awkward or prolonged? Is it okay to combine different areas of the exam, or should each system be explored as a block? Answering these questions and putting together a smooth exam can be challenging. Any approach should:

- Cover all aspects of the examination that are appropriate to the clinical situation.
- Be readily reproducible, allowing you to perform it the same way each time.
- Keep patient gymnastics to a minimum (ie, limit the number of times that the patient has to get up and down).
- Link together sections that, although disconnected physiologically, are connected spatially. For example, you'll note in the list provided that the cardiovascular exam is "interrupted" by the abdominal exam, which allows the examiner to move from the chest, to the abdomen, and then to the lower extremities.
- Allow you to be efficient and perform the exam with an economy of movement (eg, minimize the number of times that you pick up and put down instruments, move from one side of the patient to the other).

It will take time, thought, and practice before you come up with a system that works for you. You should experiment while choreographing your own moves. It may be helpful to practice by writing down the components of the exam in the order in which you plan to perform them. If you can write them from memory, you're a step closer to gaining mastery of the flow.

Recognize that when caring for patients, the exam is typically modularized, with physicians performing selected aspects (eg, cardiac, abdominal, pulmonary) to investigate particular symptoms and clinical scenarios. This is referred to as performing a hypothesis-driven exam (ie, you perform the exam that's appropriate to the clinical moment). For example, evaluation of a 20-year-old with knee pain after an injury would be limited to a detailed lower extremity assessment, as exploring other regions (eg, heart, lungs) would be unlikely to reveal important information. Conversely, an older person with a chief concern of weakness, which has many possible explanations, would require a comprehensive evaluation. Knowing which examination module(s) to apply in particular situations will come with experience and practice.

The checklist that follows includes all of the elements of a rather comprehensive exam and is a compilation of those presented at the end of most chapters. It describes an ordered flow, something you can refer to when thinking through and practicing these core elements. You can also choose to "extract" particular modules (eg, the cardiac and pulmonary exams) from this larger list, providing a road map for the flow of selected sections if you used them during specific clinical situations. **Special tests**, performed in particular clinical moments, are identified as such. History taking and ROS checklists accompany those chapters.

Pelvic, breast, male genital, rectal, dermatologic, eye, and detailed musculoskeletal exams are not included in this comprehensive checklist because they're typically performed in particular situations. See the checklists provided in those organ-specific chapters for details. Pediatric checklists are covered in the 3 chapters dedicated to examining children. Elements of a limited intuitive mental status evaluation are presented at the end, as these can be readily obtained during typical history taking.

✅ SUMMARY OF SKILLS CHECKLIST

- ❑ Clean your hands
- ❑ Integrated skin exam—be on lookout for skin cancers or other overt abnormalities while performing the rest of the exam
- ❑ Asking patient to wear a gown can facilitate optimal exposure

Vital Signs Pulse, blood pressure, temperature, respiratory rate and oxygen saturation are likely already available—taken by nursing staff on arrival

- ❑ Observe patient, noting: comfort level, interactivity, grooming/hygiene, etc.
- ❑ Measure temperature
- ❑ Measure respiratory rate
- ❑ Inspect hands, fingers and nails
- ❑ Measure pulse, noting: rate, regularity, and volume
- ❑ Measure blood pressure
  - • **Special test:** Orthostatic vital signs
- ❑ Measure oxygen saturation

Head and Neck

- ❑ Observe head, face, neck and scalp
- ❑ Assess facial symmetry, expression (cranial nerve [CN] VII), sensation (CN V)
- ❑ Assess extraocular movements (CN III, IV, VI)
- ❑ Assess spinal accessory nerve (CN XI) function
- ❑ Listen to voice, speech, and respiration
- ❑ Palpate lymph nodes and major salivary glands
- ❑ Inspect external ears
- ❑ Perform otoscopy to assess external canal and tympanic membrane
- ❑ Assess hearing (CN VIII)
  - • **Special test:** Perform Weber and Rinne tests *if* there is concern for hearing loss
- ❑ Examine the external nose and perform anterior rhinoscopy using otoscope
  - • **Special test:** Perform basic olfactory testing (CN I) *if* patient reports hyposmia or anosmia
- ❑ Palpate the frontal and maxillary sinuses
  - • **Special test:** Assess maxillary transillumination *if* concern for rhinosinusitis

❑ Inspect the oral cavity, including teeth, using light and tongue depressor or gloved finger

❑ Assess tongue mobility (CN XII), palate mobility (CN IX, X)
  - **Special test:** Gag reflex (CN IX, X)

❑ Inspect the oropharynx
  - **Special testing:** Palpate the base of tongue and tonsils *if* there's concern for tumor

❑ Observe and palpate the thyroid

Pulmonary

Observation

❑ General observation: note use of accessory muscles, general respiratory effort, ability to speak, audible noises, breathing pattern

❑ Inspect chest, noting external abnormalities and shape; note shape of spine

Palpation (Special Tests)

❑ Assess chest excursion—if concern for asymmetric ventilation

❑ Assess for fremitus—if concern for effusion or consolidation

Percussion

❑ Percuss posterior lung fields, top to bottom and comparing side to side

❑ Percuss right anterolateral chest (middle lobe) and anterior lobes (bilateral)
  - **Special test:** Identify amount of diaphragmatic descent with inhalation - if concern for diaphragmatic paralysis

Auscultation

❑ Listen with diaphragm to posterior lung fields, top to bottom and comparing side to side

❑ Listen to right middle lobe and lingula areas

❑ Listen to anterior lung fields
  - **Special test:** Assess for egophony—if concern for effusion or consolidation

❑ Listen over trachea

Cardiovascular (CV)—Examine from patient's right side

❑ Elevate head of table to approximately 30 degrees

❑ Inspect precordium

❑ Palpate left ventricle (LV); identify point of maximal impulse

Auscultation

❑ Identify S1 and S2 in 4 valvular areas with diaphragm

❑ Listen for physiologic splitting of S2

❑ Assess for murmurs

❑ Assess for extra heart sounds (S3, S4) with bell over LV

Carotid Artery (Special Tests)

❑ Palpation

❑ Auscultation

Internal Jugular Vein

❑ Assess central venous pressure

Abdomen

Observation

❑ Drape to allow appropriate exposure, patient lying flat

❑ Examine from right side of patient's body

❏ Observe and inspect abdomen
❏ Note shape, scars, color, symmetry, unusual protrusions

Auscultation (Special Tests)
❏ Listen for bowel sounds with diaphragm
❏ Listen for bruits

Percussion
❏ Percuss all quadrants
❏ Percuss liver span
❏ Percuss areas of spleen, stomach

Palpation
❏ Palpate all quadrants superficially
❏ Palpate all quadrants deeply; think about what "lives" in each area
❏ Assess for liver edge (with inspiration)
❏ Palpate region of spleen
  • **Special test:** Palpate area of aorta (if risk factors for abdominal aortic aneurysm)
  • **Special test:** Assess costovertebral angle for tenderness (if concern for pyelonephritis)

Lower Extremities (Continuation of CV)

Femoral and Inguinal Areas (Special tests)
❏ Palpate for lymph nodes
❏ Palpate femoral pulses
❏ Assess for inguinal hernias

Assess Knees (Nonmechanical Exam)
❏ Note color, swelling
  • **Special test:** Palpate popliteal artery pulse

Assess Ankles and Feet
❏ Note color, temperature, capillary refill
❏ Check for edema
❏ Observe for any skin breakdown or ulcerations (including between toes, soles)

Pulses
❏ Palpate dorsalis pedis artery
❏ Palpate posterior tibial artery

Neurologic

Cranial Nerves (those covered with head and neck exam can be omitted)
❏ CN I (olfactory): Smell
❏ CN II (optic): Visual acuity
❏ CN II: Visual fields
❏ CN II and III (oculomotor): Pupillary response to light
❏ CN III, IV (trochlear), and VI (abducens): Extraocular movements
❏ CN V (trigeminal): Facial sensation; Muscles mastication; Corneal reflex (with CN VII)
❏ CN VII (facial): Facial expression
❏ CN VIII (auditory): Hearing
  • **Special test:** If hearing decreased: Weber (assessing if lateralizes with tuning fork midline)
  • **Special test:** If hearing decreased: Rinne (bone vs air)

❑ CN IX, X (glossopharyngeal, vagus): Raise palate ("ahh")
  • **Special test:** Gag reflex (CN IX, X)
❑ CN XI (spinal accessory): Turn head against resistance, shrug shoulders
❑ CN XII (hypoglossal): Assess tongue movement

Motor Testing
❑ Observe and palpate muscle bulk
❑ Assess tone of arms and legs
❑ Assess strength of major groups: Shoulders, elbows, wrists, hands, hips, knees, ankles

Sensory Testing
❑ Assess spinothalamics (sharp vs dull; temperature as indicated)
❑ Assess dorsal columns (proprioception, vibration with 128-Hz tuning fork)

Reflexes
❑ Brachioradialis—C5, C6 Radial N
❑ Biceps—C5, C6 Musculocutaneous N
❑ Triceps—C7, C8 Radial N
❑ Patellar—L3, L4 Femoral N
❑ Achilles—S1, S2 Sciatic N
❑ Babinski response

Coordination
❑ Targeted movements (eg, finger → nose)
❑ Rapid alternating movements (eg, rapid foot taps)

Gait
❑ Observed walking
❑ Clean your hands

Intuitive Mental Status Evaluation
The following information is typically available from general history taking. If issues are identified or the clinical situation warrants, a complete mental status evaluation can be pursued (see complete checklist in Chapter 13).
❑ Appearance
❑ Behavior
❑ Speech
❑ Organization of thoughts
❑ Attention
❑ Memory

26

Thoughts for the Road

Charlie Goldberg, MD

It can be easy to lose your sense of perspective and purpose while working in the clinical environment. In fact, you may recognize this as a problem among many in the medical field. A few things to think about as you make your journey:

1. Treat patients as you would want yourself, a family member, or other loved one to be cared for. This covers the technical aspects of healthcare as well as the quality and nature of your interpersonal interactions.

2. Try to avoid viewing the medical training process solely as a means to an end. As medical education is a lifelong undertaking, you've got to enjoy the journey. If not, stop and consider why.

3. Do the right thing. This applies to patient care and your dealings with colleagues and other healthcare workers. If something feels wrong, it probably is! This can be challenging, particularly when you are fatigued, stressed, in a subordinate position, or working with others who don't have the same priorities.

4. Mistakes happen. You will likely contribute to errors during your careers. We are all human and thus all fallible. When errors occur, acknowledge them, report within your system so that underlying root causes can be identified and addressed, discuss with the appropriate parties, inform the patient, and make efforts to manage any consequences. Learn from what happened, while also remembering to forgive yourself. Being a doctor can be a humbling experience.

5. There is no substitute for being thorough in your efforts to care for your patients. Performing an appropriate exam and obtaining an accurate history take a certain amount of time, regardless of your level of experience, ability, or efficiency. In addition, get in the habit of checking the primary data yourself, obtaining copies of outside studies, mining old records for information, requestioning patients when the story is unclear, and in general being tenacious in your pursuit of clinically relevant material. This dogged search for answers is a cornerstone of good care.

6. Learn from your patients. In particular, those with chronic or unusual diseases will likely know more about their illnesses than you. Find out how their diagnosis was made, therapies that have worked or failed, disease progression, and reasons for frustration or gratitude with the healthcare system. Realize also that patients and their stories are frequently more interesting and revealing than the diseases that inhabit their bodies.

7. Become involved in all aspects of patient care. Look at the computed tomography (CT) images, talk with the radiologist, review the slides with the pathologist, watch the echocardiogram being performed. While you can't do this for every patient, create space to make this happen on occasion. This will allow you to learn more and gain insight into a particular illness/disease state that would not be well conveyed by simply reading a report. It will also give you an appreciation for how tests are performed and their limitations.

8. Make it interpersonal. Find the consultant, nurse, or others involved in your patient's care and talk directly to them. Notes or texted messages often fail to convey the full story. By speaking directly (at least on occasion), you can unpack nuance and get to the roots of certain issues. If murkiness remains, you can all go to the bedside together. This helps to build relationships with colleagues, smoothing the way for better care and allowing everyone to learn more.

9. Follow up on patients whom you care for in the emergency department or are transferred to other services, are seen by subspecialists, or are discharged from the hospital. If you don't make an effort to learn about what happens as their situation evolves, you run the risk of convincing yourself that you're a genius every day. That is, without checking back, you can develop the sense that all of your decisions are correct. Following up via the electronic medical record (EMR) will give you a better understanding of the natural history of medical conditions and allow you to confirm (or adjust) your clinical suspicions. This is particularly relevant as patients are shuttled through the system with great speed, affording us only snapshot views of what may be complex clinical courses.

10. Keep your eyes open for other interesting things that might be going on elsewhere in the hospital or clinic. If you hear about a patient on another service or team with an interesting finding or story, ask the clinicians caring for that patient if there's an opportunity for you to meet and learn from them. This approach allows you to expand your internal library of what is abnormal and promotes the need to stay curious.

11. Pay particular attention when things don't seem to add up. Chances are someone (you, the patient, the consultant) is missing something, a clue that the matter needs further investigation. Challenge yourself and those around you by continually asking "Why?"

12. Before deciding that another provider is wrong for adopting what seems an unorthodox or inappropriate clinical approach, assume that it is you who is lacking some important historical data. Give others the benefit of the doubt until you've had an opportunity to fully explore all of the relevant information. Making use of lessons learned in a manner that promotes education and growth requires a delicate touch.

13. Become comfortable with the phrases, "I don't know" and "I need help." If those with whom you are currently working are unreceptive, make use of other resources (eg, residents, fellows, students, nurses, technicians, faculty). You can learn something from anyone.

14. Be present. Multitasking in medicine often results in diminished efforts on every front. In healthcare, it's common to type notes while interviewing patients. This begs the question: What's the point of every patient interaction? To complete the documentation simultaneously with the end of the encounter or to listen, engage, and respond to the person in front of you? I've yet to read a personal statement that said: "I anticipate great fulfillment from a future focused on texting and typing." If you're typing and

clicking while at the same time trying to talk and listen, you are not being fully present, and something is getting lost.

15. Try to read something medical every day. This will help you to stay abreast of new developments and provide an opportunity to become reacquainted with things that you've learned and forgotten. Medicine is less about achieving mastery than it is about reinforcing old lessons and making incremental gains. Our individual "knowledge tanks" leak information on a daily basis. There is no way to plug the hole. Instead, you must continually replenish by adding to the top.

16. Realize that, ultimately, you are responsible for you. The quality of care that you provide is a direct result of the time and effort that you invest in the process, coupled with a willingness to work within the multifaceted team that is necessary to provide optimal care.

17. You are not automatically endowed with the historical wisdom of a particular institution merely by walking through its doors. Nor does this knowledge necessarily arrive with your white coat, degree, or other advanced title. Rather, this is something that's learned and earned, often on a daily basis.

18. Every once in a while, push yourself to become an expert in something. Firsthand knowledge is a powerful tool, one that is available to anyone willing to take the time to read through the primary literature. Become informed by delving into the original papers pertaining to a particular subject. You may find that the data are robust and the rationale for a clinical approach or treatment well grounded. Frequently, I suspect you'll find instances where the data are rather shaky, and the best path is not as clear as guidelines or expert opinions might suggest.

19. Be kind, both to others and yourself. Recognize the signs that you and/or your colleagues are struggling. Burnout, depression, substance use, and fatigue are issues that can affect anyone. The path to being better requires that we all look out for one another, offer and ask for help, and function as a truly supportive community.

20. Don't outsource caring for and about your patients. Being genuine and truly engaged in attending to your patient's needs and advocating on their behalf is a unique opportunity, one that should be a regular source of joy and fulfillment. Remember what you wrote in your personal statements and said during your interviews: "I am here to help." "I care." "I want to ease suffering and cure disease." Keep these first and foremost in your mind and periodically adjust your course so that they are always in sight.

There is magic in medicine. It does not, however, derive solely from mechanical interventions, technology, testing, or diagnostic aptitude. Rather, it often comes from your interactions with patients, a touch on the sleeve, sitting at the bedside and treating a patient as a fellow human being and not as "that person with lupus." You are all capable, right now, without additional training, of being magicians. The challenge lies in not losing track of this as you make your way through training and beyond.

BIBLIOGRAPHY

Gawande A. When doctors make mistakes. *New Yorker*. February 7, 1999, 40-55.

Index

Note: Page numbers followed by f indicate figures; those followed by t indicate tables.